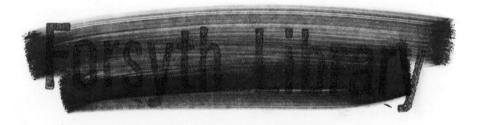

INTRODUCTION TO INSTRUMENTATION IN SPEECH AND HEARING

INTRODUCTION TO INSTRUMENTATION IN SPEECH AND HEARING

EDWARD A. CUDAHY, Ph.D.

Director of Research
The Lexington Center
Jackson Heights, New York

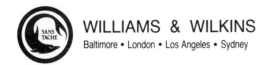

WILLIAMS & WILKINS
Baltimore • London • Los Angeles • Sydney

Editor: John Butler
Associate Editor: Victoria M. Vaughn
Copy Editor: Elia A. Flanegin
Design: Mack Rowe
Illustration Planning: Wayne Hubbel
Production: Raymond E. Reter

Accurate indications, adverse reactions, and dosage schedules for drugs are provided in this book, but it is possible that they may change. The reader is urged to review the package information data of the manufacturers of the medications mentioned.

Printed in the United States of America

Library of Congress Cataloging-in-Publication Data

Cudahy, Edward A.
   Introduction to instrumentation in speech and hearing.
   Includes index.
   1. Audiometry—instruments. 2. Speech therapy—Instruments. I. Title.
[DNLM: 1. Audiometry—instrumentation. 2. Speech Therapy—instrumentation.
WV 26 C964i]
RF87.C83 1987   617.8′0028   86-15750
ISBN 0-683-02245-8

Composed and printed at the
Waverly Press, Inc.

88 89 90 91 92
10 9 8 7 6 5 4 3 2 1

PREFACE

This book is intended to serve as a primary textbook for an introductory course in instrumentation in speech and hearing. The focus in this book is application. Although some theoretical background is given for each instrument, most of the book is devoted to describing the functions and applications of various instruments. Quiklabs at the end of each chapter provide an opportunity to acquire experience by applying the information gained from each chapter. Throughout the book, "hands-on" experience is emphasized as the way to learn about instrumentation.

The book is divided into two parts. The first part consists of an introduction to the fundamentals of electronics and test instrumentation. The second part describes instrumentation specifically for speech and hearing, including common clinical instrumentation and instrumentation that is presently used mostly in research but is likely to be used in the clinic of the future. The division is between basic information and instrumentation used to calibrate and examine other instrumentation, which is typically used by a technician servicing other instrumentation, and the instrumentation used in the clinic. This book is designed to encourage clinicians to use test instrumentation (as described in the initial portion of the text) in an effort to be time and cost efficient. In addition, this text will assist all users of instrumentation to become more comfortable and more competent with their equipment. The book begins with a basic introduction to electronics. This is followed with a chapter describing basic test instrumentation. The basic information about electronics covered in chapters 1 and 2 serves as an introduction to the world of electronics, and chapter 3 gives the tools to examine this world. Clinicians can then apply this knowledge to the instrumentation with which they are more familiar and better understand the instrumentation that they use every day. The instrumentation commonly encountered in the clinic is covered in chapters 4–7. The last three chapters challenge the students to expand their knowledge beyond current clinic instrumentation and into the future. Chapter 7 covers both clinical and research instrumentation that measure physiological parameters of speech or hearing behavior. The next chapter is devoted to the principles and use of instrumentation for signal acquisition and analysis. While the concepts discussed in this chapter are applicable to virtually all of the instrumentation covered in this book, more advanced theoretical material is covered in this chapter; therefore this chapter might be of greater interest to more advanced students or classes. The final chapter covers computer and computer-related instrumentation in the field of speech and hearing. This chapter not only covers how to use the computer as a test or diagnostic instrument but also covers some of the other applications such as word processing and record keeping. A balanced view is attempted between the limitless possibilities offered by computers and the real-world concerns of applying the computer to the problems of the clinic and laboratory.

The book is developed in accordance with the successful procedures that I have used in my instrumentation course. The target audience is graduate or advanced undergraduate students, who routinely take such a course. Instrumentation is described in terms of the context in which it is most commonly used, and hints for the use of instrumentation are frequently given. Examples of research instrumentation that may be used in the clinic are presented, especially in the physiological instrumentation chapter.

In summary, this book is intended to be used as a teaching text and also as a reference on common clinical and research instrumentation in speech and hearing. An attempt is made to encourage familiarity with instruments in order to enhance the skills and efficiency of the clinician. The book also attempts to look to the future with the chapter on computers, which seeks to encourage clinicians to take advantage of these excellent general-purpose tools. This chapter also provides a knowledge base to those unfamiliar with computers, so that they may use the strategies given in the book to more adequately make decisions with regard to computer purchase and utilization. This book focuses not only on teaching about instrumentation but also on making the reader more comfortable in that world and on encouraging applications that he or she may not have thought of before.

CONTENTS

Chapter 8
Instrumentation for Signal Acquisition, Generation, and Analysis

Chapter 9
Modular Programming Equipment and Computers

Section III

SECTION I

1

Fundamentals of Electronics

You are about to be introduced to the marvelous and fascinating world of electronics. Electricity is so pervasive in our lives that we think little about how it is used, where it comes from, or even how all the gadgets that we use every day operate. Many of us know very little about how an automobile or digital alarm clock uses electricity. We may even think of electricity as having an almost magical quality. After working through this chapter, you may feel that some of the glitter is gone, but your initial sense of awe will be replaced with sufficient understanding of electronics to appreciate how some of these devices work. In addition, increased confidence regarding your use of electronic instrumentation should also be achieved. The Quiklabs at the end of the second chapter will provide opportunities to apply the knowledge gained from this chapter and to practice new skills.

This introduction to electronics is needed to insure that a few basic facts are learned before using instrumentation to make electronic measurements. These facts will help you to understand the quantities measured and will facilitate interpretation of measurement results. Trying to use instrumentation intelligently without understanding fundamental principles of electronics is akin to trying to build a house without a foundation. Lacking this supporting structure, the "house" will eventually sag and gaps will appear in the walls of knowledge surrounding you. Likewise, without some background information regarding electronics a person stands on pretty shaky ground when trying to use electronic instrumentation; worse yet, the maximum advantages provided by electronic technology will not be available. Remember that all measurements made with electronic instrumentation operate in some way on the basis of the fundamental principles that will be discussed in this chapter.

This introduction to electronics fundamentals begins with a description of basic electrical quantities (volts, amperes, ohms, and watts) and their properties. Next, electrical components that modify and control electricity are discussed, as well as some ways of describing instrumentation setups and electrical circuits. Then, the most common part of all instrumentation, the power supply, is examined. Finally, the behavior of direct current (DC) circuits and alternating current (AC) circuits is explained. Obviously not all aspects of electronics can be included in two chapters, nor will all of the indicated topics be considered in complete detail. To do so would require a number of volumes. Rather, the intent here is to provide the reader with some of the basics that will be useful in understanding the measurements and instrumentation covered in later chapters.

What is Electricity?

Electricity is the flow of electrons, which are small atomic particles. Electrons represent energy, and it is the energy in electricity that permits its multitude of uses. Another powerful aspect of electricity is the malleability of its energy. Electricity's pervasiveness in our daily lives illustrates the many different ways in which this power source can be altered and manipulated. Electricity can flow through almost any material, but the material's nature has an impact on the behavior of the electron flow or electrical current. This interaction of electricity and materials is critical to the operation of many current electronic devices such as transistors and integrated circuits.

Ohm's Law

A fundamental rule in electronics is Ohm's law. Ohm's law is the rule that ultimately governs the behavior of electricity, and like all good fundamental rules, it is very simple. Ohm's law (Equation 1) states that the electromotive force (E) equals the current (I) times the resistance (R). A more common name for electromotive force is *voltage*. Each of these fundamental attributes of electricity will be described along with some real-world representations.

$$E = I \times R \qquad (1)$$

Electromotive Force

Lightning is a good example of electromotive force. No one denies that there is considerable force in a lightning bolt. If we fix a visual image of a lightning bolt in our minds, we note that the force travels a distance. Although the amount of distance is not critical, the difference between land and sky or low and high is important. During a storm, the sky and the land build up different kinds of electromotive force, called "positive" and "negative," which are attracted to each other.

Nature abhors an imbalance and solves the problem by using lightning to "equalize" the differences between the "negative" land and the "positive" sky. The force, in this case lightning, travels between the two points, or between land and sky. The greater the imbalance, the greater the force that must travel between the two points. The imbalance is quantified as volts, which is the difference in electromotive potential force between two points. An equivalent way to state the same thing is that voltage refers to the passage of electrons between two points of opposite polarity. Fortunately, most electrical differences do not (usually) generate lightning but behave in a much more sedate manner. These differences in electromotive force can be measured with a voltmeter, which is a measurement device discussed in the next chapter.

In general, the terms *electromotive force* and *volts* can be used interchangeably. In this book the electromotive force (EMF) will be used to describe the fundamental phenomenon that we measure as voltage potential and *voltage* will be used to describe the measurement of EMF. This is analogous to the fundamental phenomenon of height, which we measure in terms of feet and inches (or meters and centimeters).

Current

When lightning strikes, the force must get from land to sky in order to equalize the electrical differences. Electricity has been described previously as "the flow of electrons." The electrons carry the force from place to place. Current (I), the second quantity in Ohm's law, is the measure of this *flow* of electrons through a conducting point and is quantified as amperes. To give some idea of the number of electrons required to carry electrical current, 1 ampere equals 1 coulomb/s. Since 1 coulomb equals 6.28×10^{18} electrons (that is, 6,280,000,000,000,000,000 electrons), this means 6.28×10^{18} electrons/s.

One very interesting and important feature of current is the direction of its flow. Electrical potentials can be either positive or negative. Current flows from negative to positive. This occurs because electrons carry a negative potential and in the world of electricity opposites attract. Thus electrons flow toward positive potentials. This produces the interesting fact that since land is negative and the sky is positive, lightning actually goes upward, not downward, as our visual image tells us. It also means that the current flow in an electrical circuit will be from the negative portions of the circuit toward the positive portions of the circuit. This can be very important and must be kept in mind when examining or testing circuits because electricity flowing in the wrong direction at the wrong time can have disastrous results.

The statement that current can flow in only one direction represents a simplification. When electrons flow in one direction only, that is, the current flow is in one direction only, the current is referred to as direct current (DC) (Fig. 1.1*A*). When the current flow alternates direction over time, it is referred to as alternating current (AC) (Fig. 1.1*B*). The schematization represents a circuit with a power supply, and the *arrows* are the direction of current flow. Next to each circuit is a plot of the current over a period of time. For the DC circuit, the current is constant in magnitude and polarity. Recalling our earlier discussion about how electrons are attracted toward positive potentials, we can see that constant polarity will equal constant direction of current flow. In the AC circuit the current is not constant in magnitude and polarity; hence AC really refers to the fact that the circuit is constantly changing its polarity and thus its direction.

As referred to earlier, for current to flow there must be something to conduct the current flow. Another interesting feature of current is that it travels on the outside of a conductor. This feature is handy to remember for a variety of reasons, one of which can be observed if you are ever caught in your car during a lightning storm. Since current travels on the

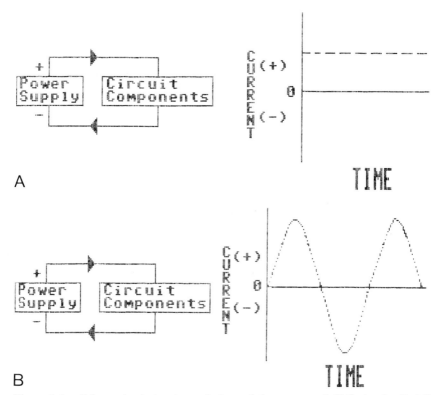

Figure 1.1. Schematized circuits and plots of the output. *A,* DC circuit. *B,* AC circuit.

outside of the car, unless you touch something connected to the outside of the car, you will not make contact with the current from the lightning. Of course, it is not recommended that you drive to a lightning storm to observe this phenomenon, but the fact that current travels on the outside of a conductor may be useful for explaining other more mundane and useful aspects of electronics and will be used later for that purpose.

Resistance

The third and final quantity in Ohm's law is resistance (R). Resistance is measured in ohms (named after . . . guess who?) and is exactly what its name implies, the *resistance* to electrical flow. The greater the resistance, the more the flow of electrons is impeded. One way to view the operation of resistance is to consider some of the consequences. When lightning strikes, we often hear a sizzling sound, and certainly lightning can produce fire when it "hits" a tree. The sizzling sound comes from the resistance of the air to the lightning bolt, and the fire comes from the resistance of the tree to current flow. In the case of lightning in air, the bolt pushes the air out of the way. But this produces friction between the air and the lightning and hence produces heat. That is, it takes energy for the bolt to force its way through the air, and this energy takes the form of heat. The reader can work through what happens when the lightning bolt is connected to a tree. The point of all this is that just as for the lightning bolt, resistance is typically generated by friction in electrical circuits.

Conductors, Semiconductors, and Insulators

Most of the time, lightning is not used to carry electricity from place to place. In addition to being somewhat hazardous, lightning requires a great deal of force to push the current. Electricity is carried by electrons, thus a medium that will permit the easy flow of electrons will require less force to carry electricity than a medium that does not permit the easy flow of electrons. Materials that easily conduct current have many "free" electrons available to "carry" the current from atom to atom and are called *conductors*. Most common conductors are in the form of metals, such as wire or metal strips on a printed circuit board. Copper, a good conductor, has about 10^{23} free electrons/inch^3. Conductors are rated in terms of their conductivity, or ease of current flow, with silver, copper, and gold having the highest conductivity of most common conductors.

All materials have some free electrons, but those with the least number of free electrons have the greatest resistance to current flow and are called *insulators*. A good insulator may have up to 10^{12} free electrons/inch^3, but insulators have their free electrons tightly bound to their parent atoms, and so there is little mobility of electrons in these materials. If sufficient force is applied to the electrons, they will eventually break free and become mobile. Thus, if sufficient voltage is applied to an insulator, it will break down and current will flow. The "breakdown" voltage is determined experimentally for different insulators and is termed the *dielectric strength*. The dielectric strengths for some common insulators are shown in Table 1.1. Dielectric strengths are tabulated either as volts per millimeter length of the insulator or in volts per mil (0.001 inch) thickness of the insulator.

There is a third group of materials that fall between conductors and insulators (i.e., they have between 10^{13} and 10^{19} free electrons/inch^3) and that cannot be properly called either conductors or insulators. These materials are very important and are called *semiconductors*. They form the basis for the integrated circuits, and the discovery of how to use them led to the current revolution in microelectronics. They will be discussed more fully later in this chapter.

Voltage Sources and Current Sources

Although lightning gets its power from the sky, the current and/or voltage in a circuit has to come from somewhere else. Therefore, all electrical circuits have sources for either current or voltage. Recall the circuit schematizations used in Figure 1.1, which had a box labeled "power supply." As we will see later in this chapter in the section on power supplies, there are a number of ways to supply circuits with power. Power supplies are classified as either voltage or current sources. For now, the important point is that circuits and some devices require either a voltage source or a current source to operate.

There are a number of other electrical phenomena that occur, and some of these will now be discussed. Most of these phenomena alter or utilize the fundamental properties already discussed and are associated with electrical components that will be described later.

Table 1.1.
Dielectric Strengths

Material	Volts/mil
Air	76
Bakelite	250–750
Glass	750–4,000
Mica	125–5,500
Polyester	250–500
Rubber	375–1,300
Paper (waxed)	1,250–1,800
Porcelain	40–400

Capacitance

Capacitance refers to the ability of a material or device to *store* an electrical charge and is measured in farads. An intuitive way to visualize charge is to think of electrons as packets of energy, each of which carries a small charge. The lightning bolt that we have been using as our intuitive tool for understanding electricity is actually the result of a capacitive discharge. The distance between the land and the sky requires not only a lot of energy to get across the distance but also a channel for the energy to flow. Thus charges, packets of electrical energy (that is, electrons), are stored up until there is sufficient charge to cross the space between the land and the sky. If a channel, such as a lightning rod or Benjamin Franklin's key is provided, then the charges are released and the process begins anew. Capacitance operates the same way and is measured by the maximum charge that can be stored. This is expressed mathematically where capacitance (C) in farads is equal to the charge in coulombs (Q, a measure of the electrons) divided by the voltage (V, a measure of the force across a distance).

$$C = \frac{Q}{V} \tag{2}$$

You will recall from our discussion of lightning that the charge was described as being built up over time. A little study of Equation 2 shows why that has to be the case. The units for coulombs are electrons per second. Thus the greater the electron flow, the faster the device will charge. Therefore, according to the equation, the amount of charge required to charge a capacitance device instantaneously would be infinite. So it always takes some finite time for a capacitor (a capacitance device) to charge. It also discharges at a finite rate (or frequency) for essentially the same reason. Frequency is introduced because of the time lags, that is, the current is not flowing all the time. It is alternating between flow and no flow. Since discharge can only occur if there is change in potential (to allow some place for the electrons from the capacitor to go) and this requires a changing voltage, capacitance is not a DC phenomenon; in fact, capacitors are used to prevent DC in an AC circuit.

Inductance

Inductance is that property that resists a change in current through a device. Inductance can be thought of as the current counterpart of capacitance. Inductance comes from the effects of a magnetic field upon an electrical circuit. The fundamental rule is that when any change is made in the magnetic field of an electrical circuit, an EMF is induced that opposes the change. Thus, when a current builds up a magnetic field (which it will do in any wire), a counter electromotive force will be generated that will oppose the current change. The greater or more rapid the change, the greater the counterforce. Inductance provides no opposition to a DC current because the current does not change. Opposition to current changes are in proportion to the inductance of the device and the amount of the current change. The greater the inductance, the more slowly the current will change. Inductance is measured in henrys and an inductance of 1 henry will induce a counter electromotive force of 1 volt when the current is changing at the rate of 1 ampere/s.

Power

Power is the amount of work done to move charge from place to place and is measured in watts. Electrical power is probably very familiar to most people because almost all electrical devices, from toasters to toys, are rated in terms of their power consumption. While lightning bolts are not generally rated in terms of their power, imagine the power required to carry large charges across open space. Power is a very important quantity to know in electrical circuits because components and devices are rated in terms of the amount of power that they can handle. Too much power will damage or destroy the device; too little power will result in poor operation. Power is measured by multiplying the current used by the device times the voltage used by the device.

Impedance

Impedance is the reaction of a system to an imposed force and is measured in ohms. Impedance is one of the most important concepts in electronics because it determines the energy transfer between devices and can be used to describe the behavior of the device itself when current is applied. Impedance will be discussed later because it is difficult to understand outside the context of circuit analysis.

Diagramming for Instrumentation

Before describing the operation of the components that use the quantities discussed in earlier sections, this chapter will present a standardized means of describing components, circuits, and instrumentation setups. Two general types of diagraming will be described: *schematic diagrams* and *block diagrams*. Schematic diagrams are used to describe instrumentation at the component level; a circuit diagram is an example. Block diagrams are used to indicate the organization of instrumentation devices or of blocks of circuits within a device.

Schematic Diagrams

A schematic diagram shows the electrical connections of an electronic device, with symbols and straight lines used to represent the parts and their connections. The graphic symbols used in a schematic represent the function of a part in a circuit, not its outward appearance. Table 1.2 gives some of the common graphic symbols for various components. In addition, there are standard class letters for various components, which are also shown in Table 1.2 next to the name of the component.

Schematic Analysis

Schematic analysis consists of determining the nature and function of an electronic circuit by separating the overall electrical picture into its parts. It is a process like anatomical analysis. A schematic is organized like the organs in a body, where the organs are individual circuits within the "body" of the device.

If done properly, schematic diagrams are easy to understand because there is a convention for laying out each circuit within a schematic. Figure 1.2 shows an example of a circuit schematic. The input signal almost invariably comes from the left side of the page, and the output signal goes out the right side of the page. This horizontal flow from the left to right takes place along two paths (Fig 1.2). The upper path is the "high" side of the circuit, and the lower is the "low" side of the circuit. The low side is the return path for the electrons and is usually considered to be at zero or ground potential, although it may not be connected to a real earth ground at all. (For an example of a real earth ground, recall our discussion of lightning and the direction of current flow.) In some circuits, connections to the low side are indicated by the ground symbol, shown in Table 1.2,

Table 1.2.
Some Schematic Symbols

Symbol	Name	Symbol	Name
—⌇—	Resistor (R)	—⌇—	Variable Resistor
—╢├—	Capacitor (C)	⏚	Ground
—▶├—	Diode (D)	—• •—	Switch (S)
—┤├—	Single cell battery	┤│├—	Battery

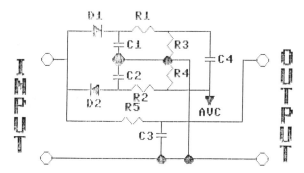

Figure 1.2. Example of circuit schematic.

rather than by drawing a line through the whole schematic to the low side, which could be extremely confusing.

As can be seen from Figure 1.2, a circuit has many elements or components, which are combined in specific ways to alter the signal in a specific manner. You will encounter examples of this in the labs in the next chapter, where electrical circuits are discussed further.

Active and Passive Elements

Elements are either *passive* or *active*. Passive elements (for example, resistors, capacitors, and inductors) are those that do not require an external source of power in order to function. Active elements (for example, vacuum tubes and transistors) use external power, which they introduce into the circuit to modify an existing signal or generate a new one.

Most circuits consist of a small number of passive elements built around an active element. The type of active element will frequently give you a clue as to the function of the circuit. A part number for each active element will be included with the schematic. Looking up the part number in an electronic parts catalog will give the function of the device, and from this the function of the circuit can be determined. Note also that each component is labeled with a class letter and number. For example, R_1 refers to resistor number 1. Such labeling is intended to aid in matching the component in the schematic to the parts table. A table provided with the schematic will usually give the values for each component according to its label, if it is not indicated in the circuit itself.

The labeling of components also serves another function. Since most circuits in current instrumentation are implemented on a printed circuit board (sometimes abbreviated as pcb), a printed circuit diagram (pc diagram) is usually provided with the instrument along with test points for troubleshooting indicated on the diagram. The pc diagram should always be included in the documentation for an instrument, but it is an imperfect world and the diagram may have been left out. If the pc diagram is not included, it is best to request it from the manufacturer of the instrument. Having the diagram available will make every one's life, especially that of the technician's, much easier. The labels on the schematic and the pc diagram should be the same and will assist in finding components on the printed circuit board and in working from the schematic diagram to the board itself.

The intent of this chapter is *not* to enable the reader to troubleshoot at the component level, except for very simple circuits. However, being able to identify the source of the problem for the technician can save time, money, and aggravation. By learning the simple circuits in this book, many of which are building blocks for circuits used in modern instrumentation, readers can do simple troubleshooting and problem identification.

Schematic diagrams throughout the text will utilize the conventions described in this section. The circuits will be simple circuits and the function of each component in the circuit will be described at the same time. After seeing several of these circuits, readers will better understand schematic analysis.

Block Diagrams

Just as a book starts with a table of contents to tell the reader where to locate the different chapters and what they are about, so does a block diagram summarize large and complex devices or instrumentation setups. Both schematic and instrumentation block diagrams have the essential units of the overall system drawn in the form of blocks, and their relationship to each other is indicated by connecting lines. These lines usually represent the signal paths and often have arrows to show direction. A typical instrumentation block diagram is reproduced in Figure 1.3.

A block diagram is useful because it gives the observer a quick overall view of the system. Where a block diagram is provided, it can be used to identify a particular circuit or instrument because the block names it. Then

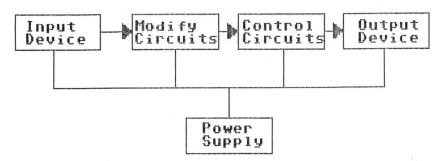

Figure 1.3. Universal block diagram.

the circuit or instrument can be located in other documentation to get a full description of its function or operation.

The intent of most instruments and instrumentation setups is to act upon some input so as to obtain a desired output. Consequently the sequence of circuits and/or instruments will reflect this fact. Thus, block diagrams have a conventional layout similar to that for schematics. The input signal(s) enter from the left and will exit to the right. Instruments and circuits will be placed in the order in which they operate upon the signal. The block diagrams used in this book will be organized according to these rules and in the manner illustrated by Figure 1.3.

Electrical Components

Examination of the inside of any electronic instrument reveals that there are a large number of components within the instrument. As mentioned before, in most current instrumentation these components are arranged on a printed circuit board. This section will cover some of the common components and describe how they alter the electron flow. Most of these components alter the electrical properties that were described in the first part of this chapter.

Resistors

All materials conduct electricity to a greater or lesser degree. All materials also provide resistance to current flow to a greater or lesser degree, but certain components, called *resistors*, are manufactured to provide specific amounts of resistance. Resistors are made from a number of different materials and operate by impeding the flow of electrons through friction. There is a change (decrease) in EMF as the current passes through the resistor because of the energy required to overcome the resistance. Recalling Ohm's law, we would measure the drop in force as a voltage change. The larger the resistance, the greater the voltage change. Resistors usually look like Figure 1.4.

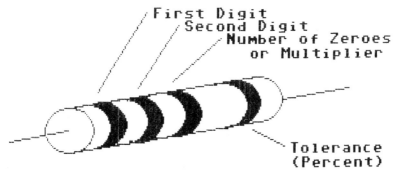

Figure 1.4. Resistor and color code bands.

Resistors are rated in terms of three quantities: resistance, tolerance, and power. The resistor's resistance is labeled directly on the resistor in the form of a color code, which encircles the resistor. Each color is associated with a digit, and each stripe has a particular meaning. The digit associated with each color is shown in Table 1.3.

The value assigned to each stripe depends upon the relative location of the stripe. Reading the color code requires that the resistor be oriented such that the group of stripes is put on the left, just as shown in Figure 1.4. The first stripe is the first digit of the resistance value for the resistor. The second stripe is the second digit of the resistance value. The third stripe is a multiplier and gives the number of zeros in the resistance value. The fourth stripe is the tolerance, which will be described shortly. For example, let us assume that the resistor in Fig 1.4 has the color code red, violet, and green. The corresponding resistance value for this resistor would be obtained by using Table 1.3. For this case the first two digits would be 2 for the red stripe and 7 for the violet stripe. The 5 for the green stripe means add 5 zeroes to the first two digits. Thus the resistance value for this resistor would be 2,700,000 ohms or 2.7 megohms.

The resistance value that is on the resistor is a nominal resistance value. That is, normally resistors are not produced with exact resistances, because of, for example, impurities in materials; however, the resistance is specified within a certain range or tolerance that is given by the fourth stripe and is expressed as a percentage of the nominal value. The silver and gold values in Table 1.3 refer to tolerances. For example, if the fourth stripe in the case just given was gold, the resistance would have been 2.7 megohms ± 5% of 2.7 megohms. If the tolerance is not 5% or 10%, it will usually be printed on the resistor. Occasionally no resistance-tolerance value is written on the resistor. These resistors typically have a 20% tolerance.

It is possible to obtain resistors with tolerances less than 5% for special applications. These resistors are called "precision resistors" and are made by coiling a fine wire around an insulating material or by an extremely precise layering technique that overlays a substrate with a thin film. Not surprisingly, the latter type of resistor is referred to as a "thin film resistor." One difficulty with coil-type precision resistors is that the coiling of the

Table 1.3.
Color Code Used for Resistors

Black 0	Blue 6
Brown 1	Violet 7
Red 2	Gray 8
Orange 3	White 9
Yellow 4	Gold 5
Green 5	Silver 10

wire can induce effects at high frequencies with regard to impedance that prohibit their use. Therefore, use of these types of resistors should be restricted to frequencies below 100 kHz.

Since the resistor impedes the electron flow through friction and thus there is energy required to overcome the resistance, a natural consequence is heat. That is, the energy in electrons is not destroyed by the resistor, it is merely changed into another form. The heat generated by the resistor must be dissipated by the material of the resistor, and there is obviously a limit to how much heat may be dissipated by any material. The temperature coefficient of the resistor determines this heat dissipation ability and is measured in watts of power that can be passed through the resistor. Thus all resistors have a power rating, which is generally printed on the resistor. The most common values are between ½ watt and 1 watt.

Some resistors have a variable resistance value that is externally adjustable. Generally these resistors have a coil that determines the range of values and a sliding contact that moves along the coil. Depending on the proportion of the coil between the input to the resistor and the slide contact, the coil has a resistance between the minimum and maximum values. The maximum value is given on the side of the resistor. Another name for a variable resistor is a "potentiometer," or "pot" for short. The adjustment of the slide contact for these resistors is usually done using a small screw on the side of the resistor. These resistors are frequently specified in terms of the maximum number of turns that the screw can make between the maximum and minimum resistance values for the resistor (for example, there is a "10-turn pot").

This variety of resistor types is a result of differing requirements for resistance. There are many cases in circuit design where a fixed value of resistance is required, and other cases where a variable resistance is required. An example of the use of a potentiometer is a tape recorder volume control. However, as discussed in the first part of the chapter, there are other ways in which current flow and electrical behavior can be changed and there are appropriate components for each case. The next component handles capacitance in circuits.

Capacitors

Just as a resistor is used to control resistance, a capacitor is used to control capacitance. A capacitor is composed of two conductors separated by an insulator, or dielectric. When a capacitor is placed in a circuit with a voltage source, the electrons from one conductor or plate of the capacitor are attracted to the positive side of the voltage source and the voltage source supplies electrons to the other plate of the capacitor. The charge collects on the foils, or plates, of the capacitor at a rate commensurate with the capacitance of the capacitor until the charge has reached the potential of the voltage source. If the voltage changes, then the capacitor discharges at a rate commensurate with its capacitance. Capacitance does not occur in a DC circuit because there is no voltage change, except "on" and "off" conditions, to discharge the capacitor. The most common applications of capacitors are in filters and to remove DC from an AC circuit. The simplest capacitor is two sheets of foil separated by an airspace; however, the dielectric is usually made of paper, mica ceramic, or plastic film. Figure 1.5 gives a schematic representation of a capacitor. The dielectric is "sandwiched" between the two conductors, and the whole capacitor is then sealed from the atmosphere. The larger the area of the foil and the thinner the dielectric, the higher the capacitance value. Some care must be taken because too high a voltage across the capacitor can ruin the dielectric and create a direct path for discharge between the two conductors, which would result in permanent damage to the capacitor. Capacitors are given a rating (the breakdown voltage) based on the voltage at which the dielectric begins to disintegrate. The thicker the dielectric, the less possibility of such a breakdown, but the capacitance is also lower. Fortunately, modern circuitry employing transistors and integrated circuits uses small voltages and capacitance values, so the problem is not severe.

The accuracy of capacitors is handled in the same manner as for resistors. That is, capacitors have tolerance ratings that are a percentage of the rated value of the capacitor. Typical tolerances are 20%, 10%, and 3%. Higher-accuracy capacitors can be obtained, but they are expensive and are seldom used. Capacitors have some temperature coefficient (due to the dielectric),

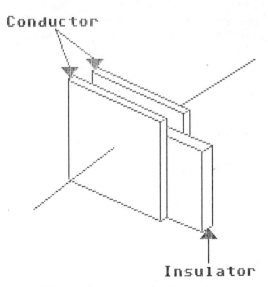

Conductor

Insulator

Figure 1.5.   Schematized capacitor.

but they do not generate much heat and thus do not have a resistance. In some cases, capacitors will "leak" current because the dielectric or capacitor construction is not perfect. If necessary, capacitors with high leakage resistance can be obtained. Since no power is dissipated by a capacitor (resistance is needed to dissipate power), there is no power rating.

There are many different types of capacitors, but they all operate on the same basic principle of separating conductors with insulators. There are "variable capacitors" and "air capacitors" (two foils separated by air). Variable capacitors operate on the principle of varying the amount of insulation in the capacitor and hence the capacitance of the capacitor. For example, this could be done by varying the distance between the foils in an air capacitor. Another type of capacitor construction is the electrolytic capacitor. An electrolytic capacitor is composed of a metal foil whose surface is covered with an anodic formation of metal oxide film. The anodized foil is in an electrolytic solution. The oxide film is the dielectric between the foil and the solution. The dielectric is so thin that a high capacitance can be obtained with a very small capacitor, which is an obvious advantage for creating miniaturized circuitry. However, the electrolytic capacitor has some disadvantages. The polarity of the circuit must always be in one direction. Reversal of current flow reduces the oxide, which removes the dielectric; gas will be produced at the cathode; and the capacitor will *explode*. The electrolytic capacitor will also deteriorate with time, as opposed to the simpler "sandwich type" capacitor.

The main considerations when choosing a capacitor for a given circuit are the value of the capacitance, the voltage rating of the capacitor, and the resistance of the dielectric (which relates to the "leakage" of the capacitor) employed. Occasionally, the space available for the capacitor is a factor. The physical size of a capacitor increases with increased capacitance and voltage rating.

Inductors

The control of inductance in electrical circuits is done, not surprisingly, by a component called an inductor. The simplest inductor is a coil of wire. Recall that inductance is based on the magnetic properties of electricity. Thus, the inductor coil is not always wound around an insulator such as air, but sometimes around a material, such as iron, that can sustain a magnetic field. In general, the larger the number of coils, the higher the inductance. The length of an inductor relative to its diameter and whether a magnetic core is used are important factors in determining the inductance of a coil. When choosing an inductor for a specific application it is necessary to consider:

1. The value of the inductance;
2. The DC resistance of the coil (the wires of the coil always have some resistance);

3. The current-carrying capacity of the coil windings (inductors melt);
4. The frequency range in which the coil is designed to operate.

For a number of reasons, including the lesser expense and the greater ease of building circuits that include only resistors and capacitors, inductors are not used as much as in the past. They are included here for completeness and to serve as an introduction to transformers.

Transformers

Transformers are devices containing two or more coils whose magnetic fields interact. The general schema for a transformer is shown in Figure 1.6. The input comes from the left, and the output is on the right; in effect there are two inductors side by side. The magnetic field generated by the first inductor (recall that inductors work through magnetic fields) creates an opposing field in the second inductor. This opposing field will react in opposition to the field in the first inductor, and a voltage will be induced in the second coil by the fluctuating current required for this fluctuating magnetic field. In this manner, energy gets transferred from coil 1 to coil 2. In order to maintain the magnetic flux in coil 1, more current will be required for coil 1, which can be used by coil 2, and so on. This schema can be expanded to more than two coils, but there is always only one input coil. The coil to which the power is supplied is called the "primary," and each coil in which current is induced is called a "secondary." Frequently, transformers are described in terms of their primary and secondary "windings." Winding is simply another name for coil. Recall that DC current does not induce fluctuating magnetic fields in inductors. Thus no current will be induced in coil 2 except for AC current, or when the current is turned on or off. Thus, transformers are excellent for isolating DC current from equipment. This isolation feature has led to the use of stand-alone

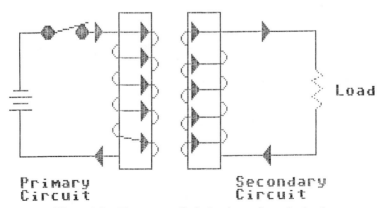

Primary
Circuit

Secondary
Circuit

Figure 1.6.   Two mutually inducting coils and a load.

transformers in biomedical applications to reduce the risk of shocking the patient.

The efficiency of a transformer is determined by the power loss between the two coils. If the magnetic coupling between the two coils is perfect (i.e., unity) and there is no power loss in the coils or coupling medium, then there is no power loss and the power in coil 2 will equal the power in coil 1. This is expressed mathematically in Equation 3, where Ep is the voltage in the primary, Ip is the current in the primary, Es is the induced voltage in the secondary, and Is is the induced current in the secondary. The equation states that with perfect coupling the power in the two coils will be the same, although the voltages and currents in the two coils may differ. Coupling refers to the fact that the two circuits are arranged such that energy is transferred from one circuit to the other. Obviously, most transformers are not ideal, but the equation still applies fairly closely.

$$Ep \times Ip = Es \times Is \qquad (3)$$

Transformers are frequently used to provide a number of different voltages from the same source. An example is a transformer for a model railroad that can output several voltages. A transformer is able to do this because of Equation 4, which states that the voltage in the second coil is determined by the ratio between the number of turns in the first and second coils (Np and Ns refer to the number of turns in the primary and secondary coils respectively; Ep and Es are the same as in Eq. 3). Equation 4 can be extended to more than two coils, and the rule remains the same regardless of the number of coils, although large numbers of coils increase the potential for power loss due to poor coupling.

$$Es = Ep \times (Ns/Np) \qquad (4)$$

It is important to remember that there is no power loss in transformers because of Ohm's law. We will use an example employing transformers to illustrate this phenomenon. Assume that the circuit is the same as Figure 1.6 with a voltage source of 240 volts AC and 3,000 turns in the primary coil. What are the consequences of coupling this coil with two different secondary coils, one with 9,000 turns and one with 500 turns? First, we will use Equation 4 to do the calculations.

Solution:
Case 1: $Ep = 240$ volts; $Ip = 1$ ampere; $Np = 3,000$; $Ns = 9,000$.
Case 2: $Ep = 240$ volts; $Ip = 1$ ampere; $Np = 3,000$; $Ns = 500$.
Using Equation 4, we calculate
Case 1: $Es = 9,000/3,000 \times 240 = 720$ volts.
Case 2: $Ex = 500/3,000 \times 240 = 40$ volts.

Transforming Equations 3 and 4 into the relation between the current and the turn ratio, we find

$$Is = Ip \times (Np/Ns) \qquad (5)$$

Using Equation 5, we calculate

Case 1: $Is = 1 \times (3{,}000/9{,}000) =$ ⅓ ampere

Case 2: $Is = 1 \times (3{,}000/500) = 6$ amperes

This example illustrates that when changing the voltage to desired values, amperage changes must be kept in mind because if the amperage is allowed to get too large, it will burn out (literally melt) the transformer. This is easy to determine because the transformer will smoke. Conversely, if the voltage gets too large, the magnetic field cannot be sustained and the transformer will break down. However, due to the fineness of the wires employed in transformers, the current limitations are usually more of a concern than the breakdown voltage.

There are a number of different types of transformers, and they are frequently used in power supplies (a topic covered late in this chapter). In general, the same limitations with regard to the resistance of the windings, the current capacity of the windings, the breakdown potential between the windings and the frame (the iron core mentioned earlier), and the response as a function of the frequency of the current apply to transformers as apply to the inductors described earlier.

The devices discussed to this point have all been based on simple materials and therefore have been used for almost a century. Recently, new materials with different ways for handling electricity have been discovered, changing the whole manner in which circuits are constructed and used. In fact, these discoveries have led to the development of state-of-the-art microcircuitry, e.g., computers and "intelligent" appliances, such as the programmable microwave ovens that are so common today.

Semiconductors

As the name implies, semiconductors are materials that are not good conductors but are also not good insulators. Two very common materials that have these properties are germanium and silicon. In fact, silicon is such a pervasive semiconductor that the area in California where many of these devices are made is called Silicon Valley. In their natural state, semiconductors are more like insulators than conductors, and so impurities are added (that is, doping) that make the material conduct better. Doping can involve either increasing the number of free electrons in the material, i.e., the number of electrons that can leave the material to conduct electricity or creating an electron deficiency so that the material will attract electrons.

The number of electrons can be increased by combining substances such as arsenic, antimony, and phosphorus with the semiconductor material. Since there is an excess of electrons and electrons carry a negative charge, the material will have a negative character. Thus such semiconductors are called *N-type* semiconductors.

An electron deficiency can be created by combining substances such as aluminum, gallium, or indium with the semiconductor material. The materials are considered to have "holes" because of the electron deficiency and conduct current through the holes. The holes can be thought of as tunnels of low resistance to the flow of current, which can carry the current through the semiconductor. The lack of electrons (removal of the negative charges carried by the electrons) gives the semiconductor a positive character. Thus, these semiconductors are referred to as *P-type* semiconductors.

There are two types of semiconductor components that are very common in instrumentation: diodes and transistors. These devices are composed of more than one type of semiconductor and are classified according to the combination of semiconductors. For example, a device that is built from a combination of *N*-type and *P*-type semiconductors is called an NP-junction device. Another common name for semiconductor devices is *solid state devices*.

Diodes

The solid state device that consists of a p-type semiconductor block joined together with an N-type semiconductor block is called a PN-junction diode. Figure 1.7 shows the composition of the device at the electron level. A diode is a two-element device that offers a low resistance to current from one direction and a high resistance to current flow from the opposite direction. If the polarity of the voltage source is the same as the polarity of the diode, that is, if positive voltage is going into the p-type end of the diode, current will flow freely through the diode [forward bias situation (Fig. 1.8*A*)]. However, if the polarity of the current is reversed, current will

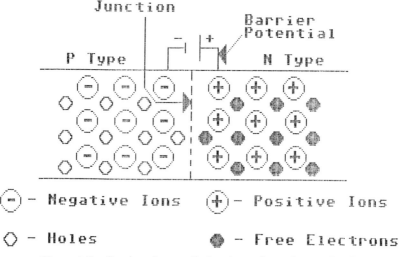

Figure 1.7. Semiconductor diode schematic at electron level.

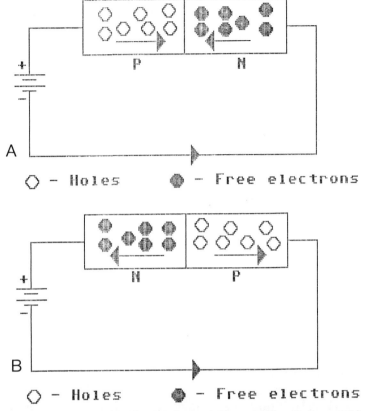

Figure 1.8. Electron flow for PN diode. *A*, Forward bias. *B*, Reverse bias.

be blocked by the diode [reverse bias situation (Fig. 1.8*B*)]. In addition, there is an effect of this unipolar response, which is called *rectification*.

A *rectifier* is a device that allows current to flow through in one direction only. (Sounds a lot like a diode, doesn't it?) For example, if an alternating current signal (which has both positive and negative current polarities) is applied to the P-type end of the device, only the positive part of the signal is sent through the device; whereas the negative portion will be blocked. This is half-wave rectification. If the negative portion of the waveform is made positive so that the whole waveform is positive, the process is termed full-wave rectification. Figure 1.9 illustrates these two types of rectification. Due to their "blocking" action, diodes are used to provide rectification in circuits.

Transistors

A transistor is a solid state device constructed of semiconductor materials and is used for amplification and/or control in electronic circuitry.

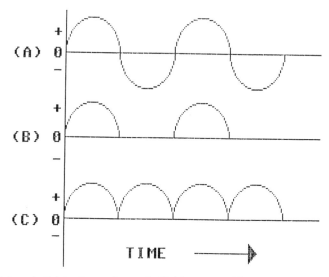

Figure 1.9.   *A*, Original waveform. *B*, Half-wave rectified. *C*, Full-wave rectified.

Since transistors are such an important component in modern instrumentation, we will devote some space to a description of their nature and operation.

Transistors perform many of the functions that vacuum tubes used to perform; they have largely replaced vacuum tubes because transistors are smaller, cheaper, require less power, and operate at low voltages with relatively high efficiency. Although diodes are also made from semiconductor materials, they do not amplify. Therefore, care should be taken not to classify all solid state devices as semiconductors, but rather as particular devices that are constructed from semiconductor materials.

To obtain amplification with semiconductors, a third semiconductor section must be added to form a semiconductor triode. Such a device is called a *junction transistor*. One type of transistor can be built by adding an N-type section to the PN diode described previously and reducing the thickness of the P-type section considerably. When the three sections are connected together, the P-type material is made common to both N-type sections. This is called an NPN junction transistor. If an N-type section is placed between two P-type sections, the transistor becomes a PNP junction transistor.

Figure 1.10 shows the general structure of NPN and PNP transistors along with their schematic symbols. Note that each transistor has three connections labeled collector, emitter, and base. The emitter and collector sections are the two outer sections, while the base is the inner section.

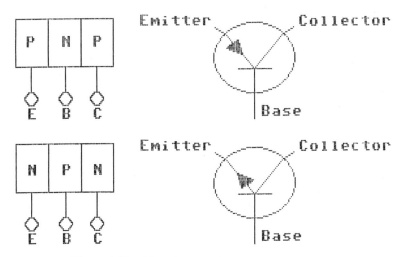

Figure 1.10.   Transistor structure and symbols.

As mentioned earlier, one of the primary uses of transistors is to amplify; that is, a small current at the input becomes a larger current at the output. Before explaining how transistors amplify and in order to better understand that aspect of transistor operation, we will describe basic transistor function.

You may recall that semiconductor devices, such as a diode, must be *biased* in order to operate properly. Therefore, a transistor can be viewed as two diodes of opposite polarity placed back-to-back, and so it is logical that two biases, of opposite polarity, are required to bias the transistor. Figures 1.11 and 1.12 illustrate the biasing of both NPN and PNP transistors and show the electron flow for each case.

Although the transistor is built as though it were two diodes placed back-to-back, the results of putting the three sections together does not produce two diodes. Rather, the result of the simultaneous presence of opposite polarity biases is to permit a heavy flow of current carriers (either electrons or holes) across the junction. The NPN transistor will be used as an example, but the same rules apply to PNP transistors. To apply the following discussion to PNP transistors, we simply replace electrons with holes and keep in mind the current flows illustrated in Figures 1.11 and 1.12.

The effect of the forward bias on the left NP section is to allow electrons to flow from the N section to the P section. Due to the reverse bias for the PN section on the right and based on the description of diode operation, it might be expected that current would be blocked by the PN section and would be sent through the base. However, the thinness of the P section does not permit it to carry much current because of the relative scarcity of holes and so little current can be carried by the base. The rest of the current

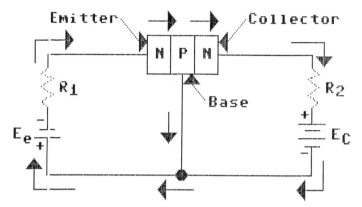

Figure 1.11. Biasing of NPN transistor.

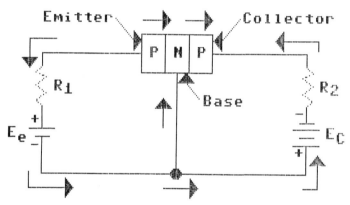

Figure 1.12. Biasing of PNP transistor.

is attracted through the N section by the positive polarity of the power supply on the right side of the transistor. Approximately 95%–98% of the electrons are attracted by the collector from the emitter. Note the similarity of name and function. For an NPN device, the emitter emits electrons and the collector collects electrons. This current flow in combination with the presence of the reverse bias at the collector is important for amplification by transistors.

Transistors as Amplifiers

To serve as amplifiers, transistors can be set up in a number of configurations; one configuration is the common-base circuit, which is shown in Figure 1.13. It can be seen that the circuit is the same as in Figure 1.11 except for two added elements: the microphone on the left, which in this case represents a signal source and a resistor placed between the collector

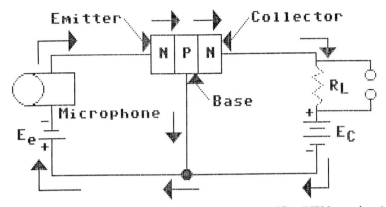

Figure 1.13. Simple common-base transistor amplifier (NPN transistor).

and the base, which represents the load resistance. To illustrate how voltage amplification is obtained using a transistor, we will describe the operation of this circuit.

Recall the discussion of how the current flows through a transistor. In this common-base circuit there is little resistance to flow through the emitter-base junction, whereas there is a large resistance to current flow through the base-collector junction. (Just as in the case of the resistors, energy cannot be "lost." Some of the energy in transistors is dissipated as heat; that is the reason for the "heat sinks" that are on printed circuits cards in computers. More about this in the computer chapter.) However, the current at the input and output stages of the circuit (Ie = emitter current and Ic = collector current) is almost the same, differing only by the very small current flowing through the base (Ib). This is represented mathematically in Equation 6.

$$Ic = Ie - Ib \qquad (6)$$

When acoustic energy is transduced by the microphone, a voltage is produced. For simplicity, let us assume a steady AC voltage of 1 volt. Let us also assume that the resistor has a value of 5,000 ohms. Now recall the very different resistances at the input and output of the transistor. A typical input resistance may be 10 ohms or less at the emitter. Ohm's law states that $E = IR$. If the emitter current is 0.01 amperes, then the collector current would be expected to be on the order of 0.0095 amperes and the base current would be 0.0005 amperes. (This is based on Equation 6 and the fact that 95%–98% of the current flows through the collector. Using a 95% ratio and the emitter current as 0.01 amperes yields $0.01 \times 0.95 = 0.0095$ amperes for the collector current. Rearranging Equation 6 gives $Ib = Ie - Ic$ or $0.01 - 0.0095 = 0.0005$ amperes for the base current.) Given a collector current of 0.0095 amperes and using Ohm's law, we find that the output voltage across the load resistor is 38 volts (0.0095 × 5,000) or 38 times the input voltage. Thus the transistor has supplied a voltage gain (output voltage divided by input voltage) of 38. The calculation is shown as

$$E = I \times R$$
$$= Ic \times \text{load resistance}$$
$$= 0.0095 \times 5,000$$
$$= 38 \text{ volts}$$

It should be noted that this output voltage is not "magic" and has to be supplied in the circuit. This is done by the DC power supply that maintains the reverse bias shown in the circuit. The power supply limits the output voltage, and the net result is that the signal source varies the output voltage by controlling the conduction of current through the transistor.

The components for the transistor described previously were passive components. However, as you may have guessed, the requirement for the presence of a power supply in order to properly bias transistor devices makes them active components.

The simple example just given shows how a transistor can provide amplification. An extension of the ability to amplify is the capability to "gate" signals. For the transistor to operate at all, some minimum voltage must be supplied to the transistor. If this voltage is not present, the transistor shuts off and will not pass any current. Thus there is a simple way to turn current on and off through a transistor, which is termed "gating." Logic devices that signal two logic states, such as "true" or "false," can be constructed of transistors; these two logic states can be given by having the transistor on or off. The ease of building circuits with transistors that can signal two logic states led to the development of digital computers and is the basis for the binary (0 or 1) logic of computer hardware.

Power Supplies

Perhaps the most critical part of a circuit is the power supply. Without power the circuit is "dead," and the most common cause of circuit failure is either a failed or improperly operating power supply. In fact, the first thing that most technicians check when troubleshooting an instrument or a circuit is the power supply. The intent of this section is to introduce different types of power supplies and a little bit about how they work.

The simplest type of power supply, which is very common, is a battery. A battery has several advantages, such as portability, ease of use, and low noise level. Most toys use this type of power supply, and all truly portable instruments employ batteries. In fact, for some applications such as physiological recording, batteries are frequently used as power supplies because of their low noise levels and because use of a battery isolates the instrument from defects in the electrical environment (such as "brownouts"), resulting from interruptions in power and fluctuations in the amount of power coming from the utility company. The main disadvantage of batteries is that their power becomes exhausted quickly, and they must be replaced frequently if the instrument gets heavy use. This can require frequent replacement of the battery in older instruments because the batteries cannot be recharged. Most current instrumentation provides rechargeable batteries whose power can be replaced from permanent power sources, considerably extending the life of the batteries. Most rechargeable batteries are good for one year, but should be replaced after one year because they do not charge efficiently and do not retain a charge well. Most laboratory and clinical instrumentation does not require noise levels as low as those required by physiological measurement instrumentation for producing accurate measurement and so does not use batteries; instead, clinical instrumentation uses the line power from a standard or three-pronged wall outlet.

It should be noted that most instrumentation employs three-pronged plugs; the third prong provides a stable ground. Unfortunately, the stability of the ground depends on how the ground wire to the third prong was installed, and many times the installation is considerably less than ideal. Another aspect of this topic is that outlets in separate rooms and labs should be isolated from one another. This is almost never done, and this can cause considerable problems when other devices that use a lot of power go on and off the line. A device that attempts to deal with this common problem is discussed later in this chapter.

Most instrumentation uses DC power internally, but the line power is AC. Therefore, the AC must be converted to DC. One method for doing this is to first convert the AC to a pulsing DC and then smooth the pulsing DC to get a steady DC current. Figure 1.14 illustrates how this conversion from AC to DC is done.

As noted previously, the term "power supply" is frequently a misnomer; a more appropriate term might be "power converter." The term power supply continues to be used because the purpose of the power supply is to provide power to the circuit at the appropriate voltages and currents. As Figure 1.14 shows, the AC current comes into the power supply as a sine wave. The wave is then rectified and smoothed. When the wave has been smoothed to a constant level, the power supply is producing DC power. The rectification is done by a diode, and the smoothing is done by a resistor-capacitor circuit. Devices supplying large voltages use tubes because of their larger current capacity, whereas most low-voltage applications use semiconductors, i.e., transistorized, power supplies. As more and more instruments use low-power devices, more and more power supplies are transistorized.

Power supplies provide appropriate voltages to circuits so that they may

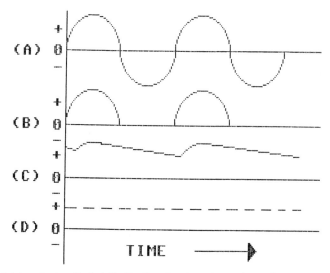

Figure 1.14. *A*, Applied AC. *B*, Conduction through a diode. *C*, Conduction through a resistor parallel with a capacitor. *D*, DC power out.

operate properly. Some applications are extremely sensitive to variations in the supply voltage, whereas other applications may be very tolerant of changes in supply voltage. These different types of requirements are reflected in regulated and unregulated power supplies. As their name implies, regulated power supplies provide exact voltages, and the power supply circuit is designed to provide compensation for changes in the voltage supplied to the power supply. [Recall from the previous discussion that power supplies get their power from the line source and so are subject to variations in this source]. The degree of regulation is dependent on the application, and regulated power supplies are more expensive than their unregulated counterparts. This does not mean that unregulated supplies are never used or are never appropriate, but merely that you should be aware that there is a difference. A regulated power supply may be required if the circuit or instrument cannot tolerate large voltage changes as in some computer devices.

Although regulated power supplies regulate the voltages internal to the instrument, instruments frequently need protection from unexpected changes in the power being supplied to the instrument from the line source. Devices that furnish this protection are line filters and surge protectors (sometimes referred to as "spike suppressors").

Line filters insure that the frequency of the current coming into the instrument is at the rated value. (Recall that the line source is an AC source and so has a particular frequency.) In the United States the standard line frequency is 60 hertz (Hz). In Europe and other places in the world the line frequency is usually different. Many instruments are designed for a particular line frequency but are frequently switchable between two or more line frequencies. If the line frequency is different from that required for the instrument, the instruments will not work properly or perhaps not at all. It is also possible that the instrument could be damaged if one attempts to use it under these conditions. A line filter insures that the power going to the instrument is at a specified frequency and does not deviate beyond specified limits. In particular, the intent is to prevent radio frequencies and other frequencies from being conducted down the line and into or out of the instrument. If you think of the power cord and power lines as antennas, you can see how this might happen. Also, many instruments use higher frequencies internally, which could interfere with the operation of other equipment. A common range for the filters to maintain is ±5% of the filter frequency.

The voltage surge protector, as its name implies, prevents large voltage changes. Just as in the case of line frequency, there is standard voltage for line power. In the United States the standard voltage is 110 volts. In other countries various voltages are used as standard, ranging from 100 (Japan) to 240 (Australia) volts. The surge protector prevents high voltages from being transmitted to the instrument and damaging it. In areas where there are large voltage fluctuations in combination with voltage-sensitive instrumentation, such as computers, voltage protectors are required. If interruption of service can be particularly damaging, then voltage surge protectors are frequently combined with line filters and a battery. Such devices are called "uninterruptable power supplies." Obviously the uninterruptable power supply provides the best protection from deficiencies in line power. The main drawback is that they are very expensive. Line filters and surge (or spike) protectors usually cost less and are sufficient for most purposes.

Chapter Summary

This chapter has introduced the basic facts about electricity. In particular, the quantities in Ohm's law have been described. Furthermore, components and power supplies as well as some of their properties, which are the parts that make up instruments, have been discussed. Some hints for proper use have been included along the way. The most critical component of most modern instrumentation, the integrated circuit, has not been discussed. However, the integrated circuit is essentially a special packaging of the components that have already been discussed, and thus is more properly explained in the next chapter on circuits.

2

Electrical Circuits

The instrumentation used in clinics and research laboratories is built from combinations of circuits, which in turn are built from combinations of the components discussed in Chapter 1. The intent of this chapter is to introduce some basics of circuit construction and analysis so that fundamental aspects of circuits may be recognized. To do this, we will explain some simple circuits and their electrical properties and derive rules for describing circuit operation. This chapter also describes integrated circuits and some basics of using integrated circuits.

The simplest circuit consists of a single component and a power supply. These simple circuits follow the rules discussed earlier for the components themselves; that is, it was assumed in the discussions of the individual components that power was supplied to the component. More commonly, circuits consist of combinations of several components. To simplify the discussion of circuit analysis, the sections on serial and parallel circuits in this chapter are restricted to cases where the components throughout the circuit are the same. In later chapters other types of circuits, e.g., resistor-capacitor (RC) circuits, will be described because their specific properties relate to topics, such as filtering, that will be discussed at that point.

Series Circuits

One easy way to build a circuit is to string together components of the same type one after the other. For example, three resistors could be attached to each other and, in turn, attached to a power supply (Fig. 2.1).

Several properties of this circuit are evident from the circuit diagram.

1. For the power supply to function properly the current must flow through the whole circuit, which means that
2. it must flow through each of the resistors in turn.

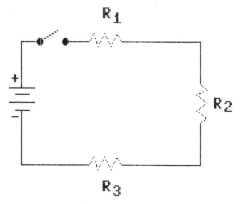

Figure 2.1. Simple series circuit.

3. All of the power comes from the one power supply, so the total voltage and total current are determined by the values for the circuit power supply.

The requirement that current must flow in order for the circuit to work suggests that if control of the circuit is desired, a method for turning the power on and off is necessary. The simplest way to do this is with a switch. (The symbol for a switch is shown in Table 1.2.) When the switch is open, no current can flow because no path is provided between the power supply and the circuit. When the switch is closed, current flows because a path has been provided. If the switch is closed, current will now flow through each of the resistors in turn. From the earlier discussion of resistors, it is evident that this will alter some aspects of the electrical signal. In particular, Ohm's law can be used to describe this circuit.

As already pointed out, the total voltage and current are determined by the power supply; therefore, the analysis of the circuit has to be focused on each of the resistors and how the changes in the parts, that is the resistors, fit into the whole. Power supplies are designated as voltage or current supplies, and after our analysis we will see why only voltage or current are specified.

Let us assume that the power supply in Figure 2.1 is a voltage supply and that it supplies 100 volts to the circuit. Furthermore, let us assume that the individual values of the three resistors are 100 ohms, 150 ohms, and 250 ohms. What is the voltage and current at each resistor? The answer involves applying Ohm's law to each of the three resistors in turn. However, before this can be done, the total current in the circuit must be determined. Since there is only one circuit path the current will be the same throughout the circuit. When the current is determined, then Ohm's law can be applied to each resistor to find the voltage for each one.

The total voltage was specified as 100 volts. Given the total resistance, Ohm's law can be used to determine the total current (I = E/R or total current = 100 volts/total resistance). In a series circuit the resistances are lined up one after the other, and so the current has to pass through each in turn. Thus the total resistance in the circuit is the sum of the resistances as given in Equation 1. For this circuit the total resistance (R_T) is 500 ohms.

$$R_T = R_1 + R_2 + \cdots + R_n \qquad (1)$$

Applying Ohm's law, we can calculate this circuit's total current to be 0.2 amperes. Given this current, knowing each resistance, and applying Ohm's law, we can calculate that the voltage at the first resistor is 20 volts (E = I × R or 0.2 × 100), at the second resistor 30 volts, and at the third resistor 50 volts. Note that the individual voltages add up to the total voltage of 100 volts. This will always be true in a series circuit. Note also that the voltage for each resistor is in the same proportion to the total voltage as the resistance for each resistor to the total resistance. For this reason, series circuits are sometimes referred to as "voltage dividers;" that is, the voltage is divided up among the resistors in the circuit. The lab exercises at the end of this chapter discuss how to measure these voltages and verify the properties of series circuits.

The components in circuits are not always laid out in series; another arrangement is to have the components in parallel. The most common situation is for instrumentation circuits to be combinations of parallel and series component circuits.

Parallel Circuits

As its name implies, a parallel circuit has the components arranged side by side rather than in a row. Figure 2.2 gives an example of a parallel circuit composed of the same components as were used for the series circuit. The switch that was mentioned for the series circuit is included in this circuit.

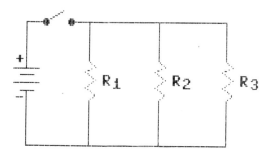

Figure 2.2. Simple parallel circuit.

It is apparent from Figure 2.2 that the most significant difference between parallel and series circuits is that the current has multiple paths in the parallel circuit while the current has a single path in the series circuit. The current will have to be divided among the branches of the parallel circuit in order for all branches to have power; thus parallel circuits can be used as current dividers. Like most things in nature, the current will be biased toward the path of least resistance (pun intended). In addition, because of the multiple paths, the total resistance of the circuit will not be the simple sum of the resistances in the circuit because the resistor impedes only a portion of the current. Equation 2 describes the total resistance in a parallel circuit. The effect of dividing the current is apparent in the equation.

$$1/R_T = 1/R_1 + 1/R_2 + \cdots + 1/R_n \qquad (2)$$

We will now go through an example of circuit analysis using Ohm's law for the circuit in Figure 2.2. Just as for the series circuit, the first step in the analysis of this circuit is to find the total resistance using Equation 2 and then to find the total current using Ohm's law. Using the values for R_1, R_2, and R_3 given for the series circuit, we find that the total resistance is 48.4 ohms. Note how much smaller the resistance is in a parallel circuit. Given the 100-volt power supply, the total current is 2.067 amperes. Recall that the current divides in a parallel circuit; therefore, we next calculate the current in each branch. Current (I) is easily calculated using Ohm's law, with R equal to the resistance in that branch and with E equal to 100 volts, giving a current of 1 ampere for the first branch, 0.67 ampere for the second branch, and 0.4 ampere for the third branch. Note the much larger currents in this circuit compared with the series circuit. This should be kept in mind when using parallel circuits because too much current will damage circuits. Go through the calculations with the values in the example circuit and then repeat the calculations with different component values to get an idea of how the quantities change with changes in component values. The lab exercises at the end of the chapter describe how to measure and verify these properties of parallel circuits.

It should be noted that not all components, when placed in parallel or series circuits, operate in the same manner as resistors. For example, capacitors perform in exactly the opposite way from resistors; that is, capacitances add in parallel circuits and divide in series circuits. Thus two capacitors of 1 microfarad will yield a total capacitance of 2 microfarads in a parallel circuit and 0.5 microfarad in a series circuit.

Integrated Circuits

The circuits that have been described thus far are combinations of discrete components. With the revolution in circuit miniaturization and the possibilities for manipulating semiconductor materials, it has become possible to integrate many discrete components into a single device called an *integrated circuit* (IC). Since integrated circuits are, in a sense, molded from a single material and then partitioned into individual integrated circuits, they are referred to as "chips."

The primary functions of integrated circuits are to amplify and to serve as logic devices. Since transistors perform these functions especially well and are constructed of semiconductor materials, transistors are the devices that are usually integrated into single components. Over the last several years the number of transistors that can be placed in a single integrated circuit has increased by many orders of magnitude. It is now possible to put about one million transistors on a single 1 mm^2 chip, and this number is certain to increase. Some of the functions and troubleshooting associated with integrated circuits will be discussed in later chapters.

Integrated circuits usually do not exist in isolation but are connected to other circuits. In addition to the rules governing behavior internal to the circuit, there are rules governing interconnections between circuits and interconnections between instruments, which is hardly surprising since instruments are collections of circuits. One very important set of rules has to do with the concept of impedance. The fundamental principles of impedance and its practical implications in terms of using instrumentation are discussed next.

Impedance

Reactance

The concept of impedance depends on the concept of reactance. We will cover two types of reactance: inductive reactance and capacitive reactance. Reactance is similar to resistance in the sense that it impedes current flow. However, reactance is different because it refers to impeding current flow without dissipating power, whereas resistors impede current flow *and* dissipate power. Recall that inductors and capacitors only operate in alternating current (AC) circuits. Thus, reactance operates in AC circuits and provides an opposition to current flow in addition to that due to resistors.

The concept of power was introduced in Chapter 1 and the general definition that power equals the voltage times the current was given. This definition will now be expanded to include both AC and direct current (DC) circuits. For DC circuits Equation 3

$$\text{Constant Power: } P = E \times I \tag{3}$$

will suffice. However, in an AC circuit the voltage and current are constantly changing, and, clearly, the power will be changing also. Thus, the appropriate measure of power in the AC circuit is the instantaneous power or the power at a given moment in time. This is defined in the same manner as the power for a DC circuit, that is

$$\text{Instantaneous Power: } p = e \times i \tag{4}$$

[Lowercase letters represent quantities that change from instant to instant (instantaneous values); capital letters represent constant or mean values.] However, instantaneous values are not very useful; therefore, we would like some measure comparable with the power for a DC circuit. A comparable measure is *effective* power. This is the sum of the powers calculated for each instantaneous value divided by the total time over which the power is calculated.

If both voltage and current are sine waves and in phase, then the effective power can be computed using the waveforms shown in Figure 2.3*A*. For the positive portion of the waveform the instantaneous voltage and current are both positive, and thus the instantaneous power will be positive. For the negative portion of the waveform both are negative, and thus the effective power will be negative.

What if the voltage and current are not in phase? Without worrying about how this might happen, let us consider an example where the current and voltage are 90 degrees out of phase. (This case is illustrated in Fig. 2.3*B*.) By going through the same analysis for the case where the voltage and current are in phase, we see that there are regions of positive and negative power. You may ask, What are positive and negative power? Positive and negative power must be considered in the context of circuits. Recall that for every circuit there is an energy source (the power supply). Positive power is when the circuit provides power to the power supply, and negative power is when the power supply is emitting power to the circuit.

The inductor, a device already described in Chapter 1, has these characteristics, namely, a phase shift and positive and negative power. Recall that the inductor operates by using a counter electromotive force (EMF) in opposition to the current. The magnetic field is proportional to the rate of change of the EMF. For a sine wave the maximum rate of change in the current occurs when the current equals zero; therefore, the maximum counter EMF or voltage will occur when the current equals zero. The end result is a 90-degree difference between the current and the voltage. It was pointed out earlier that the phase shift resulted in positive and negative power. The analysis indicated that half the time the power is positive and half the time the power is negative; the net result is no power dissipated by the ideal inductor. However, although there is no power dissipation as in a resistor, there remains an opposition to current. This opposition to current without power dissipation is referred to as *reactance*.

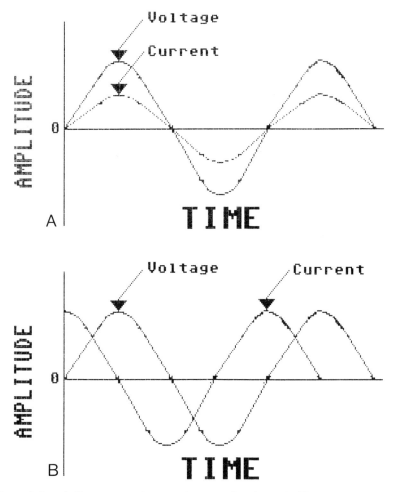

Figure 2.3.   *A*, Sine wave voltage and current in phase. *B*, Sine wave voltage and current 90° out of phase.

Since this opposition (reactance) is due to the counter EMF and the counter EMF is proportional to the change in the current, more specifically the rate of change of the current, the faster the current changes, the greater the reactance. Consequently, reactance is proportional to frequency. The actual mathematical relationship is shown in Equation 5, where XL is the inductive reactance, L is the inductance, and f is the frequency. (The factor of $2 \times$ pi comes from the fact that the waveform for the reactance is cyclical at a rate determined by f and the $2 \times$ pi factors translates the (frequency of the waveform into a magnitude. This will become clearer when vectors are discussed later in the chapter.)

$$XL = 2 \times \text{pi} \times f \times L \qquad (5)$$

The unit of inductance is the ohm, because multiplying current times reactance results in a counter EMF, which is a voltage.

Inductive reactance is one of the two forms of reactance, and the other form is capacitive reactance. Recall the earlier discussion concerning how a capacitor charges, where it was pointed out that the capacitor discharges only when there is a change in the current. If the same analysis is performed with a capacitor placed across an alternating current as was done with an inductor, we find that the current and voltage are out of phase by 90 degrees and that the power is positive and negative half of the time. One difference between the capacitor and inductor is that the 90-degree shift is in the opposite direction; that is, in the inductor the voltage leads the current by a quarter cycle (as the current starts to build up the counter EMF is at a maximum). However, in the capacitor, the current leads the voltage by a quarter cycle (the current starts at a maximum and the voltage on the capacitor builds up). Because of the split between negative and positive power and lack of resistance, there is no power dissipation in a pure capacitance.

Just as in the inductor, in the capacitor there is also a relation between frequency and reactance. Recall that the larger the capacitance, the larger the charge and the greater the current that it can accommodate; hence the "AC resistance" to the flow of current will be less. Thus, the larger the capacitance, the less the reactance, which makes reactance inversely proportional to frequency. This is expressed mathematically (again the unit is ohms) in Equation 6.

$$XC = 1/(2 \times \text{pi} \times f \times C) \tag{6}$$

where XC is the capacitive reactance, C is the capacitance, and f is the frequency (the $2 \times$ pi factor is present for the same reason as in Equation 5 for inductive reactance).

In most circuits, reactances are combined with resistance. The combination of reactance(s) with resistance is referred to as *impedance.*

Vector Representation of Impedance

Up to this point reactances have been treated in terms of the waveform. While this approach illustrates some of the underlying properties of reactance, it is a very inconvenient and awkward way to describe magnitudes and phases for the components of reactance. To determine impedance it will be necessary to combine reactances. A common way to display magnitude and phase is to use vectors, which are lines plotted on a coordinate system. This has the advantage that measures combining vectors can be shown and treated graphically. Figure 2.4 shows a typical coordinate system for a two-dimensional vector plot. Vector plots can have as many dimensions as are needed, but only two dimensions are needed for impedance. Figure 2.4 illustrates how the magnitude and phase of a vector

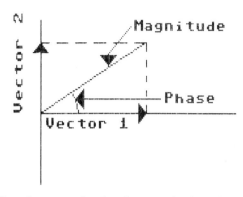

Figure 2.4. Sample vector plot showing magnitude and phase calculation.

resulting from the combination of two vectors are displayed on such a plot.

Impedance can be composed solely of resistance or of resistance along with inductive reactance and/or capacitive reactance. Each of these three cases of resistance where it combines with either one or both of the components of reactance will be treated separately. All cases will be treated in terms of input-output relationships. They are discussed in these terms because the primary influence of impedance is to alter the signal as it passes through the system. Thus, by examining how the output has changed relative to the input, we can gain an understanding of impedance and its effects.

The first case to be treated is the combination of resistance and inductive reactance. What is the output of this system for a given input? Since we are dealing with AC circuits, the simplest input is a sinusoid. Rather than dealing with the input on a point-by-point basis (which is dull, boring, and slow), we will only treat the magnitudes (which is easy, interesting, and fast). If the input is a sinusoidal voltage then the reactance will also be sinusoidal; the resistance is constant. To represent this on a vector plot, we consider everything relative to the input. The input sinusoid is considered as having a phase of zero but is not shown on the plot. The vector plot shows only the output components. As shown in figure 2.4, a phase of zero on a vector plot is represented as the positive x-axis on the plot. Since resistance is a constant, it has the same phase as the input, that is, a phase of zero. Thus resistance is represented as a vector along the x-axis with a length equal to the magnitude of the resistance. Since inductive reactance leads the input by 90 degrees (as discussed earlier), it is represented by a vector at +90 degrees relative to the resistance with a length equal to the magnitude of the reactance (Fig. 2.5*A*).

The second case to be discussed is resistance with capacitive reactance.

The rationale is the same as for the first case, except capacitive reactance lags the input by 90 degrees and, therefore, the capacitive reactance vector is drawn at −90 degrees relative to the resistance vector with a length equal to the magnitude of the capacitive reactance (Fig. 2.5*B*).

The vector plots clearly provide a much easier way to analyze reactance combinations than by using a point-by-point analysis of sine waves. This becomes even more apparent when the third case, resistance with inductive

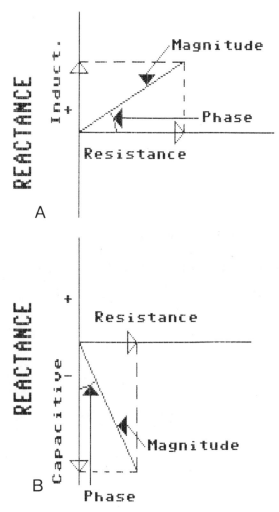

Figure 2.5.   Sample vector plots showing vector sums of (*A*) inductive reactance and resistance and (*B*) capacitive reactance and resistance.

and capacitive reactances, is analyzed. Since each of the components is represented by a separate vector, all components together can be placed on the same vector plot.

Although each component can be easily represented on such a plot, the quantity (i.e., impedance) that we ultimately want to derive is the result of the combination of these components. Fortunately, the vector plot provides an easy solution to this problem. Since each of the components can be represented by a vector, the combination can be represented by a vector combination, which in turn can be represented by a vector sum. Figure 2.6 illustrates how this can be done.

Since the two reactive components are on the same axis, their magnitudes can simply be added together, which results in another vector that can be added to the resistance. To combine two vectors that are not on the same axis, a different form of vector addition must be utilized. Vectors that both have their bases at the origin are added pictorially by drawing a line of the same phase and length as one vector from the end of the other vector and then drawing a line from the origin to the "free" end of the first vector (Fig. 2.6, *dashed line*). (Some readers may recognize the resultant shape as a parallelogram. This figure may also be familiar to those who have studied middle ear impedance or the impedance of mechanical systems.) The *dashed line* in Figure 2.6 represents the combination of all three vectors and hence the combination of all the components of impedance (resistance and the inductive and capacitive reactances). An actual numerical value for the impedance can be obtained with such a plot by measuring the length of the line.

An actual numerical value for the impedance can also be obtained from

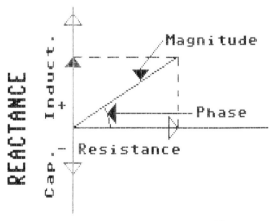

Figure 2.6.   Sample vector plot showing vector sum of inductive and capacitive reactances and resistance.

the fact that the line in these vector plots represents the diagonal from a rectangle (because the reactance components always have a 90-degree phase difference from the resistance component). The length of a diagonal for a rectangle is given by the Pythagorean theorem. Using this theorem, we get Equation 7.

$$Z^2 = R^2 + X^2 \tag{7}$$

Recall that X actually equals the sum of XL and XC and that XC has a negative sign because of the 90-degree phase lag. Thus we get Equation 8.

$$Z^2 = R^2 + (XL - XC)^2 \quad \text{or} \tag{8}$$
$$Z = (R^2 + (XL - XC)^2)^{1/2}$$

Equation 8 gives the relation between impedance (Z) and resistance, inductive reactance, and capacitive reactance. It also turns out that because of this relationship—recall that we started out with sinusoidal voltage or current waveforms—there is a generalized Ohm's law for AC circuits that simply replaces R with Z, in keeping with the concept of impedance representing an "AC resistance," namely,

$$E = I \times Z, \quad E/Z = I, \quad \text{and} \quad E/I = Z$$

where E and I may be corresponding peak values, effective values, and so forth, as long as the magnitudes for V, I, and Z are determined in the same manner.

An examination of Equation 8 raises an interesting question: What happens if XL equals XC? In this case, the magnitudes would cancel, leaving only resistance. What about phases? Since XL and XC lead and lag respectively by the same amount, the phases also cancel and the overall voltage and current are in phase as if only the resistance were present. Thus the case where XL and XC are equal is the case that will result in the maximum amount of power being dissipated in the circuit because the reactance is zero. There is another interesting facet to this particular case of $XL = XC$. If the appropriate expressions are substituted for XL and XC, then we get Equation 9.

$$2 \times \text{pi} \times f \times L = 1/(2 \times \text{pi} \times f \times C) \tag{9}$$

Note that only one value of f will satisfy this equation for any given values of L and C, that is, the circuit will act as a pure resistance only at the frequency given in Equation 10.

$$f = 1/(2 \times \text{pi} \times (L \times C)^{1/2}) \tag{10}$$

This frequency is the *resonant* frequency of the circuit, which is a very useful quantity to know because it represents the frequency at which the maximal power will flow.

It can be shown that the maximum current will occur only for this special case by using Ohm's law for current in AC circuits and the derivation for impedance in terms of reactance and resistance. Since

$$I = E/Z = E/(R^2 + (XL - XC)^2)^{1/2}$$

it is clear that the current will be greatest when XL and XC are equal, which occurs at the resonant frequency. Also note that for any other case the current will be less. This current peak in the frequency domain is the basis for resonators, which are frequently used for filtering—a topic that will be discussed in a later chapter.

We can conclude from the preceding discussion of impedance that impedance describes circuit output with regard to its input, especially with regard to the frequency of the input. This is obviously very important for AC circuits. In instrumentation, impedance has implications for interactions between instruments and provides the basis for optimum operation. As was indicated before, impedance describes the sum of the reactance and resistance components of a circuit. We have seen that circuits dissipate their maximum power when XL equals XC. When two circuits interact, the best case for power transfer will be when the two circuits exhibit the same behavior with regard to input frequency. Since impedance describes this behavior, it makes sense that two instruments interact optimally when their impedances are equal. Whenever two instruments are interconnected, every effort should be made to match the impedances of the two instruments because this will result in optimal performance.

Equation 11 is the proportion of the power of device a that will be transmitted to device b given the impedance of device a and the impedance of device b. Two important properties of combining impedances are derived from this equation:

1. If the impedances for both devices are the same, all the power will be transmitted from device a to device b.
2. If the impedances for both devices are not the same, all the power from device a will *not* be transmitted to device b; this will be the case regardless of the direction of the impedance mismatch, that is, regardless of which device has the lower impedance.

$$X = 4 \times Z_a \times Z_b/(Z_a + Z_b)^2 \tag{11}$$

Mismatches in impedance not only result in power loss between instruments as described by Equation 11 but can also result in the creation of unwanted signals. This aspect of impedance mismatches will be discussed in a later chapter when distortion is examined. The basic rule to follow is to match impedance when connecting devices.

Chapter Summary

This chapter provided an introduction to the fundamentals of electronic circuits. Some basic information was provided including a description of circuits and some simple analyses of circuits. The final topic was impedance, which is very important for describing the behavior of circuits when signals are applied and for interconnecting instrumentation. The lab exercises at the end of this chapter will permit some "hands-on" experience with concepts that have been discussed in this chapter and Chapter 1. In addition, the labs provide an introduction to some of the instrumentation that will be described in Chapter 3. The next chapter will discuss basic test instrumentation and how this test instrumentation may be utilized to measure some of the fundamental properties of electronics that were described in this chapter.

1

Series and Parallel Circuit Construction and Testing with a VOM

Introduction

*T*his lab provides hands-on experience with building simple circuits and in using a VOM (voltohmmeter) to examine the circuit after you have built it. The lab will also give you an opportunity to verify Ohm's law for yourself (to see that its does work in real life). *Be sure to read the entire description for this laboratory before doing any of the work.*

Method

Apparatus

You will receive two resistors and several pieces of wire in a box. There will also be a battery or a power supply that gets its power from the wall outlet and a soldering iron with solder to build the circuit. The final piece of equipment will be the VOM. The VOM described in this laboratory is called a "digital multimeter." This particular model is made by Tektronix, but other digital multimeters will be very similar.

Use of the Soldering Iron

A soldering iron is basically a piece of metal that is heated to a sufficient temperature to melt the solder. The solder itself is a conductive, low-melting-temperature metal similar to silver. The solder provides a way of securing components in a circuit that need to conduct electricity between them. Soldering is not equivalent to welding, that is, the solder is not intended to provide major structural support but only connective support. Therefore, do not expect the solder to hold the circuit together if any great amount of stress is placed on the circuit.

To solder a wire to a component, place the wire against the component with the tip of the solder against the wire. Place the soldering iron on the wire close to but not on the solder. The wire will heat up and melt the solder and it will flow onto the wire and the component. Use a *small* amount of solder. Using large amounts of solder leads to "cold joints," which are cases where air pockets form within the solder and act as insulators. As said earlier, air is an insulator. Do not hold the soldering iron against the wire too long because the wire will get very hot and you might burn yourself.

A little observation and thought will suggest that the means of soldering just described clearly requires at least three hands, one for each of the components and one to handle the solder and one for the soldering iron . . . well, maybe four hands. Now is the time to remember the value of preparation and cooperation. If two people do the soldering, make sure both know what they are doing. Another suggestion is to wrap the wire around the component prior to soldering so that it does not have to be held in place. This will help avoid accidents such as burns and also help insure good circuit construction.

Use of the Voltohmmeter

The digital multimeter that will be provided is a multifunction instrument (as are most VOMs) that can measure current (AC or DC), voltage (AC or DC), or resistance. For voltage, the measurement can be direct (in terms of volts) or in terms of decibels relative to 1 volt. The type of measurement is determined by the position of the rotary dial on the face of the multimeter. In addition, the range of measurement for a particular type of measurement is determined by the position of the dial. Looking at the dial, you can see that the value in decibels for a zero meter value is shown on the outside of the range indications for voltage. The meter readout itself is called a "digital readout," which just means that instead of a needle meter which has a needle pointing to position on a scale, the digital meter gives a readout in numbers. The range for meter readouts on this multimeter is between −20 and +20. It will also provide values outside this range with reduced accuracy. This "extra range" measurement is indicated by a flashing meter display. It is best to avoid this by adjusting the dial so that the reading is steady and not flashing. This meter is "3 ½ digits," which means that the last digit has some specified error. However, the meter displays four digits along with a sign.

To measure the current in amperes, you must set the meter to the appropriate type of measurement (amperes) and then to the appropriate range within that type of measurement. To get an idea of the appropriate range, look at the power supply and see what current is being provided to the circuit. This will give you an upper bound, at least for the types of circuits that you will be measuring. To make the measurement itself, you must insert the meter into the circuit so that it is part of the circuit. In the case of the series circuit, this means that the wire from the negative pole of the meter must be toward the negative pole of the power supply and the positive pole of the meter must be toward the positive pole of the power supply. You might try switching this orientation to see what happens. It will not damage the meter.

To measure voltage in volts, you must set the dial to the voltage scale and then to the appropriate range. Just as with the current measurement you can get an idea of the upper bound from the voltage being supplied to the circuit by the power supply. To make the measurement attach the meter outside the circuit from point to point using clip leads. Clip leads are wires that attach at one end to the meter and have alligator clips on the other end for attaching to measurement points. Again the negative pole of the meter should be oriented toward the negative pole of the power supply and the positive pole of the meter is oriented toward the positive pole of the power supply. As with the ampere measurement, you can try reversing the leads to see what happens. This is much easier with this measurement because the meter is outside the circuit and is attached with clip leads.

The resistance measurement is made outside the circuit just as the voltage measurement is made outside the circuit, but it is made with power off. *Caution: The meter is not inserted into the circuit.* The meter dial is set to OHMS and the range is set by looking at the code on the component. The code for the resistor is determined by looking at the color code on the resistor and then decoding it as in Table 1.3. The leads are attached on each side of the resistor and the value in ohms is read off the meter.

With regard to reading the meter and arriving at the correct units, note the scale values around the dial. In particular, note the value between the two red lines on the plastic collar of the rotary dial itself. This value is the range for that setting of the meter. Notice that at various places around the dial there are abbreviations such as "mV." These abbreviations indicate units that are not shown as part of the scale value itself. Be sure to look carefully at the scale value so that you use the correct units.

Procedure

Series Circuit

Construction.   Before constructing the circuit, measure the resistance of each of the resistors. Then measure the voltage of the power supply. To construct a series circuit, take one of the two resistors and attach a wire to each end using solder and the soldering iron. For the other resistor, solder a wire to just one end. Now solder the second resistor to one of the wires from the first resistor. Then attach the loose wire from each resistor to each of the poles of the power supply. *Do not solder the leads to the power supply.* You now have a series circuit (Fig. 2.7).

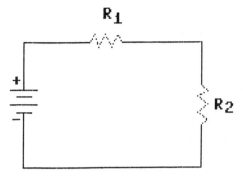

Figure 2.7. Simple series circuit.

Measurement.   After constructing the circuit and attaching the power supply, measure the voltage across each of the two resistors. Then measure the amperage at the negative end of the circuit by removing the wire from the power supply and inserting the multimeter. Now break the circuit in the middle and measure the current at that point by inserting the meter into the circuit at that point. This will finish your measurements for the series circuit. It is not necessary to reconstruct the series circuit unless you want to check some measurement, which is not always a bad idea. Look at your numbers and see if they are reasonable based on Ohm's law.

Parallel Circuit

Construction.   To construct a parallel circuit, take the two resistors and reconnect them. Take one of the wires on the end of the circuit and attach it to the opposite end of the other resistor. The circuit should now look like a square with a tail. The square should have resistors on opposite sides and wires on the other two sides. Now take the side of the circuit with one of the resistors and the tail and attach a wire to the other end of the resistor. When you are done, the two loose wires should be coming from each end of one of the resistors. The two loose wires should now be attached to the poles of the power supply. *Do not solder the wires to the power supply.* You now have a parallel circuit (Fig. 2.8).

Measurement.   The resistance values and power supply voltage were already determined during work on the previous circuit, but the power supply voltage should be checked. Now measure the voltage across each of the resistors. As before, break the circuit in each of the branches and measure the current within the branch by inserting the meter into the circuit at that point.

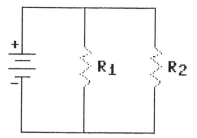

Figure 2.8.   Simple parallel circuit.

Results

Draw a circuit diagram for each circuit labeling all components along with their values. Compare the measured value of each resistor to its rated value. Prepare a table of these measured and rated values.

Use the rated value of the resistors and the known output of the power supply to compute (using Ohm's law) a set of predicted voltage and amperage values for each circuit at the measurement points that were used. Prepare a table of these predicted values along with the actual measurement values. For each circuit be sure to compute V, I, and R, that is, the total voltage, current, and resistance in the circuit respectively, and put these in your tables. Create separate tables of predicted and actual values for the series and parallel circuits.

Discussion

How well did your circuits conform to expectations? That is, how well does Ohm's law work in the real world? Support your conclusions by using the data that you have collected in this lab. What measurements are the easiest to make? What implications do you think this might have for the way circuits will be specified in terms of the measurements for checking out circuits?

Comparing AC and DC Voltage Relationships

Introduction

*R*ecall from our discussion of circuit analysis that the impedance of an AC circuit is determined by combining the reactance of the circuit with the resistance in the circuit *vectorially*. This can be done by drawing lines to scale representing the resistance and reactance to form the legs of a right triangle. The hypotenuse of the right triangle is equal to the impedance on the same scale, and the angle between the resistance and impedance lines is equal to the phase angle between the voltage and the current in the circuit.

Since the resistance and reactance must be combined vectorially to obtain the impedance, it is reasonable to expect the voltage drops across these components must also be combined vectorially. In the simple series DC circuit used in Quiklab 1, we noted that the sum of the voltage drops across the resistors equals the applied voltage (Kirchoff's voltage law). The circuit used in Quiklab 1, with two resistors, is reproduced here in Figure 2.9*A*. Figure 2.9*B* shows a similar circuit, but the second resistor has been replaced with a capacitor.

The replacement of the resistor with a capacitor has changed the circuit from a purely resistive circuit to a reactive circuit. Hence, the voltage across the resistor and the voltage across the capacitor cannot be simply added to get the supply voltage, but the two voltages must be combined vectorially. The combination is done in the same manner as for the impedance calculation. The two voltages represented by the resistive and reactive components are drawn as vectors in a right triangle, and the hypotenuse of that triangle represents the combined voltage.

This Quiklab is intended to demonstrate the relationships just discussed. The combined voltages for a purely resistive circuit and for a reactive circuit will be calculated using simple addition and vector addition and compared.

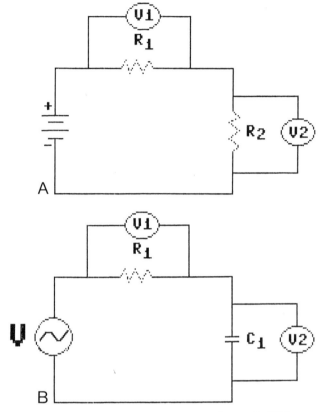

Figure 2.9. Simple series circuits. *A*, With two resistors; *B*, With one resistor and one capacitor.

Method

Apparatus

The following parts and tools are required for building the two AC circuits for this lab. Circuit 1 (a purely resistive series AC circuit) requires

1. Soldering iron;
2. Solder;
3. Wire (#16 gauge or larger);
4. Breadboard (if not using items 1, 2, and 3);
5. Three resistors (100, 200, and 300 ohms);
6. AC signal source.

Circuit 2 (a reactive series AC circuit) requires

1. Items 1–4 and 6 from circuit 1;
2. One resistor (approximately 5,000 ohms);
3. One capacitor (approximately 1 microfarad).

Circuit Construction

Use the techniques given in Quiklab 1 and the components listed previously to construct circuit 1, the purely resistive circuit. After making the measurements given next, use the same techniques to construct circuit 2, the reactive circuit.

Test Procedure and Measurements

For testing circuit 1, the purely resistive series circuit, follow these steps:

1. Measure the AC voltage drop across each resistor with a multimeter or voltmeter using the procedures given in Quiklab 1. Use the AC volts scale to make the measurement. Record each of the values.

$$\text{Voltage drop across } R_1 = V_1 = \underline{\hspace{2cm}}\text{volts}$$
$$\text{Voltage drop across } R_2 = V_2 = \underline{\hspace{2cm}}\text{volts}$$

2. Add the voltages obtained in step 1 and record the value.

$$V_1 + V_2 = \underline{\hspace{2cm}}\text{volts}$$

3. Measure the voltage of the AC voltage source and record the value.

$$V_s = \underline{\hspace{2cm}}\text{volts}$$

If everything is going well, V_s should equal the total from step 2. If not, check the circuit to make sure that it is properly constructed. Then go back to step 1 and repeat the measurements. If a measurement is not the same as before, repeat it again for verification. If all else fails, see the instructor.

To test circuit 2, the reactive series circuit, follow these steps:

1. Measure the voltage drop across the resistor and the voltage drop across the capacitor using the techniques from Quiklab 1. Record the values.

$$\text{Voltage across the resistor} = V_1 = \underline{\hspace{2cm}}\text{volts}$$
$$\text{Voltage across the capacitor} = V_2 = \underline{\hspace{2cm}}\text{volts}$$

2. Add the voltages from step 1 using simple addition and record the value.

$$V_s = V_1 + V_2 = \underline{\hspace{2cm}}\text{volts}$$

3. Combine the voltages vectorially as shown in Figure 2.10. Recall from the introduction that the same scale is used for all voltages and that the hypotenuse represents the combined voltage. Record the values.

$$\text{Vectorially calculated } V_s = \underline{\hspace{2cm}}\text{volts}$$

Before completing step 4, let us discuss how to use Figure 2.10, which illustrates the vector sum used to calculate the combined voltage for circuit 2. The vector sum can also be computed mathematically and

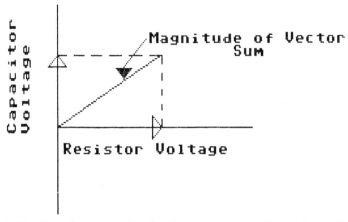

Figure 2.10. Sample vector plot showing vector sum of capacitor voltage and resistor voltage.

given the ease of the computation is clearly much easier to do than to draw figures and compute the vector from the figure. Equation 7 in Chapter 2 describes the mathematics for doing the computation. If R in Equation 7 is replaced with V_1 and X is replaced with V_2, the equation will yield V_s.

4. Measure the voltage across the AC voltage source and record the value.

$$V_s = \underline{\hspace{2cm}}\text{volts}$$

If circuit 2 has been constructed correctly and the measurements are accurate, the voltage recorded in step 4 should equal the voltage in step 3 and not the voltage in step 2. If this is not the case, follow the remedy given for circuit 1.

Results and Discussion

Tabulate your results in two tables, one for each circuit. Note the difference in results for the two circuits. Discuss why the two circuits gave different results.

3

Test Instrumentation

In the previous chapter we discussed general principles of electricity and used a voltmeter in the laboratory exercise. A voltmeter is an example of *test* instrumentation, which may be distinguished from the *clinical* and *research* instrumentation that will be discussed in section II of this book. Test instrumentation is used primarily to calibrate other instruments rather than to make experimental measurements. This does not imply that test instruments are not involved in the analysis of experimental data, but rather that the primary function and purpose of these instruments is to examine and calibrate other instruments.

It is important to note that test instrumentation must be calibrated *before* it can be used. Usually such calibration requires special equipment and has to be done by the manufacturer of the equipment. The manufacturer frequently derives his standards for calibration from the National Bureau of Standards in Washington, D.C., which develops and provides standards for accuracy. A general rule of thumb for test instrumentation is that the instrument doing the calibration measures must have significantly less error than the instrument being calibrated. For example, if the measurement accuracy of an instrument is specified as $\pm 10\%$, then the calibrating instrument should have an error of less than $\pm 1\%$. In general, test instrumentation should be as accurate as can be afforded.

Brief descriptions of the use of test instrumentation necessary for a particular lab will be covered in the Quiklabs. Instructions for use presented in the Quiklabs refer to particular instruments, but test instruments serving a particular purpose (for example, VOMs) are similar and there should be little difficulty applying the instructions to other models of the same type of instrument. While this chapter will focus on general principles of operation for the instruments, some of the particularly salient aspects of use for each test instrument will also be covered within separate sections in this chapter.

If at all possible, read these sections with the appropriate instrument right in front of you. This will enable you to try out the directions for use immediately and experiment with the instrument. There is no substitute for direct or "hands on" experience with instrumentation. There is an art as well as a science to the use of instrumentation, and the only way to develop the art is to practice the science. It is very similar to learning how to perform in the clinic. The first client is always tough, but with experience things become easier. This message will be repeated frequently throughout the book.

Voltohmmeters

The voltmeter is probably the most ubiquitous of all test instrumentation. This is because it measures the most fundamental of all aspects of instrumentation, namely, the electricity that "drives" all other instrumentation. Although there are devices that measure only voltage, the voltmeter used for circuit testing and other general troubleshooting is more properly referred to as a "voltohmmeter" (VOM). Occasionally, in manufacturers' specifications, you will see the acronyms VTVM or VTVOM. These refer to vacuum tube models, which are not used very often. Thus, when we refer to a "voltmeter" in this text it should be understood that we are referring to a VOM. The theory of operation of a VOM will be discussed before describing how to use a VOM in order to develop some appreciation for what a VOM does when we use it to make our measurements. In addition, the meter's calibration must be checked prior to use, and the procedure for doing this will be described.

There are two general models of VOM: an analog model, which uses the quantity measured to move a needle on a meter scale, and a digital model, which converts the quantity to a number and displays the number. Both types of VOM measure current and resistance using Ohm's law (see chapter 1), but the voltage measurements for the two types of VOM are done differently. *Voltage* is measured for the analog model by passing the unknown voltage over a known resistance and using the resulting current to control the movement of the meter needle. Since in this case current is directly proportional to voltage, the greater the voltage, the greater the current and the more the needle will move. Calibrating the amount of needle movement for a given amount of voltage will accurately move the needle through the conversion of voltage into current. Current is measured by passing the unknown current over a known resistance and using the voltage change to move the needle. Recall that voltage will be proportional to current, and so the greater the current, the greater the voltage, given that the resistance is constant. Resistance is measured by passing a known current over the unknown resistance and using the resulting change in voltage to move the needle. The greater is the resistance, the greater is the voltage change; hence the greater is the needle movement.

The digital model measures the voltage directly by comparing the voltage coming into the instrument to a known voltage through devices called "analog-to-digital converters" and "comparators." It is not necessary at this time to know how these devices work. The point is that the digital VOM actually only measures one quantity and that is voltage. All other measurements are derived from the voltage measurements using Ohm's law. The current is determined by passing the unknown current through a known resistance and measuring the voltage change. Resistance is measured by passing a known constant current through the unknown resistance and measuring the resulting voltage drop. The AC current and voltages are rectified (all values are made positive) and the resulting DC voltages are used. Interactions between the VOM and the instrument under test are avoided by having very high input impedances at the meter.

As an illustration of how the digital meter would work, consider how the VOM would measure DC current. Inside the meter there is a resistor for each of the settings of the VOM. We will say that the current going into the meter is 0.5 amperes and that the resistor in the meter is 1,000 ohms. Using Ohm's law ($V = I \times R$) gives us $V = 0.5 \times 1,000$ or $V = 500$ volts. If the amperage were reduced to 0.2 ampere, the voltage would be reduced to 200 volts. Working through several of these examples will show that the voltage changes in the same manner as the current if the resistance stays constant. The VOM takes advantage of that fact by using the voltage to adjust the meter reading.

An important fact should be noted with regard to making AC measurements. Many VOMs are "root-mean-square" (RMS) voltmeters. For AC measurements it is critical that the user be familiar with the difference between amplitude as measured on an oscilloscope and the reading that will be obtained on the VOM.

The term *root-mean-square* is equivalent to saying, "the square root of the mean square of the waveform deviations from zero," which sounds much more confusing than it really is. Figure 3.1 shows how the RMS calculation is done for a sine wave. In effect, a square wave with the same area as the sine wave is superimposed onto the sine wave. The amplitude of this square wave is the RMS amplitude for the sine wave. There is a constant conversion factor between the RMS aplitude and the peak amplitude of the sine wave. The RMS amplitude will always be 0.707 times the peak amplitude of the sine wave, which, as we will see, has advantages and disadvantages.

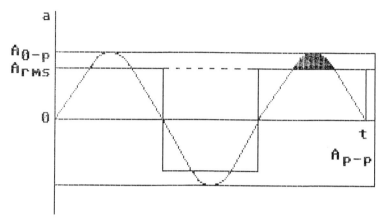

Figure 3.1. Comparison of root-mean-square amplitude (A_{rms}) to peak (A_{0-p}) to peak-to-peak amplitude (A_{p-p}).

Many VOMs take advantage of the relation between the RMS conversion factor and another conversion factor. The relation between *peak* and *average* amplitude of the sine wave after it has been rectified is that the average equals 0.636 times the peak value and is 0.9 times the RMS amplitude. VOMs that use the technique of finding the average amplitude, which is easier to instrument, are referred to as "averaging voltmeters." Voltmeters that actually measure the RMS amplitude are referred to as "true RMS" voltmeters.

Why is it important how the VOM measures amplitude? Part of the purpose of Quiklab 2 is to address this issue by comparing the measurement of a variety of waveforms by an averaging VOM with the measurement of the same waveforms by an oscilloscope. It will be seen that comparing measurements for the VOM to measurements from the oscilloscope for waveforms such as triangular waveforms can be difficult because separate conversion factors need to be determined for each waveform. That is, the relation between the average amplitude of a waveform and the RMS amplitude of a waveform is not the same for all waveforms. As a result, if you were unaware of how the VOM makes the amplitude measurement, you could easily reach an erroneous conclusion regarding the accuracy of measurement for instrumentation, such as oscilloscopes, which may measure other aspects of the waveform. The amplitude measurements for a particular waveform also would be in error if this factor is not taken into account.

Calibrating the Voltohmmeter

Prior to making any measurements with a VOM it is necessary to calibrate the meter. The meter is calibrated by using a known value to check the meter reading. It is known that if the positive and ground or negative probes of the VOM are pressed together the resistance between the probes should be zero. This provides an easy way to check the meter. Thus VOMs are typically checked by putting the probe tips together with the VOM measuring resistance. The meter should read zero, and there is usually an adjustment available to correct for small errors. If the meter is consistently in error and needs to be constantly adjusted, it should be checked for malfunction, which is best done by the manufacturer. If the meter is a portable meter, then the first thing to try is replacing the battery. A good indication that the VOM's battery is weak or dying is erratic measurements, such as not being able to get the same value on two different days for the same measurement. Replacement of the battery is a simple operation that can be done by consulting the manual.

Reading the Voltohmmeter

The VOM that will be described in this section is called a "digital multimeter." The digital multimeter is a digital model VOM and is a multifunction instrument, as are most VOMs. The rules for use given next apply to all VOMs except with regard to reading the meter, which for many VOMs is a needle meter display rather than a digital display. Figure 3.2 shows an example for both types of VOM. A digital display gives a readout in numbers rather than by means of a needle meter pointing to a position on a scale. The range for meter readouts on digital multimeters is usually symmetric about zero, e.g., between −20 and +20. The meter will also provide values outside this range with reduced accuracy. This "extra range" measurement is frequently indicated by a flashing meter display. In general, it is best to avoid this by adjusting the dial so that the reading is

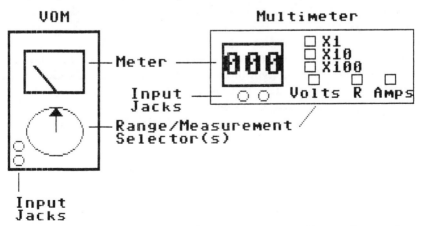

Figure 3.2. Two common forms of voltmeter. The multimeter is sometimes referred to as a "digital" voltmeter.

steady and not flashing. Meters are quantified in terms of the number of digits of accuracy; for example "3½ digits," which means that the last digit has some specified error. However, the readout would be four digits along with a sign.

A multimeter can measure current (AC or DC), voltage (AC or DC), or resistance. For voltage, the measurement can be direct (in terms of volts) or in terms of decibels (dB) relative to the midrange value (for the digital meter; the analog meter scales are usually decibels relative to one of the end points or the voltage corresponding to a reading of 1 on the meter). With an appropriate attachment the digital multimeter shown in Figure 3.2 can also measure temperature, but this is not a common attachment in hearing and speech clinics. The quantity being measured is determined by the position of the rotary dial on the face of the VOM, which can point to several ranges of measurements for that quantity. The value in decibels for a zero meter value is shown on the outside portion of the dial showing the range indications for voltage (digital) or on a scale directly above or below the measurement scale (analog).

For many VOMs the type of measurement and range is selected by a pointer dial. For others, the type of measurement and range may be indicated by LEDs in combination with the display. For example, there may be an LED lit next to the volts symbol while a millivolts symbol is shown on the display. This value on the display is the measurement unit for that setting of the meter.

With regard to reading the meter and getting the correct units, be sure to look carefully at the selected scale value so that you use the correct units. For a digital meter, the reading should be unambiguous, but if the display is flashing or otherwise indicating an out-of-range condition, note whether the overrange is positive or negative and move the scale in that direction. When using a meter with a needle display, note the same cautions as for the digital readout, namely, be sure to set the meter for the correct type of measurement and the appropriate range of measurement. Most meters have several scales shown on the display portion of the meter. At either the right or left margin of the scales there will be indications as to which scale should be used for which measurement. For example, the resistance measurements should be read off the scales with ohms or the ohm symbol next to them. The range indicated by the setting on the meter will indicate which of the set of scales on the display should be used. For example, if the range is 300 mV, then the scale going from 1 to 3 should be used; whereas if the range is 1 volt, then the scale going from 1 to 10 should be used.

An additional concern with a needle meter is "parallax," which refers to the visual phenomenon that the apparent position of the needle depends upon the angle of view. To get a correct reading, the meter *must* be viewed from directly in front of the face of the meter. If the reading is taken from the side, the angle of view will affect the reading, and thus the measurement will be erroneous and unreliable.

Measuring Current

To measure the current in amperes, set the meter to the appropriate measurement (AC or DC amperes) and then to the appropriate range. To get an idea of the appropriate range, look at the power supply and see what current is being provided to the circuit. This will give you an upper bound, at least for the types of circuits that you will be measuring. To measure the current for a circuit, the VOM must be inserted into the circuit so that it becomes part of the circuit. Figure 3.3 provides a schematic diagram showing how the measurement is made. Note that the probe from the negative pole of the meter must be toward the negative pole of the power supply and probe from the positive pole of the meter must be toward the positive pole of the power supply. (Try switching the leads, and see what happens.)

Measuring Voltage

To measure voltage, set the dial to the voltage scale (AC or DC) and then set to the appropriate range. Just as with the current measurement, you can get an idea of the upper bound by looking at the voltage being supplied to the circuit by the power supply. To make the measurement, attach the meter outside the circuit, with the circuit's power supply on, by attaching clip leads from the multimeter such that they are on either side of part of the circuit to be measured. Figure 3.4 shows the instrumentation configuration for the voltage measurement. Just as for the current measurement, the negative pole of the meter should be oriented toward the negative pole of the power supply and the positive pole of the meter should be oriented toward the positive pole of the power supply. *Caution: Do NOT insert the meter into the circuit.* Note the ease of measurement for voltage in contrast to the measurement of current because the meter is

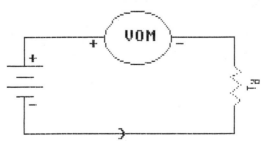

Figure 3.3.   Connecting an ammeter into a circuit.

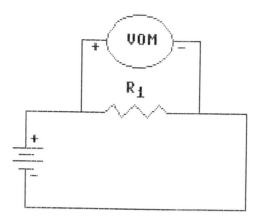

Figure 3.4.   Using the voltohmmeter (VOM) to make voltage measurements.

outside the circuit and is attached with clip leads. (Again, try switching the leads to see what happens.)

Measuring Resistance

The resistance measurement is made outside the circuit just as the voltage measurement is made outside the circuit, but it is made with the circuit power supply off. The meter dial is set to the ohms position and the range is determined by looking at the code on the component. The leads from the multimeter are attached on each side of the resistor, and the value in ohms is read off the meter. Figure 3.5 shows the instrument configuration for a resistance measurement. The code for the resistor is determined by decoding the color code on the resistor (see Table 1.2 for a description of the color code for resistors).

Signal Generators

There are many different types of signal generators, but all fall into two general classes: single waveform and function generators. All signal generators could be described as function generators because the circuitry for all signal generators is designed on the basis of the waveform function(s) it must generate, but the term *function generator* has usually been reserved for signal generators that produce several different waveforms, as opposed to the signal generators that generate only a single waveform.

Two examples of single waveform generators are DC signal generators and oscillators. An example of a DC signal generator is the triple power supply, which generates a DC (constant voltage and current) signal whose amplitude of current or voltage can be modified. The triple power supply is frequently used with computers because of the common need for more than one DC voltage in computer circuits.

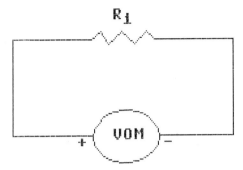

Figure 3.5.   Using the VOM to make resistance measurements.

Function Generators

The function generator is a multisignal generator in a single unit that is capable of generating several different waveforms. This is in contrast to oscillators, which only produce sine waves. Waveforms (functions) frequently provided by function generators are the sine wave, the square wave, positive or negative pulses, positive or negative linear ramps (waveforms that increase or decrease in amplitude in a straight line and then abruptly return to zero), and the triangular (sawtooth) wave. All waveforms are derived from the triangular and square waveforms.

The sine wave is generated by smoothing the shape of the triangular wave, while the ramps are generated by altering the shape of the triangular wave. The pulses are generated by, in effect, reducing the duration of either the positive or negative portion of the square wave to zero. The primary consequence of the fact that many of the waveforms are derived from other waveforms is that the derived waveforms are less exact than they would be if the circuitry had been designed to produce these waveforms directly. This means, for example, that if an application requires an extremely exact sine wave, then a function generator will not be the way to obtain it. However, for many purposes the waveforms produced by function generators are adequate.

Using a Function Generator

The waveform from a function generator is usually selected either by a rotary knob or by push buttons. The knob or push button positions are labeled by the shape of the waveform corresponding to that position. If a knob selector is used, the knob is positioned so that it points to the picture of the waveform selected; these pictographs encircle the knob. After selecting the desired waveform, it is necessary to set the amplitude and frequency.

The amplitude to the waveform is controlled by another knob labeled amplitude. The common rule for amplitude change is to turn the knob to the right to increase the amplitude and turn the knob to the left to decrease the amplitude.

The frequency of the waveform is controlled by either a pair of knobs or a knob-and-push-button combination. For the pair of knobs, one of the knobs sets the frequency range and the other knob provides fine tuning of the waveform frequency. For the knob–push button combination, the push-button usually sets the range and the knob is used for fine tuning within that range. In this case the frequency is equal to the push-button setting times the value of the knob. This is a very common arrangement on signal generators and sometimes the knob-and-push-button arrangement is implemented using two knobs. That is, the frequency is usually determined by the combination of a range setting and a fine control for setting the frequency within that range.

Many instruments have calibrated and uncalibrated modes of operation. This will be encountered most explicitly in the case of the oscilloscope, which is discussed later in this chapter but is mentioned now as a cautionary note. When operating instruments, unless there is a good reason to do so, operate the instrument in the calibrated position. Most equipment has a knob in the center of a control as a feature for providing additional flexibility in setting the control. The calibrated position is usually rotated all the way to either the right or left stop and can generally be felt as a slight click when the control is turned against the stop.

The waveform from the function generator is output continuously through a BNC or other type of connector, which is marked "OUTPUT." Many waveform generators provide a variety of outputs, such as outputs at different impedances or gating. Be sure to select the appropriate output for the application. When in doubt, consult the manual or call the technical representative for the instrument company.

Frequency Counters

Almost all frequency counters measure both the frequency and period of periodic waveforms. Some frequency counters can also count waveform cycles and can function like a stopwatch. The functions most commonly used are the period and frequency capabilities.

As for the VOM, all measurements in the frequency counter are derived from a single measure, in this case the counting of cycles. The frequency counter is basically a very fast clock with a counter and the ability to note cycle onsets and terminations. For example, if the measurement desired is the period of a waveform, then the frequency counter would note the beginning of the period and start counting. If the rate at which the clock ticks is 1 MHz (period of clock = 1 μs) and the input waveform had a period of 1 ms, then the clock would count up to 1,000 (1,000 $\times$ 1 μs = 1 ms) by the end of the cycle. Since the counter always uses the same clock rate, the period can be determined by dividing the counter by the clock rate, which is what the frequency counter does. Of course, frequency is simply the reciprocal of the period, so one measurement gives both frequency and period. The other measures such as the stopwatch function are derived similarly and are left as an exercise for the reader.

Using a Frequency Counter

The type and range of measurement for a frequency counter is selected by some combination of knobs, push buttons, and/or switches in a manner similar to the VOM. For example, the period measurement could be selected by a push button with the range in terms of time (microseconds, milliseconds, or seconds) selected with a knob. For frequency measurements, the ranges would be in terms of megahertz, kilohertz, and hertz. Just as with the VOM, the unit of measurement will usually be indicated on the display or with LEDs. Most frequency counters use a digital display. There are two other aspects of using a frequency counter that are common to almost all frequency counters: measurement time window and trigger level.

The measurement time window refers to the fact that frequency or period measurements reflect an average over some time period that is selectable by the user. The time period is measured in terms of periods or absolute time. For example, the counter could be set to the 1S or 100 period position. This setting means that the counter will update the display every 1 s for frequency measurements and every 100 periods for period measurements. Thus the frequency or period displayed equals the average frequency over 1 s or 100 periods, respectively.

The trigger level determines the amplitude at which the frequency counter will start measurement. This amplitude is usually set in combination with an attenuation setting. The attenuation switch is usually labeled "ATTEN" and attenuates the input signal in order to reduce noise, if necessary. The trigger level sets the amplitude and phase of the input signal at which the counter will recognize the occurrence of the waveform (Fig. 3.6). When the waveform exceeds the amplitude determined by the trigger level (*dashed line* in Fig. 3.6), the frequency counter will start counting. If the waveform amplitude is insufficient to reach the trigger level, the waveform will be ignored. The trigger level is adjusted with a knob that moves the trigger amplitude in the positive direction when the knob is rotated to the right or clockwise and in the negative direction when the knob is rotated to the left or counterclockwise. The trigger level and attenuation should be adjusted until a stable reading is obtained on the display.

The input to a frequency counter is an appropriate connector, usually a BNC, and has a very high impedance. Many counters have two channels that can be compared in terms of period or time of onset; in which case each channel will have an input.

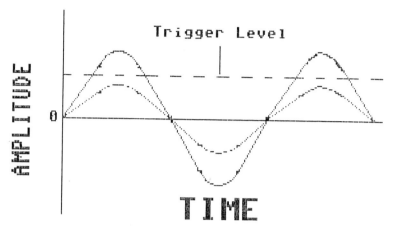

Figure 3.6. Sinusoidal signals above and below trigger level.

Oscilloscopes

Figure 3.7 shows a schematic picture of an oscilloscope with the screen, the screen controls to the right of the screen, and the horizontal and vertical amplifiers located below the screen compartment.

As can be seen from the figure, an oscilloscope has quite a few controls. Don't be intimidated. After using an oscilloscope for a while you will notice that most of the work is done with the vertical ("volts/div") and horizontal ("time/div") scaling controls. Along with position ("pos") controls, these two scaling controls are used to get a good display for visualization and measurement purposes.

The visual display (cathode ray tube, or CRT) is a raster scan display, which means that the display is generated by a beam moving back and forth across the face of the CRT that excites the phospher. The phospher is a fluorescent substance "painted" on the inside of the face of the CRT. One scan equals one time across the display. The volts/div dial controls the height of excursion of the beam per unit voltage and the time/div dial controls the rate at which the beam moves across the face of the CRT.

If you look closely at the face of the scope's CRT, you will see thin black lines in a matrix pattern across the face of the scope. The lines that cross in the middle look a little like railroad tracks, while the other lines are dashed. The entire matrix of lines is the *graticule*. Each cube or square on the graticule is 1 cm on a side. We can use the graticule to estimate the amplitude of a waveform by using the height of the waveform in terms of graticule squares and subdivisions. It should be noted that the graticule is a plate of plastic that is placed over the face of the oscilloscope and that can be removed or replaced with a different graticule. It is possible to

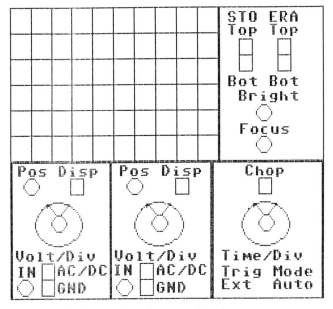

Figure 3.7.   Schematized oscilloscope.

design different graticules with different coordinates or contours for special
viewing needs.

Using an Oscilloscope

As we go through the instructions for the use of the oscilloscope, keep
Figure 3.7 in front of you because frequent reference will be made to the
figure. To begin, turn the oscilloscope on. This is done by pulling out the
rod (or pushing a button) marked "power" that is just below the focus
control shown in the figure. Make sure the scope is plugged in. The two
buttons under "store" should be out. The brightness and focus will be
adjusted later when a waveform is being viewed. The volts/div and time/
div dials are set depending on the waveform that is being viewed. The
volts/div dial usually has a lighted window in it that shows the current
setting. The number shown is the value in volts of each vertical graticule
square.

The time/div dial is similar to the volts/div dial except that the temporal
extent of each horizontal graticule square is indicated in the lighted section
of the dial. In addition to the time/div dial, the horizontal, or time base,
amplifier has the triggering controls. These controls determine what aspect
of the waveform or the oscilloscope itself will trigger a display of the current
input. Some common classifications for trigger control are: internal (INT),

which means due to the waveform itself; line (LINE), which means that it is triggered by the line frequency (once every $\frac{1}{60}$ second); or external (EXT), which means that another waveform other than the input to the vertical amplifier is used to trigger the display.

There are several trigger modes that can be used in combination with the trigger controls. Normal mode causes the display to be started whenever the trigger condition is satisfied. Automatic (AUTO) mode causes the display to start every time the previous scan is finished. The plus/minus mode determines the slope of the triggering waveform necessary for triggering. The single sweep (SGL/SWP) mode does a single scan display when triggered. This mode needs to be turned on for each sweep. Thus, after a single sweep, the display will not be triggered by future waveforms until the single sweep is enabled or the trigger mode is changed. Review the earlier description of triggering to refresh your memory of how the trigger controls work.

To display a waveform, connect the signal source to the input on the vertical amplifier and set the trigger to INT and AUTO. The trigger source, which is not shown in Figure 3.7 but is usually in the region of the time base amplifier, should be set to the vertical amplifier channel that has the signal source. On many oscilloscopes these are labeled "left" and "right" and on others as "channels 1" and "2." Now set the volts/div and time/div dials according to the amplitude and frequency of the waveform so that the waveform fits into the display. That is, set the amplitude to a value that is larger than the peak amplitude of the waveform and the time to a value that is between one and five times the period of the waveform. The vertical and time base amplifiers can then be adjusted to optimize the image for visual analysis.

There are other instruments that measure the amplitude of the waveform, but the instrument most commonly used in hearing and speech clinics is the sound level meter. This instrument is used because the amplitude is translated directly into the units most commonly used in the field of hearing and speech, namely, decibels sound pressure level. This instrument is also used frequently by industrial audiologists and by researchers to quantify sound intensity.

Sound Level Meters

The simplest description of a sound level meter (SLM) is a voltmeter that reads the output of a microphone. That is, the microphone on an SLM takes the pressure fluctuations corresponding to the acoustic waveform and transduces these into electrical currents, which the voltmeter displays. How the microphone performs the transduction process will be covered later in the text.

Sound level meters have many functions, but their primary function is to permit measurement of the intensity of an acoustic signal. This is in contrast to the VOM, which measures the amplitude of the electrical signal that goes to the earphone and makes the earphone produce the acoustic signal. There are a number of common definitions of acoustic intensity, and sound level meters are designed to provide measurements of sound within these definitions.

Using a Sound Level Meter

A "generic" sound level meter is shown in Figure 3.8. As with the oscilloscope, there are a number of controls, but most are self-explanatory and are easily mastered. The general configuration of any sound level meter matches that shown in the figure (i.e., a meter with a microphone input) regardless of its manufacturer, although other meters may have a digital display.

The range of measurement for a sound level meter is set in a manner very similar to that for the VOM. There is a rotary knob that points to the range. Most sound level meters have a range from approximately 10 dB SPL to 140 dB SPL, depending on the microphone. The sound level meter shown in Figure 3.8 has a needle meter. Generally, the scale on such a meter is from −10 to 10 dB. (Ignore the minus infinity sign at the far left; most likely you will not be making measurements at that intensity.) The value referred to by the range setting is at 0 dB on the meter display. The reading on the meter display is added to the range setting to determine the sound level read by the meter. Some SLMs have digital readouts similar to those for the multimeter. Some instruments have a convenient feature

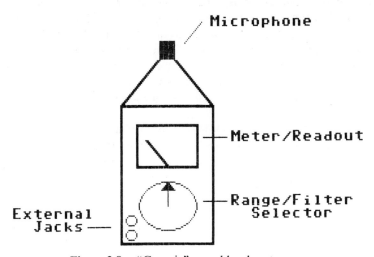

Figure 3.8. "Generic" sound level meter.

called "autoranging" that is becoming more common. This feature has the instrument set the range by examining the intensity of the signal and adjusting the range so that the signal intensity is within the minimum and maximum scale values for that range.

The classification of the sound units is usually done with a rotary knob that points to the desired classification. These classifications involve various weighting networks that are contained within the meter, or they can be contained in an external system. The weighting functions reflect scales used for analyzing acoustic signals. For example, a common classification indicator is the letter *A*, which stands for the *A*-scale. If the knob is pointing to the *A*, then the value being read off the meter is decibels (*A*). The *A*-scale weighting function means that when intensity is summed across frequency, not all frequencies are represented equally. In particular, the frequencies around 1,000-3,000 Hz are the most important determinants of the sound intensity measured by the *A*-scale. The "Lin" setting refers to a linear scale, that is, all frequencies in the input are weighted equally.

There is also a setting for external filters (Ext. Filter) that provides a way to send the output of the SLM to an external device. This capability is usually used to pass the signal through an external filter, which has particular characteristics that are important for analyzing the signal. (Commonly used filters are octave band and one-third octave band filters. Filters are described more fully in a later chapter.) This external filter capability permits the SLM to measure the intensity in the particular filter region selected.

In addition to the range and output characteristic settings there are controls for power, testing the battery, and controlling the operation of the needle meter. The power setting is obvious; it turns the meter on. The battery test function permits examination of the power remaining in the battery and is described below. There are several settings for controlling the meter display. "Fast" and "slow" refer to how rapidly the display can change its value. If there is a setting marked "imp," it provides a very fast display suitable for measuring impulsive waveforms. Some meters have the capability to measure the peak amplitude of impulses and to hold this value so that it can be recorded.

To use the SLM, first check the battery by pointing the setting knob to BAT, or a similar abbreviation. Look quickly at the battery scale on the meter; the needle should be well out of the red area on this scale. Turn the SLM off. *Do not continue the battery test for more than a very short time because it will rapidly drain the battery.* If the batteries are low, get new batteries and put them in the battery compartment of the SLM. Do not use the SLM with low batteries, as your measurements will be inaccurate and unreliable.

Calibrating a Sound Level Meter

Prior to measuring sound with the SLM, you must calibrate the meter. This is done with a pistonphone, or an actuator, which produces an exactly specified amount of sound pressure. The pistonphone is a heavy polished steel tube with a sliding button on one side and an opening in one end. Just as with the SLM, the batteries of the pistonphone have to be checked prior to use. There are three settings of the sliding button: OFF, BAT, and ON. To test the battery, put the button on BAT. If there is no sound, then the batteries are bad and should be replaced. *Do not leave the button at the BAT position for any longer than is necessary to verify the condition of the batteries because it will rapidly drain the batteries.* In general, whenever checking the battery level of any device, do not leave the device in the battery check mode for long because almost all devices will drain the battery in this mode.

The next step is to attach the microphone to the SLM. The SLM should not be stored with the microphone inserted into the SLM. *Do not force the microphone onto the SLM.* Use a slow, steady pressure after first finding the grooves, as the threads on microphones are very fine and can be very easily damaged. Place the opening of the pistonphone over the microphone of the SLM, making sure to slide it down all the way to the stop. This does not mean to *ram* it in! Set the range of the SLM to 120, and set the output characteristic to linear. Set the meter characteristic to SLOW NORM, and turn on the pistonphone. The meter should read approximately 124 dB. See the side of the pistonphone for the exact value. There is also a correction for atmospheric pressure. This correction can be obtained from the barometer, which is included in the pistonphone box.

Measuring With the Sound Level Meter

In the sound field. Set the range of the SLM and the output and meter characteristics to settings that are appropriate for the measurement that you wish to make. For example, to get decibels sound pressure level put the dial on LIN. Set the meter to SLOW NORM. Adjust the range setting until you get a reading between 0 and 10 on the meter. The reading on the meter plus the range setting is the decibels sound pressure level for that signal.

Measurements in sound field require that you know the source of the sound. While this is not always possible to establish with certainty prior to making a series of measurements, some attempt should be made to do so. After selecting the sound source for measurement, the face of the microphone should be held perpendicular to the sound source. Then adjust the meter as described above. Figure 3.9 gives an example of how the meas-

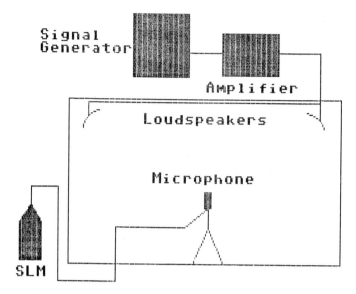

Figure 3.9.   Sound field measurement with a sound level meter.

urements should be made. When making sound field measurements it is a good idea to make up a chart showing where the measurements were made and also showing the location of the sound source(s) measured.

From earphones.   Figure 3.10 shows the instrument configuration for measuring sound coming from an earphone. Measurement of sound intensity for earphones requires the use of a coupler. The purpose of the coupler is to simulate the response of the earphone when it is placed on the ear. A common coupler is the National Bureau of Standards (NBS) 9A coupler, which is the standard 6-cc coupler. It should be noted that another coupler has been developed and is described briefly in the next chapter. To use the coupler, it is necessary to take off the microphone and attach the coupler to the microphone connector. *Attach the coupler gently and firmly. Do not overtighten.* The microphone and microphone connector threads are very fine and easily stripped. The microphone is put in the coupler. To do this, unscrew the top of the coupler and attach the microphone to the microphone connector. Screw the top back on. Place the earphone on top of the coupler with the diaphragm facing the microphone. Then clamp the earphone to the coupler with force of 0.5 kg. The sound intensity can now be read using the same techniques as for the sound field measurement.

Chapter Summary

This chapter has covered a variety of test instrumentation that will be used to examine and calibrate the measurement instrumentation to be

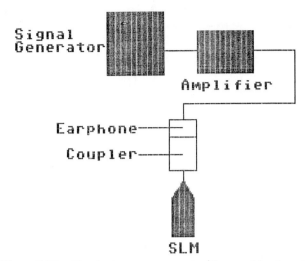

Figure 3.10. Earphone measurement with sound level meter.

described in section II. The VOM and oscilloscope will be used frequently in laboratory exercises throughout the book. The Quiklabs for this chapter are designed to give some experience using test instrumentation and to show the limits of measurement for some types of instrumentation. This chapter focused on how-to information rather than on a theoretical treatment and should be referred to during the lab as the various instruments are tried. For a more theoretical approach, most manuals that come with test instrumentation have a theory-of-operation section. In some cases, there are separate manuals for maintenance and use of the instrument, and so the theoretical treatment of the instrument may be in a different manual than the user section. The equipment and procedures covered in this chapter are basic to using instrumentation to examine events. The principles of careful calibration of instruments, recognition of the limits of measurement, and the art of using instrumentation will be returned to throughout the next chapters.

3

Measuring a Sine Wave with an Oscilloscope

Introduction

The primary purpose of this lab is to provide some hands-on experience with an oscilloscope. While a signal generator, frequency counter, and VOM will be used in this lab, they will be used perfunctorily. The lab will give experience measuring amplitude and period (frequency) of a sine wave on an oscilloscope.

Method

Apparatus

An oscilloscope, voltmeter (digital multimeter or VOM), frequency counter, and signal generator (function generator) are provided, along with appropriate connectors and cables. Refer to the text for descriptions of how to use the instruments.

While the directions for use of the frequency counter given in the text are adequate for use in this lab, there is one small change in the use of the VOM. Since the signal generator is not a circuit, the output of the signal generator is sent directly to the VOM and the measurement is made at the appropriate AC volts setting. The only other note is that adapters may have to be used to connect the cables to the various instruments.

Procedure

The primary task in this lab is to measure the amplitude and frequency of a sine wave. This will be done for three amplitudes at 1,000 Hz and for three frequencies at 1 volt. The three amplitudes will be 0.5, 1, and 2 volts. The three frequencies will be 100, 1,000, and 5,000 Hz.

Amplitude

Use a 1,000-Hz signal for all amplitude measurements. Start with the function generator set to sine wave, then follow these steps.

1. Measure the frequency of the sine wave using the setup shown in Figure 3.11 and the description for the use of the frequency counter given in chapter 3.
2. Set the voltage of the waveform to 0.5 volt using Figure 3.12 and the description for the use of the voltmeter given in chapter 3. Recall that the voltmeter measures in volts RMS.
3. Display the waveform on the oscilloscope using Figure 3.13 and the description on the use of the oscilloscope given in chapter 3.
4. Measure the amplitude of the waveform using the graticule in conjunction with the setting on the volts/div dial.

Repeat steps 2–4 for 1- and 2-volt sine wave signals.

Frequency

Perform all the frequency measurements with a 1-volt signal. Start with the function generator set to a 1,000 Hz sine wave, then follow these steps.

1. Set the waveform amplitude to 1 volt using Figure 3.12 and the description on the use of the voltmeter given in chapter 3.
2. Set the frequency of the signal using Figure 3.11 and the description of the use of a frequency counter given in chapter 3.
3. Display the waveform on the oscilloscope using Figure 3.13 and the directions for an oscilloscope given in chapter 3.
4. Determine the period of the waveform on the oscilloscope using the graticule in conjunction with the setting of the time base amplifier.

Repeat steps 2–4 for 1,000- and 5,000-Hz sine waves.

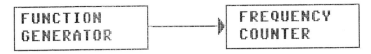

Figure 3.11. Block diagram of frequency measurement.

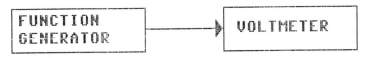

Figure 3.12. Block diagram of amplitude measurement using a voltmeter.

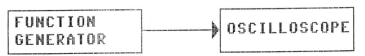

Figure 3.13. Block diagram of amplitude measurement using an oscilloscope.

Results

Make up tables of your data. The tables should show all of your measurements made on the test instrumentation and the measurements from the oscilloscope. Convert the period measurements on the oscilloscope to frequency ($f = 1/P$). Put all the amplitude data in one table and the period data in another table.

Discussion

Discuss your estimation of the accuracy of frequency and amplitude measurements on the oscilloscope. Discuss the use of the oscilloscope in terms of its potential for visualization of waveforms.

4

Calibration Check of Oscilloscope with Voltmeter, Signal Generator, and Frequency Counter

Introduction

*T*his lab is intended to provide some hands-on experience with oscilloscopes and test instrumentation. A voltohmmeter (VOM), an oscilloscope, a signal generator and a frequency counter will be used. This lab will give experience measuring amplitude and period (frequency) on an oscilloscope for various waveforms. In addition, this lab will provide some experience regarding the accuracy of an oscilloscope for making amplitude and period (frequency) measurements.

Method

Apparatus

An oscilloscope, voltmeter (digital multimeter, or VOM), frequency counter, and signal generator (function generator) are provided, along with appropriate connectors and cables. The use of these instruments was described in the text.

The calibration will be checked using the VOM and the frequency counter. While the directions for use of the frequency counter in the text are adequate for use in this lab, there is one small change in the use of the VOM. Since the signal generator is not a circuit, the output of the signal generator is sent directly to the VOM and the measurement is made at the appropriate AC volts setting. The only other note is that adapters may have to be used to connect the cables to the various instruments.

Procedure

The primary task in this lab is to check the calibration of the oscilloscope for amplitude and frequency using a square wave. This will be done for three amplitudes and three frequencies. The amplitudes will be 0.5, 1, and 5 volts and the frequencies will be 100, 1,000, and 10,000 Hz. Amplitude and frequency measures will be made in separate phases of the lab, with the amplitude phase being done first. For purposes of comparison, one amplitude and one frequency measure will be made for a sine wave and for a sawtooth (triangular) wave.

Amplitude

Use a 1,000-Hz signal for all amplitude measurements. Start with the function generator set to square wave, then follow these steps.

1. Measure the frequency of the square wave using the setup shown in Figure 3.14 and the description for the use of the frequency counter given in Chapter 3.
2. Set the voltage of the waveform to 0.5 volts using Figure 3.15 and the description for the use of the voltmeter given earlier. Recall that the voltmeter measures in volts RMS.
3. Display the waveform on the oscilloscope using Figure 3.16 and the description on the use of the oscilloscope given in this chapter.
4. Measure the amplitude of the waveform using the graticule in conjunction with the setting on the volts/div dial.

Repeat steps 2–4 for 1- and 2-volt square wave signals. Then set the function generator to sine wave and do steps 2–4 for a 5-volt sine wave. Do the same for a 5-volt sawtooth wave.

Frequency

Do all the frequency measurements with 1-volt signal. Start with the function generator set to a 100-Hz square wave, then follow these steps.

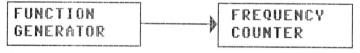

Figure 3.14.   Block diagram of frequency measurement.

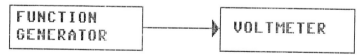

Figure 3.15.   Block diagram of amplitude measurement using a voltmeter.

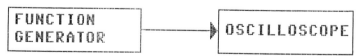

Figure 3.16.   Block diagram of amplitude measurement using an oscilloscope.

1. Set the waveform amplitude to 1 volt using Figure 3.15 and the description on the use of the voltmeter given in Chapter 3.
2. Set the frequency of the signal using Figure 3.14 and the description of the use of a frequency counter given in Chapter 3.
3. Measure the period of the signal using Figure 3.14 and the description of the use of a frequency counter given in this chapter.
4. Display the waveform on the oscilloscope using Figure 3.16 and the description of the use of an oscilloscope given in Chapter 3.
5. Determine the period of the waveform using the graticule in conjunction with the setting of the time base amplifier.

Repeat steps 2–5 for 1,000- and 10,000-Hz square waves. Then set the function generator to sine wave and repeat steps 1–5 for a 1,000-Hz signal. Do the same for a 1,000-Hz sawtooth wave.

Results

Make up tables of your data. The tables should show all of your measurements made on the test instrumentation and the measurements from the oscilloscope. The tables should also include the error of the oscilloscope in absolute and relative terms. Put all the amplitude data in one table and the period data in another table.

For the purposes of computing error, assume that the test instrumentation has no error. For absolute error, compute the difference between the amplitude or period as measured by the test instrumentation and the amplitude or period as measured by the oscilloscope. Keep the sign. For the relative error, take the absolute error for amplitude or period computed and divide by the amplitude or period as measured by the test instrumentation. Drop the sign and multiply by 100. This will give you the error of the oscilloscope in percent.

Discussion

Discuss the accuracy of the oscilloscope in terms of its potential use for calibrating other devices, such as oscillators or audiometers. Discuss the use of an oscilloscope in terms of its possible applications with regard to visualization of waveforms. Discuss the use of the voltmeter to measure the amplitude of waveforms other than sine waves.

Building an Operational Amplifier Circuit

Introduction

T his lab should only be done if Quiklabs 1 and 2 have been completed, as the measurements and circuit construction will build upon the techniques learned in the previous labs. The purpose of this lab is to not only demonstrate amplification with an operational amplifier but also to show how to build a simple oscillator by using an operational amplifier. Furthermore, this lab provides an opportunity to use all the skills developed up to this point.

The operational amplifier ("op amp") chosen for this circuit is the model 741, but other op amps will do as well. Model 741 is widely available and cheap and comes in an integrated circuit package. This lab assumes an amplifier with similar operating characteristics and similar packaging.

An oscillator is a *high-gain* amplifier with regenerative feedback. To look at the amplification properties of the 741 op amp, we must connect it as an oscillator. The basic circuit is shown in Figure 3.17. Note that the feedback circuit (R_1 and R_2) returns the output signal to the noninverting amplifier input. Oscillation occurs when the output signal is returned *in phase* with the input signal. At the noninverting input terminal the input and output signals are in phase.

When the circuit is first energized, the output voltage (at pin 6) rises. This rising positive voltage goes to pin 3, where it is amplified. The output at pin 6 becomes more positive as it is amplified, and the op amp goes into *saturation* very quickly. "Saturation" refers to the fact that the output voltage of the amplifier can no longer rise when the input voltage increases.

Capacitor C_1 starts to charge to the positive output voltage (recall the discussion of capacitors in Chapter 1). The voltage at pin 2 rises as the capacitor charges. When the voltage across the capacitor at pin 2 becomes more positive than the voltage at pin 3, the op amp output goes negative very quickly. Capacitor C_1 starts to discharge. When the capacitor voltage is less than the voltage at pin 3, the output goes positive again.

The overall result is a square-wave output voltage. The square wave produces sound in the speaker. The oscillator is called a "multivibrator" because its output is a square wave and its frequency depends upon the rate of charging and discharging of a capacitor. Recall that the rate of charging (and discharging) is dependent on the capacitance and thus the frequency, which depends on this rate of charging and discharging, will change with the capacitance of C_1. Another way to control the charging rate is to control the voltage going to the capacitor and this can be done through the variable resistor R_2. Increasing R_2 decreases the flow into the capacitor which increases the amount of time that it takes for the capacitor to charge. This increases the time between discharges as well, and therefore the system does not cycle as quickly and the frequency of the square wave will go down. Decreasing the resistance does just the opposite: it increases the frequency of oscillation.

Note the path from the output back into the inverting input. There are two resistors in this path, R_3 and R_4; there is also R_5 going to ground. This path is the *feedback* path and controls the amount of amplification provided by the op amp. Since R_3 is a variable resistor, it will control the amount of feedback going into the op amp and can be used to control the amplification. If the amplification goes down, then the volume will go down because the output voltage will be less.

Method

Apparatus

The following circuit components and tools are required for building the oscillator circuit for this lab:

1. Soldering iron;
2. Solder;
3. Wire (#16 gauge or larger);
4. Breadboard (if not using items 1–3);
5. Six or seven resistors (various values from 1,000 to 100,000 ohms);
6. Variable resistor (10-turn potentiometer in the range indicated in item 5 would be best);
7. Two or three capacitors (in the microfarad range);
8. Model 741 operational amplifier or equivalent;
9. Integrated circuit chip socket (if desired);
10. Power source (9-volt battery or power supply).

Circuit Construction

Use the techniques given in Quiklab 1 and the components given in the preceding list to construct the circuit shown in Figure 3.17. Note that there appear to be extra components. Arrange the components into two or three groups, depending on the amount of time available for the lab. Then make the measurements given in the next section. There are several measurements that require changing one of the circuit components, and so a breadboard is recommended for this lab.

Results

The measurements for this circuit are used to verify the operation of the circuit and to observe how component changes affect the output. Each result consists of measuring amplitude and frequency of the output for a set of circuit components. In addition, the oscilloscope is used to visualize the output waveform.

After building the circuit with the first set of components, use the techniques from the previous labs in this chapter to measure the amplitude with the voltmeter (keeping in mind the lessons learned in the previous labs). Measure the frequency of the output with the frequency counter and display the waveform on the oscilloscope. When observing

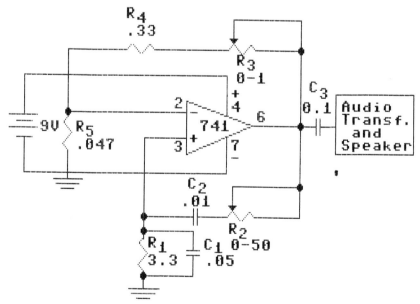

Figure 3.17.   A simple oscillator circuit using an operational amplifier.

the waveform, note the amplitude and period and try to describe the waveform shape.

Repeat this series of measurements for at least one other combination of circuit components. If possible, repeat this for three or more component sets, varying both the resistance and capacitance values in the circuit. Display all results in a table. Be sure to include the circuit component values in the table as well as the results of the measurements specified in this section.

Discussion

Examine the results to see if they obey the rules given in the lab introduction with regard to changes in frequency and amplitude as a function of changes in circuit components. Did this circuit produce a desirable waveform? That is, could this circuit be used as a signal source. Answer this question and give some of the limitations of the circuit.

SECTION II

4

Transducers for Sound and Vibration: Microphones, Earphones, and Accelerometers

A common element among instrumentation used for clinical and research purposes in speech and hearing is a device called a *transducer*, which transforms acoustic, or sometimes vibrational, energy into an electrical signal that can be manipulated by electronic instruments. Transducers can be defined generally as devices that transform energy from one form into another. This chapter will restrict itself to discussing transducers for which the input is acoustic or vibration energy and the output is electrical energy. The most common transducers that deal with acoustic energy are microphones, earphones, and speakers. In the field of underwater acoustics there are hydrophones, which are the underwater equivalent of speakers, but they will not be discussed in this chapter because of their specialized use. They operate very similarly to speakers except for their medium, which is water rather than air.

Microphones are discussed first to maintain the pattern of starting with input and ending with output. In addition, since many of the principles associated with microphones are the same as those for earphones or speakers, which also transduce acoustic energy, the discussion on microphones provides a natural introduction to these next two topics. Finally, a discussion of accelerometers is also included.

Microphones

Microphones transduce acoustic energy to electrical energy and serve as input sources to many of the instruments used in the field of speech and hearing. Microphones have evolved over time from unreliable and environmentally sensitive devices to highly accurate, reliable, and stable transducers. They have also benefited from the tremendous advances made in the miniaturization of components and in materials science. A high-quality microphone is essential to any acoustic measurement system because any analysis or use of an acoustic signal can only be as good as the electrical representation of that signal. Thus an important requirement for any laboratory or clinic is a high-quality microphone.

There are many different forms of microphone construction and many different models of microphones within a particular type. However, microphones can be grouped into some broad categories based on their construction. Some examples of different types of microphones are *carbon, dynamic, condenser,* and *electret.* Within any of these classifications there are other differences, such as a microphone designed to be more sensitive in a given direction or a microphone designed for a special environment. Due to the diversity in available microphones, the specifications describing the microphone's characteristics should be carefully examined to determine if the microphone performs the appropriate transduction and if the accuracy meets the desired measurement criteria.

A Brief History

The carbon microphone, invented during the 1890s, was the first device used to transduce an acoustic signal, but it did not produce an electrical signal itself. This microphone depended on a carbon granule, which vibrated in response to the acoustic signal. The microphone was sensitive to both humidity and sharp movements and had a very small dynamic range in terms of frequency, but was very inexpensive and with proper care lasted decades. Some (very few) of these microphones are still in use on hearing aids manufactured in the 1930s.

The crystal microphone, which came into common use in the 1930s, was developed next. This microphone not only transduced the signal but produced an electrical signal as a result of acoustic stimulation. The typical crystal microphone consists of a diaphragm connected to the crystal with a wire connecting a crystal to an amplifier (Fig. 4.1). The diaphragm is deformed by the acoustic signal and this in turn deforms the crystal.

The crystals are special crystals that exhibit a property called the "piezoelectric effect." Two examples of piezoelectric crystals are quartz and Rochelle salt. The piezoelectric effect is the property of a crystal exhibited by the generation of a voltage when pressure is applied. What this means is that if a piezoelectric crystal is deformed, it will produce an electrical signal that is proportional in amplitude to the degree of deformation. Since the deformation of the diaphragm mirrors the acoustic pressure applied to its surface, the crystal will be deformed in the same

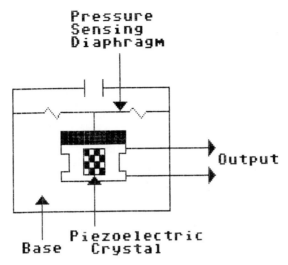

Figure 4.1. Piezoelectric microphone.

way as the diaphragm because of the rigid connection to the diaphragm; thus a small electrical signal that mirrors the acoustic pressure will be produced. This signal has to be amplified in order to be used by other instrumentation.

Crystal microphones were a significant advance over the carbon microphone in terms of frequency range, lower sensitivity to movement, and immunity to dust and dirt. However, such microphones continued to be sensitive to humidity and temperature. They also produce a high impedance output, which makes them more difficult to use with current solid-state equipment. In addition, crystal microphones do not recover rapidly after a severe shock.

Crystal microphones were improved by the introduction of ceramic technology during the 1940s. Ceramic materials are synthetic crystals that exhibit piezoelectric properties. In addition to increased immunity to humidity and temperature, the ceramic transducer has the advantage that its properties may be tailored to a specific need (one application is in hydrophones as well as in microphones.). Thus, ceramics should not be thought of as a single type of material but rather as an extremely flexible transducer. Piezoelectricity is also involved with the new integrated circuit sensors, which will be mentioned at the end of this chapter.

With the advent of the transistor, microphones that operated on a magnetic principle became popular because transistorized devices required a low-impedance source. These magnetic microphones were quickly supplanted by the condenser microphone, which is currently the microphone design of choice. Because the overwhelming majority of microphones in current use are of the condenser type (or electret, which operates on the same transduction principles as a condenser), the rest of the discussion about microphones will be primarily concerned with the condenser microphone. It should be kept in mind, however, that many of the basic principles described for the condenser microphone also apply to other types of microphones. This is because the basic description of a microphone is a diaphragm that drives a transducer. The transducer produces an electrical signal. Thus the complete transduction process involved for microphones is from acoustic to mechanical to electrical. The final electrical signal is usually amplified for use by an instrument such as a tape recorder or signal analyzer.

Condenser Microphones

Condenser microphones have many positive features, which include a broad frequency response, resistance to humidity and temperature, relative insensitivity to movement, and good absolute sensitivity. It should be noted that the resistance to humidity has limits for all microphones. In particular, no microphone designed to measure air pressure will measure sound appropriately in a condensing (raining) environment. This is because the rain forms a conductor that disrupts the designed electrical properties of the microphone. The water will also damage the diaphragm through rust deposits, altering the properties of the diaphragm and microphone. Obviously, microphones must be stored in a dry place to prevent these problems.

The condenser microphone has a very thin diaphragm of metallic material stretched very tightly across the face of the microphone. The diaphragm is separated by an airspace from a polarized flat plate. The diaphragm itself is also polarized. This construction should remind the reader of a capacitor, which is discussed in chapter 1. The two plates made up of the diaphragm and the fixed plate are part of a capacitive circuit that will pass a charge proportional to the distance between the plates. Since the outer plate (diaphragm) is driven to air pressure (in particular, sound pressure) the movement of the diaphragm will be translated into a change in charge that is an electrical analog of the signal driving the diaphragm.

The advantages of such a system are that the microphone can be made very durable by use of appropriate materials and by protection of the most sensitive part of the microphone, namely, the diaphragm. The protection of the diaphragm is done through the use of a protective cap that passes sound for the effective frequency range of the microphone. The primary disadvantage of the condenser microphone is the need for an external power supply.

Materials used to construct the diaphragm of a condenser microphone have been the subject of intensive investigation since the 1950s, when the condenser microphone was introduced. During the late 1960s, diaphragms were constructed of prepolarized materials, obviating the need for an external power supply. Such microphones are referred to as "prepolarized" or "electret" microphones.

Several advantages accrue from the lack of a power supply. One is the capability of making very small, high-quality microphones, such as those used in hearing aids. Another advantage is the elimination of a power pack for the microphone itself. The power pack is required because the condenser microphone configuration does not provide amplification by itself, as is the case for piezoelectric microphone construction, and does require power for the polarization of the plates. Thus, the transduced signal from a condenser microphone must always be amplified. The new electret condenser microphone still requires a power source to be useful, but the problem of power consumption shifts from the microphone stage to the amplifier stage when an electret condenser type of microphone is used.

A microphone on a chip was produced very recently, which may open up a whole range of new microphone applications. In the field of speech and hearing such a microphone would be especially useful for hearing aids. In addition, this type of microphone may have applications for experimental monitoring of speech levels since it would make possible the construction of extremely small (0.25 × 0.25 inch or 0.6 × 0.6 cm) microphones that include the amplifier. Interestingly, some of these microphones utilize the piezoelectric effect (recall the discussion of crystal microphones and ceramic materials), which was largely supplanted by the condenser microphones. The piezoelectric effect has been employed because the transduction process occurs within the material, which results in considerable savings in terms of circuitry and hence bulk. These new microphones may provide not only a size advantage but also a cleaner signal as a result of the short signal path between the microphone and the amplifier. There are also some exciting possibilities in terms of having special purpose signal-processing chips integrated with the microphone without a significant increase in the size of the total package.

How to Use a Microphone

The basic principles of operation of a microphone were discussed in the preceding section. Microphones are used in a number of settings, and these settings do not require the same microphone or even the same rules of operation with a similar microphone. Therefore, this section will describe some of the different ways to use a microphone and also will discuss a select number of microphones within the microphone types discussed earlier.

In addition to the types of microphones discussed earlier, there are different implementations of the same type of microphone. Microphones may differ in terms of their frequency response, absolute sensitivity, stability in the face of temperature, pressure or climate fluctuations, directional sensitivity, and/or distortion characteristics. Thus it is important to consider all of these factors when selecting a microphone for a particular need.

Microphone construction has a large impact on stability and sensitivity, but other factors also play a role. The most important of these factors is size. Microphone size is defined by the device and is measured in inches or centimeters (occasionally in millimeters). Microphone size not only affects sensitivity but plays a role in frequency response and directional sensitivity as well. Most of the effects of size can be understood in terms of the diffraction properties of a microphone interacting with sound. Due to the importance of understanding how microphone size determines microphone properties, the next section will be a brief discussion of diffraction.

Diffraction

Diffraction describes the manner in which waves of energy interact with an object. In this particular case, it describes the way sound energy interacts with a microphone. To gain some understanding of diffraction, recall the sine waves described in chapter 1 on electronics fundamentals. The fundamental waveform for sound is the sine wave. The concept of sound will be expanded considerably in the next chapter, but for present purposes only the concept of wavelength is introduced.

Sound travels and has some finite velocity, i.e., sound takes time to get from place to place. Also, sound has a finite frequency range because of the limited frequency range of human hearing. The range of interest for hearing is approximately 20 Hz to 20,000 Hz, although many people do not hear over this broad a frequency range. Thus sound not only takes time to get from place to place, but also cycles over a finite time. The combination of these properties leads to the measure of wavelength, which is the distance covered by sound during one cycle or period. This relationship is described by Equation 1, which states that wavelength is inversely proportional to the frequency. Thus, high-frequency sounds have short wavelengths and low-frequency sounds have long wavelengths.

$$\text{wavelength} = \text{speed of sound/signal frequency} \qquad (1)$$

Diffraction is determined by the relation between wavelength and the size of an object, in particular, the cross-sectional size of an object. The inverse relation given in Equation 1 for frequency and wavelength means that diffraction also describes the relation between frequency and the size of an object. The fundamental properties of diffraction in relation to size and wavelength are shown in Figure 4.2, where, for simplicity, *straight lines* are used to show the location of the peak of the waveform and the distance between the lines show the wavelength. The figure reveals that when the wavelength of the sound is long, relative to the size of the object, then the sound will travel well around the object. However, when the size of the object is large, relative to the wavelength of the sound, then the object will effectively block the sound.

The description of diffraction effects in terms of frequency is very straightforward. Recall that wavelength and frequency are inversely related. Thus, the diffraction effects described here and in Figure 4.2 can be restated: high-frequency sounds tend to be blocked by objects, whereas low-frequency sounds are not. The relation could also be stated in terms of the objects, i.e., the smaller the object, the higher the frequency of the sound that will be blocked by that object.

Some thought about the relations described here will reveal that diffraction has several implications for microphones. First, for small microphones, the frequency range over which the microphone will interact with the sound field will start at a higher frequency. Thus, the size of the microphone has an impact on the directional characteristics of the microphone. Second, the frequency response of the microphone will be affected because the smaller microphones will tend to block less high-frequency sound coming from different directions than the larger microphones. Third, size will affect sensitivity. This is due to the relation between the diameter of the diaphragm and the effective surface area of the microphone. However, there is another phenomenon that can also impact microphone performance, namely, resonance.

Resonance

Resonance has been discussed previously in terms of electrical properties, but it also has implications for sound and refers to the fact that the interaction of sound with an object depends on the length of an object.

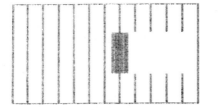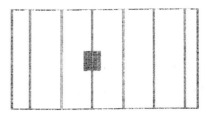

Figure 4.2. Relation between wavelength (*distance between lines*) and diffraction effects.

Perhaps the best example of this is the case of strings such as piano and violin strings. The rule of resonance for strings is that a string will resonate if the length of the string is equal to twice the wavelength of the sound that is oscillating the string. Thus short strings will resonate at higher frequencies than long strings, i.e., the resonant frequency of a string is inversely proportional to its length.

The same general rule holds true when the diameter of a round plate, such as a microphone diaphragm, is used as the length of the vibrating object. Therefore, the smaller the diameter of the microphone diaphragm, the higher the resonant frequency. Since resonance is an undesirable property in microphones (resonance in the microphone will not permit accurate measurements), smaller-diameter microphones have a broader frequency response because higher-frequency measurements can be made without resonance.

The smaller microphone has the advantage of a broader frequency response, but there is also a disadvantage to the smaller diameter. The disadvantage is that as the diameter of a circle is decreased, the area also will decrease. Sound pressure is measured per unit area, but the threshold sensitivity of a microphone is determined by the sound pressure summed over the surface of the microphone. This will be determined by the area of the microphone. Thus smaller-diameter microphones have poorer threshold sensitivity than larger-diameter microphones. This factor needs to be considered when determining which microphone is best suited for a particular need.

Directional Microphones

The most common microphone is omnidirectional, that is, sound coming from all directions is treated the same. However, there is frequently a need for a microphone whose sensitivity is greater in a given direction. Such microphones are called directional microphones. Not all directional microphones are alike. Just as omnidirectional microphones have differing sensitivities, directional microphones have differing directional response patterns. The directionality of the microphone will be indicated on the calibration sheet supplied with the microphone (using such terms as "cardioid" or "hypercardioid"). There should be a diagram depicting the response field of the microphone. In addition, the microphone will be specified in terms of a front-to-back ratio, typically given in decibels. This ratio refers to the difference in sound-pressure sensitivity of the microphone between equal intensity sounds presented in the most sensitive position in the sound field and the least sensitive position in the sound field.

Directional microphones are used for those situations in which the sound source of interest is in a specific location surrounded by noise. The intent is to focus on that signal to the exclusion of surrounding sounds.

Hence the primary applications are in the sound field, rather than in earphone listening. Common applications include radio and TV, especially for reporters in the field. The applications in speech and hearing are for hearing aids and for speech recording under noisy conditions.

Probe Microphones

There are a number of situations in the field of speech and hearing that require the ability to make measurements at a specific location with great precision. While directional microphones are good for measuring sound coming from a particular direction in a sound field, this does not imply that they are always the microphone of choice for measuring sound in a particular restricted area. Usually the primary requirement for a probe microphone is small size because the microphone should not intrude on the measurement. An example of use for a probe microphone is to measure sound at the entrance to the ear canal or perhaps even inside the canal. The special requirements for these microphones have led to some exotic designs, which are more appropriately referred to as "microphone systems"—a topic that will not be covered here. These designs include sound tubes called "waveguides" and special construction of the tubes to produce appropriate impedances at specific points in the microphone system. A more mundane example is the probe microphone to measure sound at the entrance of the ear canal or for a hearing aid response, which will be discussed here.

Ear Level Probe Microphones

There are two types of microphones used to make measurements for hearing aids: ear level probe microphones and ear canal probe microphones. The ear level microphone is covered here, and the ear canal microphone is discussed in the next section.

Ear level probe microphones are placed close to the location where the sound is expected to be picked up by a hearing aid microphone or at the entrance to the ear canal if no hearing aid is involved. These microphones are actually just miniature condenser microphones and follow all the same rules regarding their performance as described previously. Their primary advantage is the ability to measure sound at the location of interest.

The disadvantage of ear level microphones is the difficulty of calibrating them. Ear level microphones are often not round in shape and hence do not fit well into standard couplers for calibration measurements. This means that an adapter must be used, which will be discussed later in the section on microphone calibration. Another concern is how to place the microphone and how to ensure stable measurements.

The microphone should be placed as close to the entrance of the ear canal as possible if making measurements without a prosthesis. If a prosthesis is involved and you wish to monitor the input to the prosthesis, then the microphone should be placed as close as possible to the prosthesis microphone, which does not mean on top of the prosthesis microphone, but rather side by side. Some interaction effects can arise from this placement at high frequencies, but these frequencies are much higher than generally used. The face of the microphone should be oriented in the same direction as the prosthesis microphone. If there is no prosthesis involved, the face of the microphone should be facing out from the patient. To ensure stable and reliable measurements, the microphone should be taped in place. As would be expected from the discussions of diffraction, the orientation of the microphone is most critical at high frequencies. For the typical ear level probe microphone, these frequencies would be above 4,000 Hz.

Ear Canal Probe Microphones

Several companies have recently developed commercial systems for ear-canal probe microphone measurements. Previously, these microphones were used only in the laboratory. While the commercial systems still are not as sophisticated as the more advanced laboratory models, they are very useful, especially for determining the actual frequency response of a hearing aid.

A canal probe microphone, as the name implies, makes measurements in the ear canal. The systems currently available use a probe tube in combination with a miniature microphone. The probe tube is placed into the ear canal, either with or without a prosthesis present, and the sound pressure at the entrance to the probe tube is determined. It is important to point out that this is not the same as an absolute measurement of sound pressure in the ear canal because a number of factors such as the size and shape of the cavity as well as the location of the probe tube tip in the cavity are not determined. However, if proper precautions are taken to ensure that the probe tube is not moved between measurements, these probe tube systems are excellent for measurements of frequency response and relative differences between hearing-aid gain functions. Both of these are extremely important in hearing aid fitting and are the primary justification for these systems.

There are some cautions that should be observed in using a canal probe microphone system. First, care should be taken when inserting the probe tube. The probe tube should not be inserted to the point where it is touching or abutting the tympanic membrane. Not only will this be uncomfortable for the patient, but the measurements could be rendered inaccurate. The probe tube should be inserted into the canal cautiously and after looking into the canal to be sure there are no obstructions. Second, remember that the probe tube is just that, a hollow tube. If the tube is bent the effect will be similar to crimping a water hose, i.e., the pressure will be reduced. Although the tube is designed to withstand deformity to some degree, inserting the probe tube in places where canals with sharp bends can crimp the tube will invalidate the measurements. Finally, read the manual and be prepared for "a longer learning curve" than for other types of microphones. These systems are generally computer-based to assist in making the measurements and will take more time to master. In addition, the use of the probe tube system itself is more complex, and the user should take advantage of any training that is available.

Regardless of the application or the type of microphone, the microphone must be calibrated, at least with regard to intensity, prior to use. There are several methods for calibrating microphones, but the method most commonly used involves a transfer standard, which will be described next. In addition, calibration of some other parameters of microphone performance, such as phase and transient response, will be very briefly described.

Microphone Calibration

Since microphones provide the basis for calibration of devices such as audiometers and sound level meters, they must be calibrated to very precise standards. These standards depend on the use of the microphone and are specified in the context of the instrumentation that contains the microphone. An example in speech and hearing is the calibration of a sound level meter. Recall that the sound level meter was described as a voltmeter reading a microphone. Thus, the focus for the calibration procedure was calibrating the microphone. The technique described used a transfer standard. Each of the aspects of that procedure are discussed next.

Microphone calibration involves measuring the absolute sensitivity of the microphone at a single frequency and the frequency response to a single amplitude. The combination of the two allows prediction of the response of the microphone to a large range of conditions. Some special applications require further information, such as the phase or transient response of the microphone.

Usually calibration is restricted to measuring sensitivity at a single frequency, as described earlier for the sound level meter calibration, but it is desirable to measure the frequency response as well. There are three methods for measuring the sensitivity response:

1. The reciprocity method;
2. The comparison method;
3. The transfer method using a calibrated sound source.

The first method requires expensive equipment and is time consuming. The second method requires having a second calibrated microphone as well as making two sets of measurements and calculations. The third method usually requires only a calibrated sound source. All methods can require the use of couplers and accessory equipment to make the measurements, although this is usually minimal in the case of the transfer method. Based on these considerations, the method of choice for clinical purposes has been the transfer method, and instrumentation companies have designed appropriate sound sources for use in this method. Since this is by far the most common method used to calibrate microphones, it is the only method that will be considered here. (For information about the other methods see Seippel, RG: *Transducers, Sensors, and Detectors.* Reston Publishing, 1983.)

There are two types of calibrators used in the transfer method, the pistonphone and the vibrator. Both calibrators are extremely accurate (within approximately 0.25 dB) and easy to use. The pistonphone operates on the principle of a piston oscillating within a known cavity size, which permits the calculation of the exact sound pressure produced in the cavity. The vibratory source uses a piezoelectric driver element that vibrates a metallic diaphragm and causes the pressure in the cavity. The advantage of vibratory sources is that they can be driven at higher frequencies, such as 1,000 Hz, which is an appropriate frequency for calibrating weighting networks. The pistonphone, however, due to its mass requirements, can only be driven at low frequencies, such as 250 Hz, which is well below the frequency regions most commonly used in audiological, clinical, and research work.

Both devices are used similarly; A cavity in one end of the calibrator is used to fit the microphone into it (Fig. 4.3). In general, it is better if the microphone can be made stationary and the calibrator fitted over the microphone. This will avoid problems with movement of the microphone, which may cause slippage of the calibrator and hence alteration of the cavity size. Since the cavity size is an integral part of the calibrator and must be constant for accurate measurements, this is not a trivial concern. The effects of altering the cavity size can be seen by turning on the calibrator and moving it around while making the measurement.

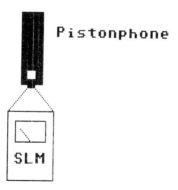

Figure 4.3. Calibration of a sound level meter using a pistonphone.

Once the microphone is fitted into the calibrator, the calibrator is turned on and the output voltage of the microphone is adjusted to match the intensity of the sound source. For a sound level meter, this means adjusting the display on the meter until it reads the intensity specified for the calibrator.

These measurements give the sensitivity of the microphone at the frequency of the calibrator, and because of the general stability of microphone frequency responses, these measurements also give the sensitivity at other frequencies in accordance with the previously measured frequency response. The microphone frequency response itself is normally measured using the electrostatic actuator method, which is also used for phase and transient response measurements. The electrostatic actuator method gives the microphone *pressure response*, i.e., the response of the microphone to the sound pressure actually acting on the diaphragm. The free-field response (namely, the response of the microphone in a sound field where the microphone can interact with the sound) was discussed earlier in this chapter. This response can be determined from the pressure response by applying the appropriate free-field corrections, which are given by the manufacturer for each type of microphone, or by measuring the response in an anechoic room. Given the cost and availability of anechoic rooms, applying free-field corrections is the method of choice.

The frequency response is measured by attaching the actuator as shown in Figure 4.4. A constant AC excitation voltage is applied to the actuator and is swept in frequency. A graphic level recorder, which is synchronized to the sweep frequency generator, records the output voltage of the micro-

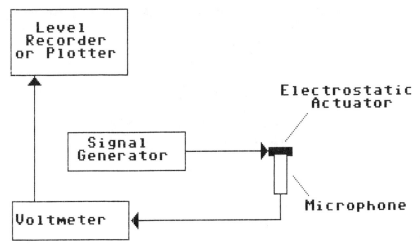

Figure 4.4. Instrumentation configuration for microphone frequency response calibration.

phone as a function of the frequency of the excitation voltage. As mentioned before, this method gives the pressure response of the microphone, and if the free-field response is desired, the appropriate free-field corrections should be added.

It is sometimes necessary to determine the phase and/or transient response of a microphone. This is a desirable measure when, for example, making electrophysiological measurements where the signal may be a click and hence a specification of the transient response of the microphone is necessary in order to specify the sound pressure produced by the click. The calibration is done using the electrostatic actuator method. For the phase measurements the signal from the microphone is compared with the excitation signal. The greatest accuracy is achieved if these signals are sent to a phase meter and the output of the phase meter routed to a graphic level recorder operating in the same manner as for the frequency response measurements. It is also possible, but not as accurate, to make the measurements using an oscilloscope and observing the interaction (lissajous) patterns on the scope when the microphone output and the signal source output are sent to the x and y inputs of the oscilloscope. Lissajous patterns will be described in more detail in a later chapter.

The transient response measurements are made in a similar manner, except the signal used is a pulse and the signals are usually compared on an oscilloscope. The critical comparison here is in terms of the comparability of the waveform shapes. An example of such a comparison is shown in Figure 4.5. Note that the microphone is unable to duplicate the square corners of the input pulse, as would be expected because of its inability to transduce the very high frequencies necessary to produce the square corners.

It is generally the case for microphone calibration that only the sensitivity is measured routinely and the frequency response is measured less often. The phase and transient responses are measured by those with special needs. Microphone calibration should be part of the regular routine of any clinic or research laboratory.

Microphones are not the only transducers used in speech and hearing; two other groups of transducers are loudspeakers (earphones) and accelerometers. The former are used to do the opposite of a microphone, namely, to output sound rather than to input sound. As might be expected, many of the principles for loudspeakers are similar to those for microphones, with some important differences. Therefore, loudspeakers are covered next, with accelerometers as the final topic for the chapter.

Loudspeakers

Almost everyone has a stereo system at home, and thus many people are greatly interested in the sound that comes from the system. Many

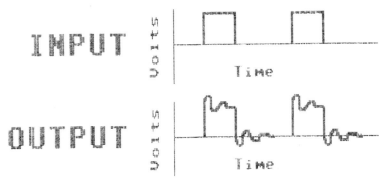

Figure 4.5. Example of microphone transient response.

stereo system owners fail to realize that the primary determinant of the sound quality is usually not the tuner or amplifer, which are usually more than adequate. The critical components of the system are the loudspeakers, which are frequently much more limited than the rest of the system.

It is interesting to note that while it is possible to get a very accurate electrical representation of sound with a single microphone, it is impossible to make a single cone speaker that will handle the broad frequency range with sufficient power to be heard over a large space. To get some idea of what is required, let us look at some considerations for speaker response. This discussion is not intended to be a design course for speakers, but rather a discussion of acoustic characteristics to be considered in selecting and understanding loudspeakers.

The first and most obvious considerations in speaker selection are frequency response and sound power. Recall the discussion of microphone size and its relation to frequency response and activity. The same considerations can be applied in reverse to speakers. A small-diameter speaker will produce high frequencies better than low frequencies because the resonant wavelength will be short, and the large-diameter speaker will reproduce low frequencies better than high frequencies for the same reason. It is also obvious that the large-diameter speaker will be able to move a greater volume of air within a single cycle than the small speaker because of the greater surface area of the large speaker. Thus low-frequency speakers can "blow you out of the room," as some may have experienced at rock concerts or other places where large speakers have been used.

It is obvious from a discussion of just these two factors that speaker designers are faced with a difficult problem: To get high frequencies, small-diameter speakers are required; to get low frequencies, large-diameter speakers are required. Furthermore, low-frequency speakers can dominate the sound because of their greater power, so this must also be taken into consideration.

These considerations have forced designers to construct most stereo speakers not as a single speaker but as a speaker system. Such a system consists of a mixture of speakers linked together with a specific weighting network, commonly referred to as a crossover network, which is designed to overcome the problems just discussed. Each of the speakers in such a system are used to reproduce a specific range of frequencies. In order to do this, the signal sent to the speaker is filtered so that the correct signal is sent to the appropriate speaker in the system. Some of the speaker designs are extremely complicated and may include 6 to 10 speakers in a single loudspeaker enclosure. As might be expected, the electronics can become quite complex in linking the speakers together. Therefore, both acoustic and electrical engineering are disciplines involved in the design of speakers. This is not to imply that good speakers are necessarily expensive but rather to indicate some considerations in speaker design.

Another factor that affects the use of speakers is diffraction. Recall that low-frequency sound easily avoids barriers that block high-frequency sound. One of these barriers is air, that is, high-frequency sound does not travel as well through air as low-frequency sound. Thus the measurement of sound coming from a speaker must always consider this factor when estimating the frequency response of a speaker. The frequency response is not constant as a function of distance. The further from the speaker the measurement is made, the less is the power at the high frequencies.

Sound Field Measurement

Since further discussion of the sound from a loudspeaker depends on some understanding of how the sound is measured, the measurement of sound in a sound field is addressed first. The most obvious aspect of the sound field is that there are numerous other factors to consider aside from the sound itself. These other factors are mostly tied to the disposition of objects in the sound field, although the boundaries of the sound field are also an important consideration.

The behavior of sound in regard to objects is called *diffraction* and has been discussed earlier. It is important to keep diffraction effects in mind when trying to measure sound in a sound field. This is especially true when attempting to calibrate the sound level in a sound booth for threshold or other testing. The obvious object here is the subject's or patient's head. The head can have considerable effect on the sound arriving at the ear because of its shape and size in combination with the frequency and angle of incidence of the sound. The effect is most manifest at frequencies above about 800 Hz, and is unaccounted for in one of the two most common methods of calibrating sound in a sound field.

The two most common methods for calibration in a sound field are the substitution method and the probe microphone method. With the advent of the KEMAR (Knowles Electronics Manikin for Auditory Research) manikin, there is an alternative method that is a combination substitution-probe method. However, the KEMAR manikin is expensive, and many facilities cannot afford this method, which is described last in this section.

The substitution method, which is the easiest and the fastest in terms of sound measurement technique, also requires the most correction in order to be useful for frequency-specific measurements (Fig. 4.6). This method places the microphone at the location that represents the center of the measurement area. For speech and hearing, this location is the expected center of the subject's or patient's head. The sound pressure at this point is used as the estimate of the sound pressure for all subsequent measurements. It is obvious that this procedure does not take into account head diffraction effects. An additional procedure that can help overcome this problem is to use published data on head diffraction effects and integrate them into the data. Since corrections already have to be applied to the microphone measurements based on frequency, angle of incidence, and microphone size (as discussed earlier), the additional corrections may not represent much extra labor. In fact, all corrections could be integrated into a single correction factor and handled by a computer.

The second most common method for calibration in a sound field is to

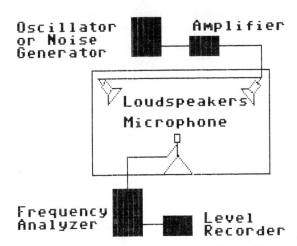

Figure 4.6.   Substitution method of sound field calibration.

use a probe microphone. As mentioned earlier, a probe microphone is simply a small microphone placed at the specific point of measurement. In the case of a sound field with a human, the most desirable location is open to question. Would it be better to describe the sound at the tympanic membrane, or is it best to describe the sound at the entrance to the ear canal? The answer depends on the specific application for the measurement. For hearing aids, the best location may be at the tympanic membrane, if it is desirable to specify the characteristics of the entire aid system, including amplifier characteristics, microphone and receiver characteristics, filtering, and the acoustic properties of the tubing or other acoustic treatments present. However, if knowing the input to the aid is essential, then the best location would be at the microphone of the aid. For the probe microphone, it is important to keep in mind the characteristics of the microphone and to be sure that these effects are compensated for in the measurement. The advantage of the probe microphone method is that since the microphone is at the location of interest, effects of environment variables prior to that location are included in the measurement and do not have to be added in post hoc.

KEMAR, which provides an alternative method of measurement, is a manikin representing the head and shoulders of a human; the manikin's dimensions are based on researched dimensions of the human body. It has a microphone at the location of a tympanic membrane. Furthermore, the microphone is housed in a coupler that represents the response of the outer ear. Since the microphone is fixed in place, measurements are repeatable with respect to the microphone location and environment.

KEMAR presents an opportunity to do a specific type of sound field measurement in a standardized way. Standardization of sound field measurement is very difficult. The substitution microphone may not be at the exact center of the head or even in the same place for every sound field measurement; the same is true for probe microphone measurements. In addition, the manikins permit different laboratories or clinics to have a standardized way to make the sound field measurement. As noted earlier, due to their precision nature and manufacturing requirements, the manikins are expensive and not easily affordable by most clinics.

Measurement of the sound field is clearly difficult, but with appropriate care, accurate measurements can be made. These measurements permit accurate assessment of other aspects of speaker performance with an impact on sound quality. These aspects are

1. The placement of the speakers and listener in the sound field;
2. The frequency response;
3. The distortion of the speakers.

Speaker and Listener Placement in the Sound Field

The placement of the listener and orientation of the speakers is important because the specification of the sound at the listener depends upon these factors. Each of these factors can impact the utility and flexibility of sound field testing for both clinical and research purposes. Before listener and speaker placement are described, an issue that affects both these factors, the number of speakers employed to generate the sound field, will be discussed.

At least two speakers should be available for use in a sound field test situation. A minimum of two speakers is required so that techniques based on sound localization in both clinical and research procedures may be used. Furthermore, a third speaker located midway between the other two speakers can be very helpful for a variety of reasons:

1. A clear reference for the listener for a midpoint in a localization task;
2. A third point in the localization space in sound field testing;
3. A reference point for balancing the output of the speakers.

The placement of the listener is important because of the need to ensure that sound from each speaker is represented equally at each ear. The listener also must be placed a sufficient distance away from both speakers so that he or she is placed in the reverberant field. That is, it is desirable that the listener not be in the near field, the area where each sound source is treated as a point source. Recall that speakers are *not* single source devices, i.e., there are generally two or three speaker cones in a speaker. In effect, what happens in the near field is that each of the speaker cones acts as a separate sound source rather than being treated as the desired single sound source. The primary difficulties arise for complex sounds such as speech, which will have output on all of the speaker cones in the speaker system. Since the speaker cones are usually displaced in the vertical plane, short and tall people would not receive the same sound from the speakers.

The placement of the listener should be at the point of intersection equidistant from the two speakers, at least 1 m from each speaker. Once this point has been determined, the spot should be marked; if a particular chair is to be used to seat the listener, the location of the legs of the chair should also be marked. All measurements should be made at the presumed location of the subject's head in the sound field using one of the techniques described previously for sound field measurement.

The orientation of the speakers must be considered when setting up a sound field system. This is important because of the difference in directionality for different frequency sounds. Low-frequency sound is omnidirectional, and high-frequency sound is highly directional due to the dif-

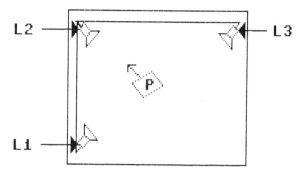

Figure 4.7.   Speaker arrangement in test room. Loudspeakers (L1–L3); patient or test subject (P).

fraction effects discussed earlier. While speaker manufacturers are aware of the problem and provide diffusers to make the speakers as omnidirectional at high frequencies as possible, no solution is perfect. Thus, the examiner/researcher must ensure that the face of the speaker is perpendicular to the listener in order to reduce the effects of directionality.

Figure 4.7 shows the speaker arrangement recommended to meet all of these requirements. The three speakers are equidistant from the listener, with a minimum distance of 1 m. One speaker is directly in front of the listener. Two side speakers are placed facing each other on either side of the speaker facing the listener and at a 90-degree angle relative to the middle speaker. Note that the walls are not equal in length and that all speakers are placed in corners of the room. In order to understand this arrangement a brief discussion of room acoustics is necessary.

Most sound-treated rooms in audiological test areas are square and have parallel walls. While this is the most economical and easiest room to construct, it is not desirable in terms of sound because of the possibility of setting up resonance in the room. When there is a match between the dimensions of the room and some multiple of the wavelength of a sound introduced into the room, this match creates a resonance. Thus, the amplitude of sound at that frequency will become amplified. When presenting complex sounds, this becomes a serious problem.

The simplest way to get around the problem is remove the parallel relation between the sound source and the walls. The best way to do that is to have nonparallel walls. Unfortunately, this is a very expensive solution in terms of construction. The means of reducing the resonance problem illustrated in Figure 4.7 is the most common. Corner placement of speakers generates a nonparallel relation between the face of the speaker and any wall. As a result, any sound will go through several reflections before it can start oscillating between the parallel walls.

Most speaker arrangements in clinics consist of one or two speakers. In the single-speaker case, the speaker should be placed in a corner of the room. In the two-speaker case, the speakers should generally be placed in the corners of the room at a 45-degree angle to the listener. (Note that such a speaker arrangement was shown in Figure 4.5 describing sound field calibration procedures.)

Once the speaker system is set up, it must be balanced. This simply means that the sound from each speaker reaching the location of the listener must be matched as closely as possible in intensity, frequency content, and time of arrival of the sound. If the speakers have been placed using the above criteria, all of these needs will be met. However, one additional complicating factor is the general rule that no two instruments are ever identical, which is true of speakers as well. The two or three speakers used to generate the sound field will not be identical with regard to frequency response, sound output relative to input, or distortion characteristics. Furthermore, the speakers will have to meet some general performance criteria with regard to these factors. To ensure that *all* factors are considered, the speakers must be matched.

The matching of loudspeakers is done by measuring the speaker characteristics that are most important to a particular application. The speakers are then selected, based on those that match most closely with the criteria of interest. At a minimum, these criteria would be the input/output relation, the frequency response, and the amount of distortion. Phase response and linearity are additional measurements that might be made. To get as good a match as possible, it is recommended that the manufacturer match the speakers prior to purchase based on your specifications. What if you already have a set of speakers and wish to test for their degree of match? The measurements are not difficult, although they are time consuming. They are the same for microphones, earphones, speakers, and, in fact, any sound source. The only difference is in the placement of the microphone and the coupling system used. However, before any extensive measurements are done, it is advisable to look at the speakers specifications to determine if the speakers meet the minimum criteria for the intended application.

All manufacturers will provide at least general speaker specifications with regard to the above-mentioned factors. In examining these specifications, look for distortion as low as possible combined with a smooth frequency response. In addition, look for output sufficient for the expected application in combination with a large (>70 dB) signal-to-noise ratio.

A smooth frequency response will usually assure that a distortion measurement at a single frequency will adequately reflect the distortion characteristics at other frequencies. An example of the potential problem is having the measurements made with a 1,000-Hz tone and having severe resonances exist in the speaker response. These resonances, as indicated by peaks in the frequency response, may not be at harmonics of 1,000 Hz. Thus, the 1,000-Hz measurement would lead to spuriously low distortion values, which would not be realized if a different frequency tone were to be employed as a test signal.

The high amplitude output/high signal-to-noise ratio combination is important to ensure an adequate dynamic range for presentation of complex sounds that may have components over a range of intensities. Be sure to check the amplitude of the signal used to make the signal-to-noise ratio measurement because that amplitude represents the amplitude needed to attain the maximum signal-to-noise ratio for that speaker. It is also important to check the absolute noise level for the speaker when no signal is present but when the amplifier feeding the speaker is turned on. This noise level will not change with the intensity of the signal, and thus represnts an absolute lower bound on the intensity domain. If the generation of low-level sounds is desired, this noise level is especially critical. As with all other instruments, while needs dictate specifications, availability and cost determine the limits of compromise.

Earphones can be treated as a special class of loudspeakers; namely, a single-diaphragm speaker. The primary difference is that earphones, as the name implies, are meant to be placed on the ear, whereas speakers are placed in a sound field at a distance from the listener. While most of the principles discussed earlier apply equally well to speakers and earphones, especially with regard to frequency response, distortion, amplitude, and signal-to-noise ratio, the placement of the earphone creates a special situation, which has some unique features.

Earphones

Earphones permit the controller of the sound to place the sound in a very well-defined place, which therefore has some advantage over speakers in terms of the specifications of the sound field relative to the listener. A simple example of this is that earphones can maintain a relatively constant sound field as the listener moves, which is difficult or impossible for speakers. Thus earphones are the preferred instrument for sound presentation by audiologists when such specification is critical to the conclusions drawn from the measurements.

Calibration of Earphones

Just as with all other instrumentation, earphones must be calibrated prior to use. As a result of their frequent use as part of the instrumentation for measuring hearing in humans, there have been some specialized instruments developed in response to standards for hearing measurement. The primary example of this is the earphone coupler.

The standard coupler was developed by the National Bureau of Standards and is referred to as the NBS-9A or 6-cc coupler due to the volume of the cavity in the coupler. The intent of the coupler is to mimic the acoustic properties of the sound field as produced by the earphone and thus obtain an estimate of the sound pressure in the ear canal. The coupler is used with a sound level meter or frequency analyzer to measure the response of the earphone. It should be noted that this coupler was designed to be used with a supra-aural (on top of the ear) cushion such as the MX41/AR cushion, which is the most common earphone cushion used for audiometric testing. The coupler will give erroneous results when used with a circumaural cushion such as is used for many stereo headphones. For this type of cushion a different technique must be employed.

The first calibration technique to be described assumes a supra-aural earphone cushion. To calibrate the earphone, remove the earphone from the headband and place the earphone with its cushion on the coupler. In order to simulate the pressure exerted by the headband, the earphone must be pressed against the coupler with a specified amount of force. The force specified in the standard (ANSI, 1973) for audiometers is 500 grams. While this represents a reasonable average for headbands, complete accuracy would require that the force of the particular headband to be used for that earphone be measured and that force be applied to the coupler. Unfortunately, headband force varies depending on the person wearing the headband. Since measuring the force exerted by the headband for a particular

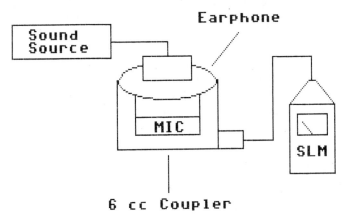

Figure 4.8.   Configuration for earphone calibration, with earphone in coupler and output of coupler going to sound level meter (SLM).

individual is not a trivial task, it is just not practical to do this for the large variety of expected wearers; hence, the standard force is 500 grams.

The dimensions of the cavity, which is basically a 6-cc cylinder, are specified in the standard. However, the method of attaining the required force is not specified by the standard, and a number of designs have arisen. The instrumentation configuration shown in Figure 4.8 is based on the 6-cc coupler. As is shown in the figure, the earphone is attached to the coupler, which contains a microphone, and the output of the microphone is sent to the measuring instrument. In the typical calibration of an audiometer this could be a sound level meter, a frequency counter, an oscilloscope, or a distortion analyzer. For research purposes, a spectrum analyzer could be attached.

Although there is a standard coupler, there is considerable controversy with regard to how well the coupler reflects the acoustic properties of the outer ear. In addition, the coupler was developed only for supra-aural earphones, whereas no comparable standard coupler has emerged for the circumaural earphone although some have been developed. Thus the method suggested here is a way to do the calibration for circumaural earphones that has been reported recently in the hearing literature.

The instrumentation configuration for calibrating a circumaural phone is the same as for the supra-aural phone except for one addition. The addition is a flat metal plate made of heavy anodized aluminum, with a hole cut into the plate of the same diameter as the opening in the 6-cc coupler. The plate is placed with the hole in the plate over the coupler opening, and the circumaural earphone is placed on the flat plate. From that point on the calibration procedure is exactly the same as for supra-aural earphones.

How often should earphones be calibrated? As with any other instrument, this depends on its use. In many audiology clinics, the intensity calibration for the earphone is done every day because of the heavy use of the earphone. In an active research facility, the same is also true. More detailed calibrations of the earphone, which include a distortion check, are generally done less frequently at intervals ranging from 1 week to 3 months, depending on the amount of use. Of course, if there is any potential problem, the calibration must be done immediately. In general, modern earphones are very stable and accurate instruments.

Other Factors in Earphone Use

In addition to the calibration issues just described, there are some other factors that should be considered when using earphones. Among these are care of the earphones, directionality effects, and matching of earphones. The first is specific to earphones, while the latter two are straightforward extensions of concepts that have been discussed in connection with loud-speakers.

Earphone care is fairly simple. A good pair of earphones will last many years if appropriate care is taken. There are really three components included in the typical earphone: the transducer itself, the cushion, and the earphone cord. The transducer should be kept dry, cool, and clean. *Do not use solvents to clean the earphone.* Simply removing the cushion and wiping with a lint-free cloth will suffice. The cushion itself should be washed with a solvent appropriate to the cushion material. Be aware that if alcohol is used as a cleaning solvent, which is a common practice, most cushion materials will dry out and crack. Thus, the cushions should be checked for structural integrity before being replaced on the transducer. This is important because the acoustic properties of the earphone depend on the integrity of the cushion. Finally, the integrity of the earphone cord(s) should be checked frequently.

The most common problem with earphones is a loosening of the connection between the cord and the transducer. To test the cord, flex it firmly but not with excessive force at the junction between the cord and the earphone and at various points along the cord, as well as at the junction between the cord and the connector on the other end from the transducer. This should be done while a continuous tone is input into the earphone. The tone should not interrupt nor should there by any crackle. If either of these symptoms manifest themselves when the junctions are tested, then reconnect the junctions. If the problem occurs only when the cord itself is flexed, replace the cord. Do not try to repair earphone cords between the junctions because if a problem occurs, it usually means that the cord has many potential trouble spots and the observed area is merely the first to fail. These points summarize the main features of caring for earphones. If they are followed faithfully and supplemented by frequent calibration to ensure the integrity of the transducer, the earphones should be reliable for many years. In my personal experience, earphones have remained within 1 dB of their original performance for a period of 7 years or more.

Directionality is a problem with earphones just as it is with speakers. One additional factor for earphones is that the earphone interacts with the acoustic characteristics of the ear canal. This means that at high frequencies, (above about 3,000 Hz) an earphone becomes highly directional with respect to the ear canal. The effects of this directionality, combined with earphone placement, can be as large as 10 dB at 4,000 Hz. Since it is generally impossible to ensure that earphone placement is repeated exactly each time, the best policy is to make all measurements with a single placement of the earphones if the measurements involve frequencies above 3,000 Hz.

Again, just as with speakers, the sound from each earphone must be matched as closely as possible in intensity, frequency content, and time of arrival of the sound. Recall from the discussion of loudspeakers the general rule that no two instruments are ever identical. This is true of earphones as well. Thus the earphones will not be identical with regard to frequency response, sound output relative to input, or distortion characteristics. Furthermore, the earphones will have to meet some general performance criteria with regard to these factors. In order to get as good a match as possible, it is recommended that the manufacturer match the earphones based on these factors. There are manufacturers who will do this, although it is more costly. The only other option is to buy many earphones and to do on-site matching, which is not practical. However, before buying any earphones, it is advisable to look at the specifications for the earphone to determine if the earphones meet the criteria for the expected application(s).

All manufacturers will provide at least general earphone specifications with regard to the factors just described. In fact, quality earphones come with a specification sheet for each earphone. These specifications should always be examined. In examining these specifications, look for distortion as low as possible combined with a smooth frequency response. In addition, look for output sufficient for the expected application in combination with a large (>70 dB) signal-to-noise ratio.

The final transducer instrument to be discussed is the accelerometer, which is used for the measurement of vibration in the field of speech and hearing. The primary users are industrial audiologists and speech-science researchers, but as clinical techniques are developed in the laboratory, more and more speech-language pathologists will be using accelerometers to make clinical measurements. Since sound is vibration, some of the considerations involved in the use of the accelerometer, such as distortion and frequency response, are the same as for the acoustic devices discussed earlier. However, there are some unique features associated with the use of accelerometers, and these will be highlighted in the next section. Since accelerometers are not yet in widespread use, the discussion here will serve only as an introduction to the topic.

Accelerometers

Accelerometers are used to measure vibration. Vibration is measured relative to a resting state, i.e., the parameters of vibration are measured relative to some position. The accelerometer is employed when measurement of the motion of a structure is desired. Examples of vibrating structures are a tuning fork, rotating gears, and vocal folds. Accelerometers measure the three major components of vibration analysis, namely, amplitude, velocity, and acceleration. As indicated by the examples just given, an accelerometer is used by a variety of disciplines, such as mechanical engineers, industrial audiologists, and speech-language pathologists.

Three measures are used to quantify the amount of vibration; displacement, velocity, and acceleration. Metric units and either peak or root-mean-square (RMS) values are employed for all measurement parameters; most modern vibration meters provide all three quantities. The *displacement* is the amplitude of the motion relative to a fixed reference point. The *velocity* is the speed of vibration or the displacement over time. Velocity can be calculated by multiplying the displacement by a factor proportional to the frequency of vibration. The *acceleration* is the change in velocity over time and has the unit g, which is the same unit as is used to measure gravity. It can be calculated by multiplying the displacement by a factor proportional to the frequency of vibration.

The accelerometer transduces the vibratory motion to an electrical signal. As with microphones, there are a variety of transduction elements and amplification is required. The most common accelerometers use piezoelectric materials. Recall that piezoelectric materials emit an electrical signal when deformed. To generate the deformation in response to vibratory motion, the general design requires that a mass apply a force to the piezoelectric element when the accelerometer assembly is vibrated. Figure 4.9 shows a schematic representation of one of the two most common configurations of mass and piezoelectric element used to generate the deformation.

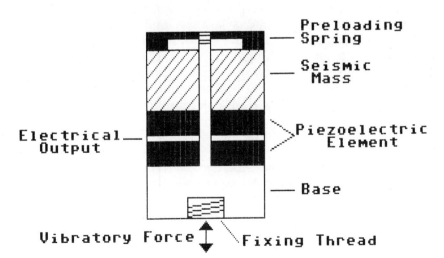

Figure 4.9.   Essential elements for an accelerometer to transduce vibratory motion to an electrical signal.

The two accelerometer configurations use either a compression or shear design. As can be seen from Figure 4.9, for the compression type, the mass exerts a compressive force on the piezoelectric element, distorting its shape and producing an electrical output proportional to the compressive force applied to the piezoelectric material. An example would be if the accelerometer were suddenly accelerated vertically. It can be seen that the accelerometer will be relatively insensitive to sideways movement because this will not force the mass toward or away from the piezoelectric material. The same is true of the shear design, although the method of transmitting the force to distort the piezoelectric material is different. For the shear design, the mass exerts a force at right angles to the piezoelectric element, which generates the alteration of material shape that results in an electrical output.

Accelerometers come in a variety of shapes and sizes for both the compression and shear configurations. This assortment is required because of the diversified application for accelerometers. Three important factors determining the accelerometer chosen are: accelerometer placement, frequency response required for measurement, and mass of mounting structure.

Vibration is frequently measured on machinery in order to monitor the state of the machine. For this purpose, the accelerometer may be mounted permanently in a very small place, and a small-size accelerometer would be required. In another case, the vibrating structure may have an unusual shape, and the mounting surface may have to mirror this shape. In still other cases, as in a special environment such as space, the mounting location may be inaccessible, and so a special casing may be required. While these examples illustrate factors that may determine the shape of the accelerometer, the most important consideration determining the size of the accelerometer is the frequency response required for the measurement. The frequency response of the accelerometer is primarily determined by its resonance properties. This relation between resonance and accelerometer size is discussed next.

It was shown previously that the frequency of resonance is inversely proportional to the mass of the object. Since accelerometers are primarily masses reacting to motion, the size of the accelerometer mass will obviously have an effect on the resonant charcteristics of the accelerometer. For example, a small (10 g) accelerometer may be able to measure up to 10,000 Hz, whereas the useful measurement frequency response for a large (1 kg) accelerometer will be limited to below 1,000 Hz. Thus, the expected frequency range of vibration must be determined before selecting an accelerometer.

An additional factor affecting accelerometer selection is the mass of the structure upon which the accelerometer is to be mounted. The mass of the accelerometer becomes important when measuring light test objects. Additional mass can significantly affect the vibration levels and frequencies at the measuring point because of the loading to the test object with accelerometer mass. As a general rule, the mass of the accelerometer should be less than $1/10$ the mass of the vibrating part onto which it is mounted.

Other factors affecting accelerometer response are the mounting position, the method of mounting, and the environment. First, the closer the accelerometer is placed to the source of the vibration, the more accurately the measurement will reflect the source characteristics. Second, the more permanent the method of mounting, the more accurately the motion of the accelerometer will reflect the motion of the mounting surface. Third, the environment can influence the measurement in a variety of ways, ranging from nuclear radiation to acoustic noise. Each of these will introduce its own effects and should be considered in the selection and use of an accelerometer. The effects of the first factor are obvious, but the effects of the latter two factors require the following brief descriptions.

Mounting an accelerometer involves considerations discussed earlier, such as mass considerations, issues of permanence, and type of mounting surface. If a permanent mounting is desired, the accelerometer is usually attached with a screw mount. This provides a permanent and repeatable mounting position with high measurement accuracy while permitting the removal and replacement of the accelerometer if necessary. For a less-permanent need, beeswax is an excellent mounting material, which has high adhesion to almost all materials and permits a very broad range of measurement frequencies. It also allows easy removal of the accelerometer when the measurements are completed. Magnetic attachment can also be considered, but is inappropriate in many situations and frequently does not permit as accurate a measurement as the beeswax material.

The type of mounting surface can also be important. For example, the same mounting material cannot be used for human skin as for steel. In fact, not all human skin can use the same mounting material. For steel and similar materials, the mounting methods and materials described earlier can be used. For speech science experiments where human beings are used as subjects, there are a number of bonding materials that have been developed for mounting accelerometers on human skin. Skin sensitivity should be considered and monitored when using these materials due to individual differences in skin sensitivity. This is especially true when working with children. For these cases, the trade-off between the need for accurate measurements and the applicability of a particular mounting material must be considered.

Accelerometer Calibration

Accelerometer calibration is similar to microphone, earphone, and speaker calibration in that the primary calibration measurements are sensitivity, dynamic range, and frequency response. A high-quality accelerometer will be accompanied by its own calibration sheet, which looks very similar to calibration sheets supplied for microphones and other sound-generating systems. These specifications should be examined carefully when deciding upon the appropriateness of a particular accelerometer.

The same variety of techniques used for microphone calibration, such as matching to a standard, can be used to calibrate an accelerometer. Usually, other methods are used by manufacturers or those individuals needing very high-precision calibration of their instruments. Accelerometer calibration is done most easily by using a calibrated vibration source in much the same manner as a calibrated sound source is used to calibrate a microphone. The calibrator has a small built-in shaker table that can be adjusted to vibrate at precisely 1 g (9.81 m/s^2). The sensitivity of the accelerometer is checked by fastening the accelerometer to the table in a specified manner and measuring the output when the calibrator is activated. Just as with microphones, the frequency response of the accelerometer will almost never change without a change in sensitivity; thus sensitivity calibration is enough to verify the satisfactory operation of the device. To measure the frequency response of an accelerometer, a variable frequency shaker table is required.

How often should accelerometers be calibrated? As with any other instrument, this depends on its use. In a research facility, the calibration is done before every use. However, even in everyday use it is possible to subject an accelerometer to very high accelerations without realizing it. For example, when an accelerometer is dropped from hand height onto a concrete floor, the shock transmitted to the accelerometer may be many thousands times gravity. Complete calibration of an accelerometer should be done annually by sending the accelerometer to the manufacturer. Of course, if a potential problem arises, the calibration should be done immediately. In general, modern accelerometers are very stable and accurate instruments.

Chapter Summary

This chapter discussed transducers for sound and vibration, namely microphones, earphones, and accelerometers. Hydrophones were not discussed, however, the principles of operation of such transducers are very similar to the transducers described in this chapter. The main foci for the chapter were the use and calibration of acoustic and vibration transducers. Methods for calibrating sound fields and the sound from earphones were discussed. The need for consideration of factors such as resonance and diffraction, as well as environmental factors, was noted for all types of measurement and transducers. Some of the accessory instrumentation required to do calibration and to use the transducers was identified. Further description of the accessory instrumentation and their uses and a further examination of the uses for transducers of sound and vibration are found in later chapters.

6

Microphone Calibration

Introduction

T he purpose of this lab is to give some experience using and calibrating microphones. The most common transducers that deal with acoustic energy are microphones, earphones, and speakers. Many of the acoustic principles associated with microphones are the same as those for earphones or speakers; the calibration principles are also similar.

Microphones transduce acoustic energy to electrical energy and serve as input sources to many of the instruments used in the field of speech and hearing. There are many different forms of microphone construction and many different models of microphones within a particular type. The microphone used in this lab is a *condenser microphone*. Prior to this lab, the specifications describing the microphone's characteristics should be carefully examined to determine the microphone's performance. Check for specifications on sensitivity and frequency response.

The condenser microphone has many positive features: a broad frequency response, resistance to humidity and temperature, relative insensitivity to movement, and good absolute sensitivity. The basic principles of operation of a microphone were discussed in the chapter. Microphones may differ in terms of their frequency response; absolute sensitivity; stability during temperature, pressure, or climate fluctuations; directional sensitivity; and/or distortion characteristics. A complete calibration, such as would be done at the factory, should consider all these factors.

Regardless of the application or the type of microphone, the microphone must be calibrated, at least with regard to intensity, prior to use. There are several methods for calibrating microphones, but the method most commonly used involves a transfer standard, which is the method that will be employed in this laboratory.

Method

Apparatus

The instrumentation used for this lab will depend on which of the two procedures described below is employed. These are potential instruments:

1. Sinewave oscillator;
2. Calibrated sound field system;
3. Test microphone;
4. X-Y plotter;
5. Spectrum analyzer;
6. Broadband acoustic noise source;
7. Attenuator;
8. Sound attenuated room (audiometric booth or equivalent);
9. Anechoic sound room;
10. All necessary cables and power supplies.

Procedure

Microphone calibration involves measuring the absolute sensitivity of the microphone at a single frequency and the frequency response to a single amplitude. The combination of the two allows prediction of the response of the microphone to a large range of conditions. Some special applications require further information, such as the phase or transient response of the microphone.

Calibration is usually restricted to measuring sensitivity at a single frequency, as described earlier for the sound level meter calibration, but it is desirable to measure the frequency response as well. Three methods for measuring the sensitivity response were described in the chapter: the reciprocity method; the comparison method; or the transfer method. The transfer method requires only a calibrated sound source and will be used here. All methods can require the use of couplers and accessory equipment to make the measurements, although this is usually minimal in the case of the transfer method.

There are two types of calibrators used in the transfer method, the pistonphone and the vibrator. Both calibrators are extremely accurate (within approximately 0.25 dB) and easy to use. Both devices are used similarly. There is a cavity in one end of the calibrator, and the microphone is fitted into this cavity (Fig. 4.3). In general, it is better if the microphone can be made stationary and the calibrator fitted over the microphone as this will avoid problems with movement of the microphone, which may cause the calibrator to slip and hence alter the cavity size. The cavity size is an integral part of the calibrator and must be constant for accurate measurements.

Once the microphone is fitted into the calibrator, the calibrator is turned on and the output voltage of the microphone is adjusted to match the intensity of the sound source. This means that the output of the microphone must be attached to a voltmeter. A sound level meter is a device that is essentially a microphone attached to a voltmeter; therefore we will use a sound level meter for our microphone-voltmeter combination. Thus, adjust the display on the meter until it reads the intensity specified for the calibrator.

This measurement gives the sensitivity of the microphone at the frequency of the calibrator. The frequency response and linearity of the microphone must also be measured in order to translate this value across frequency. The microphone frequency response itself is normally measured using the electrostatic actuator method, which is also used for phase and transient response measurements. The frequency response of the microphone can also be measured using an anechoic room and a calibrated sound source. Each of the above methods will be described, and either can be used for this lab depending upon available instrumentation.

Measuring the Frequency Response Using the Actuator.   The actuator is attached to the microphone as shown in Figure 4.4. A sinewave excitation voltage is applied to the actuator using the oscillator and is swept in frequency. A graphic level recorder, which is synchronized to the sweep frequency generator, records the output voltage of the microphone as a function of the frequency of the excitation voltage. As mentioned in the chapter, this method gives the pressure response of the microphone and if the free-field response is desired, the appropriate free-field corrections should be added.

Measuring the Frequency Response in a Sound Field.   This method is best employed in an anechoic chamber, but a standard, sound-attenuated room can be employed to simplify the measurement. The key to doing this measurement is to get a calibrated sound source. There are two possibilities: The first is to use a speaker system with a known frequency response; the second is to use a broadband noise source in combination with a spectrum analyzer. The first option will be described here. The student should be able to extrapolate how to do the second option by examining the signal analysis lab (Quiklab 12).

The sound delivery system should be set up in the configuration that gives a known frequency response. The microphone should be placed in the sound field at the appropriate location. The signal should be from an oscillator, and several frequencies should be chosen. The ideal situation is to have the output of the microphone connected to an *x-y* plotter and to sweep through the frequency range from 20–20,000 Hz. If this is not possible, use discrete frequencies. Select frequencies to insure a representative sample of the frequency range under test. (The total number of frequencies tested should not be more than 10.) The instrumentation configuration for doing this measurement is shown in Figure 4.10.

Measuring the Linearity of the Microphone.   The final measurement should be the linearity of the microphone. This measurement gives the relation between input and output at several intensities. The instrumentation configuration is the same as for the frequency response

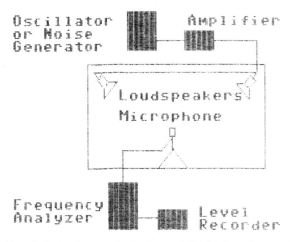

Figure 4.10. Substitution method of sound field microphone calibration.

measurement, with the exception that an attenuator is placed between the oscillator and the sound system. The linearity of the sound system must be known for this to work. Intensity, rather than frequency, is the parameter that is varied. Select 5–10 intensities, ranging from the maximum to the noise floor of the environment or the microphone, whichever is greater.

Results

The results for the sensitivity, the frequency response, and the linearity measurements should be recorded on a data sheet. For the frequency response, use either the plot, if available, to estimate the frequency response of the microphone or use the discrete measurements to plot the frequency response and make the estimate from that plot.

Discussion

Discuss the various measurements in terms of the intended applications for the microphones. Is it satisfactory? What applications are appropriate for the microphone under test? What are the limitations of measurements made with this microphone?

A lot of the points above should sound familiar. Most of this information is presented in the chapter. However, I hope that this lab leads to a better understanding of the application of the principles described in the chapter and to the ability to extrapolate those principles to new sound presentation systems.

5

Audiological Measurement Instrumentation

Clinical audiologists use a number of instruments to measure hearing and the status of the auditory system. The two primary clinical instruments are the audiometer and the oto-admittance meter or impedance bridge, which are the focus for this chapter. Audiometers are discussed first, and then impedance measurement instruments. There is a large body of literature on both of these devices, and this chapter is not meant to replace that literature, but rather to discuss major features of these instruments.

Other instruments used in audiological practice are tape recorders, microphones, loudspeakers, and, more recently, computers. Microphones and loudspeakers were discussed in the previous chapter and will be referred to in this chapter only in relation to their usage with audiometers or middle-ear measurement devices. Tape recorders are covered in the next chapter, and computers are discussed in the last chapter. Tape recorders and computers will be referred to only relative to their usage with other instruments.

Audiometers

In addition to audiologists, other professionals, such as physicians, nurses, audiometric technicians, and speech pathologists, also use audiometers. Each of these professionals has different needs, and audiometers with capabilities specific to those needs have been developed. In addition, there are many cases where it is necessary for the audiometer to be portable, and such audiometers are available. Although in the past, portability required removal of features, the development of microprocessor-based audiometers eliminates most limitations. Thus, portable units can have all the capabilities of desktop models.

This discussion should make it evident that the variety of audiometers is based more on number of features rather than on large functional differences. Audiometers that are truly programmable and permit enhancements through the addition of modules may permit true changes in the functionality of the units, but at the present time this technology has not been truly demonstrated in the marketplace. Even if the technology is applied soon, there will be a considerable lag before such audiometers become commonplace. Hence this chapter describes audiometers in terms of functions rather than in terms of features such as portability. When appropriate, it will be noted that certain functions are implemented in a certain way on a particular class of audiometer.

Components of Audiometers

Audiometers really refer to a multifunction, multicomponent instrument. Audiometers are able to present sound via earphones, loudspeakers, and bone vibrators. Potential sources contained within the audiometer are oscillators and noise generators. External sources that can be routed through and controlled by the audiometer include tape recorders, and microphones. In addition, the sound can be shaped in the frequency domain, the intensity altered in fixed steps and at various rates, and the signal timing varied. All of these can be done for each of two channels, or both channels can be combined. Communication capabilities between patient and clinician are also built into the audiometer.

This multiplicity of functions makes the audiometer a difficult instrument to master quickly and is somewhat intimidating initially. However, the functions on an audiometer form logical groups, and if these groupings are kept in mind, it is possible to use any audiometer. How fast a particular measurement can be made will depend upon familiarity with the particular instrument, which is due to the fact that different manufacturers have different ways of selecting audiometer functions. The key is to learn the various functions and not worry about how they are arranged. While speed is desirable, this can always be gained with practice.

Some of the components just mentioned should already be familiar to the reader. In particular, microphones, earphones, loudspeakers, oscillators, and noise generators were discussed in previous chapters. The attenuators, which vary the intensity of the signal, should also be familiar, although they were previously presented in different guises. Examples of attenuators that have been described previously are at the input to the frequency counter and oscilloscope (V/cm dial). Bone vibrators are simply accelerometers in reverse, i.e., instead of the mass being vibrated by the surface being measured, the mass is vibrated and it applies the vibratory force to the surface being vibrated. In summary, the basic principles for all of the basic components of an audiometer have been introduced previously, with the exception of computerization.

As noted before, audiometers will become completely programmable instruments. This programming capability will permit software upgrades to the audiometer, which will probably consist of a combination of programs on a chip and programs on some storage medium such as a disk. It is already the case that audiometers can relatively easily be connected to and communicate with computers.

Another significant change that will result from the transfer of digital or computer technology to the audiometer is the manner in which the signal is produced. The new audiometers will use digital signal paths rather than the current analog signal paths. The difference between analog and digital signal paths will be elucidated in a later chapter, but the key difference here is that a lot of the calibration will be built into the audiometer. However, as noted before, there will be a considerable lag before such audiometers become common in the marketplace, and even then some calibration will need to be done external to the audiometer.

Audiometers will now be discussed in terms of their primary applications: air-conduction threshold testing, bone-conduction threshold testing, and prepared material testing. Some of the measurements appropriate to using the instrument for each of these applications and the calibration requirements will be discussed.

Air-Conduction Measurements

There are many clinical aspects to threshold testing, in addition to the instrumentation aspects. It is not the intent here to describe techniques for measuring the threshold of hearing, but rather to describe the instrumental aspects of using an audiometer to test hearing. There are many treatments of threshold testing from the clinical point of view. The principles of hearing measurement should be known before testing a patient with an audiometer.

The audiometer components involved in air-conduction threshold testing are the oscillator(s), noise generator(s), attenuator(s), switch(es), earphone(s), and loudspeaker(s). The communication system between the tester and the patient is also employed. Figure 5.1 gives a simple block diagram of the audiometer components involved in basic threshold testing for a single channel.

Figure 5.1 shows that there are a number of optional configurations possible by selecting various combinations of components. For example, standard pure-tone air-conduction threshold testing would employ an oscillator, an attenuator, a switch, and an earphone. If masking was necessary, the noise generator and the other earphone would be added.

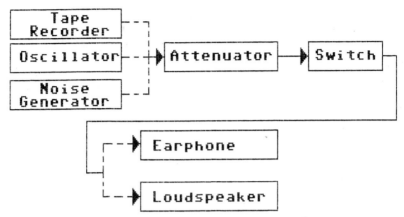

Figure 5.1.   Components of a one-channel audiometer.

Standards have been developed for audiometers so that clinicians and researchers can judge whether these instruments are appropriate and sufficient for the task.

Standards were discussed in a previous chapter that described sound level meters. The general comments in that section with regard to standards apply to the present discussion. The current standard was promulgated by the American National Standards Institute (ANSI) in 1973, although frequent reference is made to earlier standards such as International Standards Organization (ISO) 1964 and ANSI 1969. These three standards are relatively comparable. The last large change in audiometric test standards was from the ASA 1951 standard to the ISO 1964 standard. Thus data reported from instruments calibrated to the ASA 1951 standard should be adjusted to reflect the newer standards.

Audiometer standards cover intensity at threshold, accuracy of attenuators, sine wave signal distortion, acceptable ambient noise levels, and rise/fall times of switches. As has been the case with sound level meters, many of these standards reflect what is already on the market, as well as the results of research data on these aspects of an audiometer. Table 5.1 lists the standard values, as taken from the ANSI 1973 standard, for the aforementioned factors.

These standards are important when calibrating an audiometer, which will now be described along with some rationale for why a particular parameter is set within certain bounds. The discussion here will be brief because issues such as distortion and energy spread will be discussed further in a later chapter when discussing signal analysis. It should be noted that audiometer calibration will require the use of test instrumentation described in chapter 3. Review this instrumentation now if necessary because the following discussion assumes familiarity with these instruments.

Table 5.1.
Brief Summary of ANSI Calibration Values

| Test Frequency, Hz | *Air-Conduction Thresholds* | | |
| | dB SPL in TDH-39 Re 0.0002 Microbar | Maximum Range | |
		Frequency	Amplitude, dB
125	45	121–129	±5
250	25.5	242–258	±3
500	11.5	485–515	±3
1,000	7	970–1,030	±3
1,500	6.5	1,455–1,545	±3
2,000	9	1,940–2,060	±3
3,000	10	2,910–3,090	±3
4,000	9.5	3,880–4,120	±4
6,000	15.5	5,820–6,180	±5
8,000	13	7,760–8,240	±5

| *Other Parameters* | | | | |
| ON/OFF Switch | | | | |
Rise Time	Fall Time	ON/OFF Ratio	Distortion	Attenuator Step Size
0.02 s to rise from −20 dB to −1 dB of full amplitude	0.005–0.1 s to fall 20 dB from full amplitude	output in OFF at least 50 dB below output in ON	SPL of any harmonic of test frequency at least 30 dB below full amplitude	error for each 5 dB step size not to exceed 3/10 of interval (1.5 dB); if step size <3 dB, error must be <1 dB

Audiometer Calibration for Air-Conduction Testing

A quick examination of Table 5.1 indicates that the standards and hence the calibration involve all of the components used for air-conduction testing. The primary instrument employed to calibrate an audiometer is a sound level meter. The earphone is placed on the coupler as described in chapter 3, and the measurements are based on the sound coming through the coupler and the sound level meter. The standards assume that the earphone coupler is a standard 6-cc coupler similar to the National Bureau of Standards 9A coupler. There are also corrections available if it is decided to use the Zwislocki coupler, which gives a better measure of real ear response than the 6-cc coupler.

There are several phases to air-conduction calibration. The phases include measurement of the noise floor, measurement of signal frequency, measurement of the tone intensity at a specified level and for several settings of the hearing level (HL) dial, measurement of rise/fall time, and measurement of the distortion produced by the tonal signal. All of these measurements, with the exception of the frequency and distortion measurements, can be made with a sound level meter and an octave-band filter set. An octave-band filter set is included with most current sound level meters. The frequency measurement requires a frequency counter and the distortion measurement requires a distortion analyzer or spectrum analyzer in addition to the sound level meter.

The rise/fall time measurement is seldom made, but should be checked periodically. This measurement requires an oscilloscope and a sound level meter. It should be noted that an alternative instrumentation configuration for making all of the measurements mentioned here, with the exception of the distortion measurement, is an oscilloscope coupled to a sound level meter, although this is not the best method.

The most common set of measurements made when doing regular calibrations of an audiometer are checking the frequency of the tonal signal, the intensity of the tonal signal, and the linearity of the HL dial. This makes sense because these are the measurements made most frequently in the clinic, as well as being the easiest to check. This set of calibration measurements are discussed next.

Tonal Frequency Calibration

The frequency of the signal produced by an audiometer can be measured by attaching the output of the audiometer directly to the input of a frequency counter. Figure 5.2A shows the instrumentation configuration for this measurement. The earphone can be ignored for this measurement because earphones will rarely, if ever, introduce a frequency shift in a puretone signal. The test signal frequency is selected, and the output is set to be continuous. The signal frequency is selected either with a dial, with a number pad, or with arrow keys that adjust the frequency of the signal up and down. These controls will be on the front of the audiometer. To make the signal continuous, lock the test switch in the on position. In general, start with the lowest frequencies, and move toward the high frequencies because that is how the calibration sheets are generally set up. The

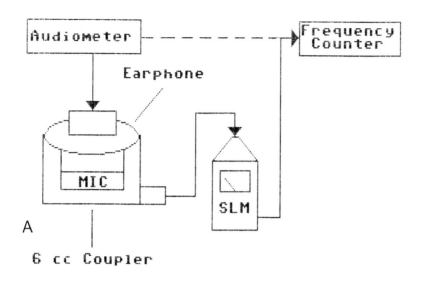

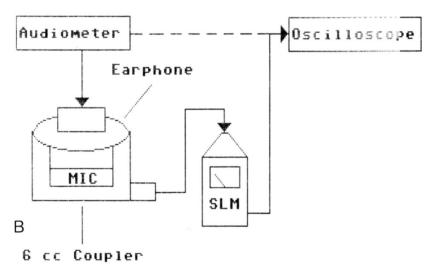

Figure 5.2. Frequency calibration of an audiometer using (*A*) a frequency counter and (*B*) an oscilloscope.

frequencies to be measured and the permitted error bounds are shown in Table 5.1.

It is also possible to calibrate an audiometer for frequency using an oscilloscope. However, the oscilloscope's accuracy for period measurement must be checked as described in the test instrumentation chapter (chapter 3) prior to using this method. Typical manufacturer's specification for accuracy of temporal parameters on an oscilloscope is about 2%–3%, which is insufficient for audiometer calibration. In order for the oscilloscope to be used, the verified error must be 1% or less. The instrumentation configuration is shown in Figure 5.2*B*. The output of the audiometer is connected to the input of the oscilloscope.

The procedure for measuring the frequency is to measure the period for each signal frequency on the oscilloscope using the methods described in Quiklab 4 on oscilloscopes. The reciprocal of the period is the frequency. Provided the oscilloscope meets the necessary requirement for accuracy (error <1%), this method will work.

Tonal Intensity Calibration

Measurement of intensity values requires the use of a sound level meter. As mentioned earlier, the procedure for doing this is discussed in chapter 3. It is important to remember one of the cardinal rules of instrumentation use; namely, whatever is connected must be capable of being disconnected. Instrumentation is designed to go together with reasonable ease and does not require excessive force on connections. If you are using too much muscle power to connect and disconnect, you are trying too hard.

The intensity calibration configuration using the sound level meter requires that the earphone be attached to a 6-cc coupler, with the coupler attached to a sound level meter. After the earphone is attached to the sound level meter, the first intensity measurement is usually the sound intensity of 70 dB HL. Set the audiometer to this intensity and to continuous output. The output intensity is indicated either on the adjustment control or on a digital readout panel of the audiometer. Be sure that the earphone under test has been selected for the channel being manipulated. This can be verified by checking the front panel controls to make sure that the earphone and channel are correct. For each of the frequencies given in Table 5.1, measure the sound intensity and verify that it is within the bounds indicated in the table. If the intensity is outside of the bounds, then it will be necessary to make up a correction sheet for the audiometer.

A correction sheet, more properly called a "correction table," is a tabulation of the intensity errors of the audiometer. If the intensity is in error by 5 or 10 dB at no more than two frequencies, then a correction table is appropriate. If the errors are larger or more frequencies are affected, then it is time to repair the audiometer because some of the basic components of the audiometer are defective. It is important to note that the table should not only give the errors but tell the user how to use the error. For example, take the number in the table and add it to HL in order to make the measurement correct. It is not critical whether the table represents a subtraction or an addition, as long as it is clear how the correction is to be applied.

Attenuator Linearity Calibration

The calibration procedure just described would suggest that the audiometer has a variable intensity oscillator, with intensity varying as a function of frequency. However, oscillators in an audiometer actually produce a fixed intensity signal so the appropriate intensity by frequency function is produced by two linked attenuators. The HL control on an audiometer is actually a variable attenuator. This dial is in series with another fixed attenuator inside the audiometer. The fixed attenuator is set as a function of the signal frequency. The amount of attenuation produced by the fixed attenuator is implemented in various ways. For example, one audiometer uses a plastic rotor with varying diameters attached to the frequency control. An arm rests on the rotor, which is connected to a variable attenuator. The amount of attenuation is proportional to the position of the arm. By shaping the rotor properly, one obtains the desired intensity by frequency function. Modern digital audiometers use a table of appropriate values that are similar to those in Table 5.1 to set an electronic attenuator. The electronic attenuator then functions as the fixed attenuator and is in series with the HL control.

The fixed attenuator is not accessible, but it is the basis for the fixed-level calibration described here. The inaccessibility and difficulty of repairing the fixed attenuator results in the requirement that if errors get too large, the attenuator must be replaced. The variable attenuator (HL control) also needs to be calibrated. The primary rationale for this calibration is that using this attenuator should not obviate the calibration of the fixed-level attenuator. That is, as the HL control is employed to change the signal intensity, the error due to the HL control must be small enough that the intensity difference specified by the HL control is correct relative to the fixed-level calibration.

Since the attenuators are in series, the total error due to the two attenuators is the sum of the errors for each attenuator. Furthermore, there are two factors in the HL control error. First, there is the error between each step on the control. For the HL control this usually means a 5-dB step size. The expectation that a 5-dB change on the control results in a 5-dB change in the signal level is referred to as "linearity." Second, over the total range of the HL control, which can be as large as 135 dB, there will be some cumulative error. Both of these contributions to error must be considered when doing a linearity calibration.

Linearity calibration of the HL control(s) on an audiometer is very straightforward. The sound level meter is set up as for the fixed-level attenuation calibration described before and the HL control is changed in 5-dB steps. As the control is changed, the change in signal level is recorded. This is done for a single signal frequency (the variable attenuator is not frequency specific) and for one or two HL controls depending on the audiometer. It is important that each HL control be measured separately because each is an independent attenuator, and it is quite possible for one attenuator to be perfect and the other to be abominable. The difficulty in the calibration arises when the HL control approaches 0 dB HL. At these low signal levels, the noise in the audiometer system and the environment can interfere with the measurement. The permissible limits of linearity error are given in Table 5.1. If the error exceeds these values, the audiometer should be repaired. Unlike the static error for the fixed intensity calibration, errors exceeding the standard in the linearity calibration should not be put on a correction sheet.

Noise Floor Measurement

Noise in measurements is a ubiquitous problem. The sources for the noise can be either in the instrumentation or in the environment. Noise is specified in terms of voltage output without any input signal. All instrumentation has some noise; there are no noiseless instruments, only instruments with degrees of noise.

Environmental noise in the measurement, which is defined here as "all sources other than the desired signal source," is not an irremediable problem. There are some strategies that will permit accurate measurements in this situation. The first strategy is to make the measurement at a sufficiently high level that the noise cannot affect the measurement. This strategy can be employed when the signal intensity is not critical to the meaurement, for example, when measuring frequency; or when it is assumed that the measured property will not be affected by a change in intensity, for example, when measuring rise/fall time. Note that these assumptions must be verified in some manner.

Calibrating an audiometer requires that the intensity-by-frequency calibration be performed at 70 dB HL, yet all threshold measurements should be referenced to 0 dB HL. This extrapolation assumes that the attenuators are linear, that is, when the control is turned to 0 dB HL the measured level will be reduced by 70 dB. The need to verify this assumption requires determination of attenuator linearity. Noise creates problems in that it obscures measurements at the very levels that we most want to measure. Therefore, a different strategy must be employed to make measurements at these intensities. This strategy requires that the noise be reduced in some way.

A common strategy employed to reduce measurement noise is to filter the signal. The filter is centered on the signal with a narrow bandwidth to exclude all noise except that at the signal frequency. This is not always the desired strategy because filtering has effects other than just eliminating energy outside the filter band, however, these effects do not intrude upon the intensity measurements and will be discussed later.

Current sound level meters provide octave-band filters as either a built-in or optional accessory. These filters are an important accessory and will frequently prove useful because noise is such a pervasive problem. When the signal is filtered, it is possible to measure down to intensities close to 0 dB HL in a very quiet sound-treated environment. Of course, if the noise has considerable energy at the signal frequency, this will obviate the filtering strategy. To determine if this is the case, it is necessary to measure the noise floor.

The noise floor should be known in any hearing measurement situation, not just for audiometer calibration. The ANSI standard has specified permissible noise levels for audiometric measurement, which are given in Table 5.1. These levels are such that the noise permits screening audiometry. The noise is specified in terms of octave band intensities. The noise floor is measured in the same manner as the measurement of signal intensity, except that no signal is presented and the signal channel is filtered by an octave-band filter. Therefore, the instrumentation setup is exactly the same as that described previously for the intensity-by-frequency calibration except for the octave filter, which is inserted in between the microphone and the sound level meter (Fig. 5.3). Incidentally, the same setup can be used for the linearity measurements if filtering is required, which usually is the case.

The noise floor measurement is made using the configuration shown in Figure 5.3. For each measurement frequency, the center frequency of the octave band filter is adjusted to the desired measurement frequencies. *Do not turn on the signal generator.* For audiometric measurements the center

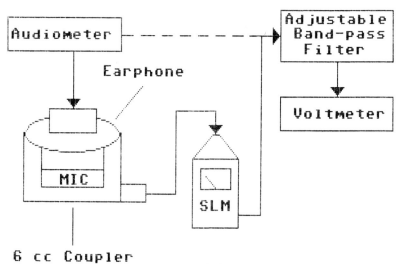

Figure 5.3. Audiometer calibration (noise floor) using a filter.

frequencies are indicated in Table 5.1, but for other measurements the center frequencies are the desired signal frequencies. The intensity measured in the absence of the signal at each center frequency represents the noise in that octave band.

Noise floor information is useful in three main ways. First, the correspondence with permissible levels can be checked. Second, the limit of signal intensity measurement using filtering is determined. For accurate measurements, that is, an error of <1 dB, no signal measurements should be made <10 dB above the noise floor. Third, the limit of audiometric measurement can be determined based on the noise level and known data about thresholds within octave bands of noise. It should be noted that in some cases the environmental noise will be below the instrumentation noise, in which case the instrument specification should be used to see if the noise is excessive for that instrument.

Total Harmonic Distortion Measurement

Noise represents one factor that can affect audiometric measurement; however, another factor is distortion in the signal itself. That is, the signal is an "impure" tone. There are two types of distortion, "harmonic distortion" and "intermodulation distortion," but this discussion will be restricted to the measurement of harmonic distortion. The ANSI standards specify the amount of permissible distortion in an audiometer. For research purposes, the standards are rather lax; more stringent criteria should be applied; namely, the intermodulation distortion should also be known.

The standard specifies total harmonic distortion at specific frequencies. This type of measurement is most easily made with a distortion analyzer, although some other methods are possible (Fig. 5.4). One other possible method will be discussed along with the distortion-analyzer method.

Figure 5.4 illustrates the instrumentation configuration for measuring total harmonic distortion. The output of the audiometer is sent to the distortion analyzer, which provides a readout corresponding to the total harmonic distortion in the signal. There are two basic parts to a distortion analyzer: a voltmeter and a band-reject filter. When the distortion analyzer is set to a desired measurement signal frequency, the center frequency of the band-reject filter is set to the same frequency. Thus this frequency is maximally rejected by the filter, leaving only the distortion products. Since total harmonic distortion is the ratio between the intensity at the signal frequency and the intensity at all other frequencies, the distortion analyzer must be able to measure the intensity both at the signal frequency and at all other frequencies. This is done by having a voltmeter in the analyzer measure the intensity both before and after the band-reject filter and then taking the ratio of these two values.

An easy error to make with a distortion analyzer is to forget that the

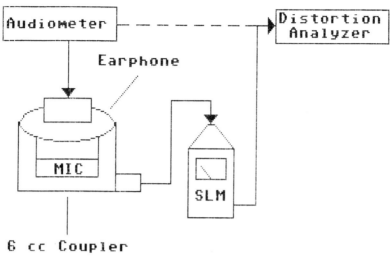

Figure 5.4. Audiometer calibration with a distortion analyzer.

analyzer does not actually measure each distortion component and then to take the sum of these components as the denominator in the ratio. Attempting to measure total harmonic distortion when the signal is close to the noise floor or in the presence of considerable noise will give erroneous values because the analyzer will measure all noise not at the signal frequency as distortion and hence calculate the ratio incorrectly. Total harmonic distortion should always be measured with the signal intensity near the top of the dynamic range of the instrument or sufficiently above any noise floor (ideally 60 dB) to avoid contamination of the measurement by the noise.

Total harmonic distortion, as was noted in the test instrumentation chapter (Chapter 3), is reported in two ways: as a percentage or as a number of dB below the signal intensity. The discussion in Chapter 3 should be reviewed at this point to reinforce an understanding of what is being measured. Another way of specifying harmonic distortion is in terms of the maximum intensity distortion component relative to the signal intensity. The difficulty with this specification is that it does not give the overall distortion level. In the unlikely, but possible case that all of the distortion components were the same amplitude, this type of specification could considerably understate the total distortion in the signal, because the sum of the distortion components would be well above the level given for a single distortion component.

Rise/Fall Time Measurement

Distortion in the generation of the signal is one way of generating unwanted signal components. Inappropriate switching of the signal can also create undesirable signals. In this case, the difficulty arises because signal energy at frequencies in addition to the signal frequency are generated if the signal is switched on too abruptly. For audiometric purposes, "too abruptly" translates into a rise/fall time <10 ms. A more theoretical treatment is provided in a later chapter, but the basic problem is that to turn a signal on rapidly requires frequencies that are contained in a click, and a click has frequencies across the entire spectrum. The more rapidly a signal is turned on, the more the signal spectrum at onset resembles that of a click. If the test is attempting to measure threshold at a single frequency, it is clearly undesirable to have signal energy at other frequencies.

This problem can be eliminated by turning the signal on slowly; this is done by switches in audiometers. The standard is very conservative in this area and requires a rise/fall time >30 ms. The audiometer manufacturer will specify the rise/fall time for the particular model of interest, but all models can be calibrated using the following technique.

Figure 5.2B shows the instrumentation setup for this measurement, which requires an audiometer and a storage oscilloscope. The rise/fall time is a temporal measurement and should not be dependent on amplitude. To help make the measurement easier and more accurate, I recommend that the measurement be made with a high-intensity signal (>90 HL) from the audiometer. The rise/fall time should not change with frequency either, but this can be checked relatively easily.

The output from the audiometer is routed to the oscilloscope, and the amplitude display is adjusted to place the waveform symmetrically in the vertical dimension around the center graticule line. The waveform display should be as large as possible vertically, while still keeping the maximum and minimum portions of the waveform on the screen. Some oscilloscope graticules have percentages visible; in this case the peak waveform amplitude should be adjusted to match the 100% lines on the graticule. After the waveform amplitude is adjusted, the tricky part begins.

The waveform must be displayed so that the change in waveform amplitude from 10% to 90% at onset or termination is visible. In the case of waveform termination, this is relatively easy. The oscilloscope is placed in storage and single-sweep modes, and with a little experimentation it is possible to catch the termination of the waveform. Remember that the single sweep must be reset after each sweep. (I have missed a waveform many times because of forgetting to reset the sweep.)

Catching the onset of the waveform is more difficult and requires adjusting the trigger level so that the waveform triggers appropriately. The oscilloscope should be in storage and single-sweep modes. One suggestion is to move the waveform horizontally so that it starts away from its normal starting point at the left boundary of the graticule. This will permit easier visualization of the waveform. This will not be as helpful for viewing the termination portion of the waveform. The calibration is made by determining the time it takes for the waveform to change from 10% to 90% of waveform amplitude, unless the specification says otherwise. Some manufacturers specify the rise/fall time on the basis of other amplitude ratios, and this should be checked prior to the calibration. The time base on the oscilloscope must be set to sufficient resolution to make an accurate measurement. For example, if the rise/fall time is supposed to be 30 ms, the time base should be set to 5 or 10 ms/division. Quiklab 7 will provide an opportunity to practice this measurement.

Warble-Tone Calibration

How to measure threshold in a sound field is a continuing issue in audiology. The difficulty comes from the resonance properties of the typical audiology test booth. Recall the discussion in the previous chapter about how square spaces with flat, reflecting surfaces can repeatedly reflect sound and create standing waves. There has been considerable discussion in the literature about what is the best stimulus in this situation. The two primary candidates are narrow-band noise and warble tones.

Since narrowband noise has been discussed before and the calibration of the intensity of narrowband noise is done with narrowband filters in the same manner as for pure tones, these two topics will not be discussed separately. The measurement of the frequency characteristics of a narrowband noise requires a spectrum analyzer, and that discussion will be reserved for a later chapter. It will be obvious how to do a complete calibration of a narrowband noise when that discussion has been completed. Warble tones, on the other hand, will not be discussed extensively later, and so will be covered here.

A warble tone is a frequency-modulated (FM) tone with a modulation width from 3 to 10% and a modulation rate from 2 to 8 Hz. An FM tone is a tone whose frequency (not intensity) is varied over a specified range at a specified rate. Figure 5.5 shows the time waveform for a sample FM tone. It can be seen that the period of the waveform changes over time, but the intensity does not change. This fluctuation in frequency reduces the standing wave problem because the frequency is never at the resonant frequency of the chamber long enough to generate stationary standing waves.

While the frequency variation is useful for avoiding resonance effects, it creates difficulties for calibration. As long as the modulation width is small, i.e., <10% of the test frequency, the intensity can be calibrated with an octave-band filter in the same manner as for a pure tone because (the intensity is constant and) the frequency of the tone will stay within the bandwidth of the measurement filter and thus, the intensity is constant. The difficult part of the calibration is measuring the modulation width and rate.

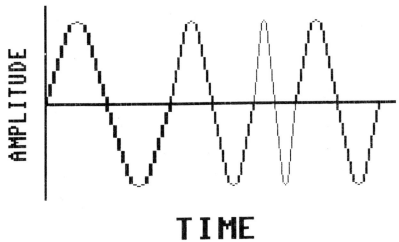

Figure 5.5.   Time waveform for a frequency modulated (FM) signal.

The best instrument for making these measurements is a modulation meter. Good meters will permit measurement of both amplitude-modulated (AM) and FM signals. However, such meters are expensive and are generally purchased only by firms either that do calibration as part of their business or that have so much instrumentation that all their calibration is done in-house. Radio engineers also use such instruments. Thus some alternative to a modulation meter would be helpful. Unfortunately, while the method to be described will work, it is cumbersome and does not offer much accuracy. If there is a real need to have an exact calibration of the modulation width and rate, have it done by a professional with appropriate instrumentation. The method described next will help determine if these parameters are significantly in error. Keep in mind that a third method, which should always be used first, is to listen. The ear is a sensitive instrument and is not to be ignored when troubleshooting.

The instrumentation setup for the alternate method of measuring modulation width and rate uses an oscilloscope and is the same as for rise/fall time (Fig. 5.2*B*). The oscilloscope must be a storage scope with a single-sweep capability. This is necessary because the technique requires extensive viewing of portions of the waveform.

The procedure for both modulation widths is to store the waveform using a single sweep with sufficient time resolution to measure the periods. The lowest possible warble tone center frequency should be used to aid in visualization. The longest and shortest periods displayed are measured. After this has been done for several sweeps, approximately 10 to 15, there will have been a reasonable sample of waveform periods to permit estimation of the modulation width.

The procedure for the modulation rate is to make the time resolution poor enough so that the period oscillation from longest to shortest is displayed. This will require some adjustment and visualization. The storage and single-sweep modes are employed for this measurement. When satisfied that the complete oscillation has been captured, you can then measure the duration of this oscillation.

The time resolutions that are necessary for each measurement can be estimated from the specifications for the warble tone. For example, if the center frequency of the warble tone is 250 Hz, the modulation width is 10% and the modulation rate is 5 Hz; the periods should vary between approximately 3.6 and 4.4 ms, with the interval between the shortest and longest period being 200 ms. Thus the time-resolution setting for the modulation-width measurements should be 1 or 2 ms/division, and for the modulation rate measurements the setting should be 20 to 50 ms. In general, a ratio of about 1 to 4 is needed for accuracy. Remember that many sweeps will be needed to get a reasonable estimate.

This measurement procedure should only be used for diagnostic purposes when something seriously wrong is suspected. It will not work well enough to detect small errors. For accurate calibration, a modulation meter must be used. Some of the newer instruments have calibration checks built in, and one of them may check for errors in one or both of the modulation indices. It should be noted that this calibration technique is employed rarely and only when there is a good reason to believe something has gone wrong. It is not part of the regular calibration procedure.

Warble tone calibrations, as noted before, will be made infrequently, unless the clinic is heavily involved in sound field testing, such as that required for fitting hearing aids. The calibrations of pure-tone signals will be made frequently.

The next section discusses another calibration technique that should be employed regularly since audiometric thresholds are commonly measured via bone conduction and bone vibrators are an integral part of most audiometers.

Bone-Conduction Measurements

Bone-conduction measurements are frequently used in the clinic as an adjunct to air-conduction measurements. The theoretical basis for their use is that vibratory stimulation provides a means of stimulating the inner ear directly, bypassing the middle ear. Thus any threshold loss due to pathologies that affect the middle ear can be differentiated from threshold loss caused by inner ear pathologies.

The extent to which bone-conduction measurements reflect middle ear disease is still a subject of research, but the basic principles of bone-conduction testing are well understood. A vibratory force applied to the mastoid area drives the skull, in particular the temporal bone that houses the cochlea. The resulting vibrations are transmitted to the cochlea and drive the fluid surrounding the basilar membrane. Due to the properties of the basilar membrane, this force is treated in much the same way as if the cochlea were stimulated through the acoustic modality. Hence, it is possible to do frequency-specific testing using a bone vibrator.

The introduction to this chapter pointed out that a common accessory for an audiometer is a bone vibrator. This bone vibrator is used to do bone-conduction testing. Just as with all other audiometer components, this vibrator must be calibrated.

Audiometer Calibration for Bone-Conduction Testing

The audiometer bone vibrator is an accelerometer in reverse; that is, instead of responding to the vibrations of a driving force, the vibrator is the driving force, much like the accelerometer calibrators discussed in the transducer chapter (chapter 4). It would seem that the straightforward way to calibrate the bone vibrator would be to attach an accelerometer to the vibrator and measure the output. Unfortunately, it is not that easy.

When bone-conduction measurements are made, the measurement situation is not as "neat and clean" as in a machinery vibration measurement situation for various reasons: First, the bone vibrator is attached to the patient's head with a flexible band. Second, for obvious reasons, nothing is used to make the vibrator adhere to the surface of the skin. Third, skin thicknesses vary. The first and third factors mean that the amount of force applied by the headband and the amount of attenuation due to skin thickness must be known. The second factor requires some way of specifying the adhesion of the bone vibrator. These factors collectively affect the amount of force applied to the bone and are referred to as "loading factors." It is clear that these factors cannot be easily measured. However, there is a device called an "artificial mastoid" that attempts to account for these factors.

The artificial mastoid is a specially designed accelerometer that attempts to simulate the mastoid area, including such factors as skin adhesion and thickness. The headband force is assumed to be a certain value, and the bone vibrator is mounted on a large pink pad that is composed of a specially formulated material simulating the skin area in the region of the mastoid. By accounting for these factors, in combination with measurements of bone-conduction thresholds, the artificial mastoid is intended to calibrate the bone vibrator to the force necessary for detection threshold in a young normal listener.

While the artificial mastoid is an excellent idea, in practice, the measurement is not as exact as the pure-tone calibration measurements and is very time consuming. In addition, the difficult and exacting production techniques required to produce an accurate simulation of the mastoid area make the artificial mastoid extremely expensive. As a result, most clinics do not calibrate their bone vibrators using instrumentation but rather use a biological calibration technique.

Biological Calibration of Audiometers

Biological calibration is useful not only for bone vibrators but for pure-tone calibration as well. However, the ease and accuracy of pure-tone calibration makes instrumental calibration of pure tones the recommended procedure. But the difficulty and expense of bone-vibration calibration with the artificial mastoid makes biological calibration of bone vibrators the recommended procedure.

Biological calibration, as the term implies, involves using a biological instrument to do the calibration. Because they are the most available biological instrument and because of their extensive sensory apparatus, humans can be very reliable and accurate calibration tools, given some training and practice. In this case, known auditory sensitivity is used to calibrate the bone vibrator.

The biological calibration procedure involves the selection of an individual with normal hearing, as verified by an independent audiogram. This person should also have no known or suspected middle ear pathology, including the common cold. The audiometer is set up just as it would be for regular bone-conduction testing. The bone vibrator is attached to the individual with known hearing, and the intensity at threshold as a function of frequency is noted. The resulting table represents the calibrated values for that bone vibrator. As in the case with earphones, each bone vibrator should be calibrated separately. If the bone vibrator is moved to a different audiometer, the calibration should be repeated.

The calibration should first be done when the bone vibrator is new. If there are large deviations from 0 HTL, then the vibrator should be replaced. The calibration should then be repeated on a daily basis in a clinic that has testing on a daily basis. Otherwise, the calibration should be done as frequently as there is testing or any time that there is suspected trouble. The requirement for daily testing is necessary because bone vibrators are notorious for suddenly malfunctioning. Thus spare bone vibrators should be on hand in a busy clinic.

The basic components of an audiometer have now been described, along with the calibration procedures for these components. As mentioned at the beginning of this chapter, an audiometer is one of the two most frequently used instruments in an audiology clinic. The other one, the impedance bridge, is covered next.

Impedance Bridge

Measurement of the impedance of the middle ear is a very useful clinical tool, and several generations of impedance measuring instruments have arisen to meet the need. Just as with an audiometer, the impedance bridge is a complex instrument that can be very intimidating at first, but is organized functionally and can be used with relative ease once the functions have been understood. To aid in this understanding, some of the principles of impedance measurement will be discussed and then the components of an impedance bridge will be described and related to the theoretical discussion. Calibration of an impedance bridge will then be briefly described. (This topic is treated in great detail in many texts, and the interested reader is referred to these texts.)

Acoustic Impedance Measurement

The function of an impedance bridge is to measure acoustic impedance. The measurement of electrical impedance was described in the chapter on the fundamentals of electronics (chapter 1). The principles of acoustic impedance are directly related to the principles of electrical impedance, and the reader should review the section on acoustic impedance if the details have gotten a little fuzzy.

It should be noted at the outset that the quantity measured by current electroacoustic impedance bridges is not impedance, but rather the absolute magnitude of the impedance. In fact, many bridges are labeled as *admittance bridges.* However, since admittance is just the reciprocal of impedance, the following discussion applies to both types of bridges. There are a variety of reasons for this: the magnitude is clinically useful, easier to measure, and primarily determined by only one component of impedance for the normal middle ear. Thus the term "impedance" is inappropriate. But the term has become so ingrained in the nomenclature of the speech and hearing professional that it is useless to call the measurement anything else, especially something as awkward as the "absolute vector magnitude of impedance," which is more correct terminology. In the interest of simplicity, sanity, and social strictures, the term *acoustic impedance* will be applied to mean the measurement that is made by an electroacoustic impedance bridge.

The basic principles of measuring acoustic impedance for the middle ear arise from mechanical descriptions of the action of the middle ear. Therefore, understanding the acoustic impedance being measured by an impedance bridge requires first understanding the concept of mechanical impedance because the middle ear has as its primary function the transfer of acoustic energy from the environment to the inner ear. To do this, the middle ear serves as a mechanical impedance matcher, matching the low impedance of the air with the high impedance of the fluids in the inner ear in order to get as efficient an energy transfer as possible.

Recall that impedance is the resistance to the transmission of force by a system, and that maximal energy transfer occurs when the source and the receiver have the same impedance. It is apparent that air has very little resistance to force, and hence has a low impedance. The fluids in the ear have approximately the same consistency as sea water and will clearly have a fairly high resistance to force. (Did you ever try to quickly move a mass of water about the same size as yourself?) It is also clear that air will need to have considerable force in order to move water.

The middle ear supplies the necessary force by multiplying the pressure (force per unit area) of the air. This is done by focusing the force over the area of the tympanic membrane onto the much smaller area of the oval window (Fig. 5.6) and through lever action by the ossicular chain. At the same time, the middle ear is providing an impedance match between the air and the inner ear fluids. The match is not perfect, but overcomes a surprisingly large portion of the difference between the two media.

The problem with this simple description is that the effects of frequency are not included. Recall from chapter 1 that impedance has three components, two of which are frequency dependent. In addition, the sound pressure that the ear is transducing has a frequency range from approximately 20–20,000 Hz. Not surprisingly, the impedance of the ear is

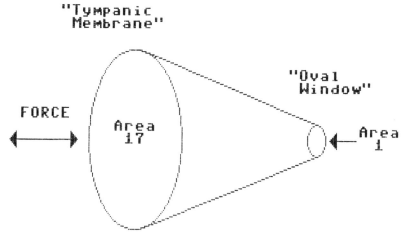

Figure 5.6.   Middle ear acts as mechanical impedance matcher by focusing the force. This is accomplished through the area differential between the tympanic membrane and oval window.

frequency dependent. Why are impedance measurements not made at several frequencies? To understand the answer, the components of electrical impedance described in the first chapter must be related to mechanical impedance components in the ear.

Mechanical Impedance

The three components of impedance are added in a vector sum to get the magnitude and phase of impedance. The three components, in electrical terms, are inductive reactance, capacitive reactance, and resistance. The reactance components are frequency dependent. The middle ear, however, is mechanical rather than electrical. The aforementioned electrical components of impedance can be related to mechanical components of impedance by matching the effects of mechanical components on force transmitted through the system to the effects of the electrical components on electromotive force transmitted through a circuit.

Recall that inductive reactance is directly proportional to frequency and capacitive reactance is inversely proportional to frequency. Resistance is friction and is not frequency dependent. Examination of the middle ear, or indeed any mechanical system, reveals that there are three components to impedance for this system also: mass, stiffness, and friction. Mass is a familiar concept, and it is obvious that the middle ear has mass, although the mass is very small. The stiffness component comes from the ligaments and muscles of the middle ear. The friction comes from the structures rubbing against each other and is also very small.

What is the relation of mass, stiffness, and friction to frequency? The last component is the most obvious. Since resistance and friction are the same thing, friction is not frequency dependent. So mass and stiffness, or more properly mass reactance and stiffness reactance, are frequency dependent. The next brief discussion on the properties of mass and stiffness will provide the correspondence to inductance and capacitance.

A mass at rest, when no force is applied, just sits there like a box resting on a shelf. If sufficient force is applied, like a swift push, the mass will move. However, there is an opposition to motion due to the mass. This property is referred to as "inertia." A better understanding of the relation between the movement of a mass and frequency of the applied force can be gained if we think of trying to shake a box. If the box is light, we can shake it rapidly. If the box is heavy, it can be shaken, but more slowly. Thus the larger the mass, the slower the rate of motion. In other words, the opposition of mass to the frequency of the applied force increases as mass increases or, mass reactance is directly proportional to frequency.

Since mass reactance is the component of impedance that is directly proportional to frequency, by default, stiffness reactance must be indirectly proportional to frequency. The basis for this will be described to aid in understanding middle ear impedance. Stiffness is a measure of elasticity, or how easily something is stretched. A simple example might be two metal rulers: one floppy and one very rigid. Just as with mass, if there is no force applied, the rulers will not move. If the ruler is held firmly in one hand and the other end bent and released, the ruler will oscillate back and forth. This principle is frequently applied by children in classroom antics. If the floppy ruler is bent and released, the oscillation will not be very fast, whereas the rigid ruler will oscillate rapidly. If this experiment is tried, it will also be noted that more force is needed to bend the rigid ruler the same distance as the floppy ruler. Both of these properties are due to the greater stiffness of the rigid ruler. What if you wanted the rulers to move slowly? To make the rigid ruler oscillate slowly would actually require holding onto the ruler and restraining its motion. In summary, as mass is increased, an object tends to move more slowly; as stiffness is increased, an object tends to move more rapidly. Thus the relation between frequency and stiffness reactance (Rs) is the opposite of the relation between frequency and mass reactance (Rm). Hence stiffness reactance is inversely proportional to frequency. By corollary with electrical impedance, the mechanical impedance (Zm) would be calculated by this equation.

$$Zm = ((Rm^2 + Rs^2) + R^2)^{1/2}$$

It turns out, for reasons not discussed here, that the stiffness reactance component is by far the largest component in the impedance of the middle ear. The effect of this on the vector representation of the impedance of the middle ear is shown in Figure 5.7. Since mass reactance is small at low

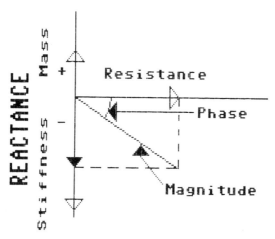

Figure 5.7. Vector plot illustrating larger stiffness component of middle ear impedance.

frequencies and stiffness reactance will be large at low frequencies, and since mass reactance is generally less important than stiffness reactance in middle ear impedance measurements, it makes sense to make the measurements at a low frequency. The frequency that is most frequently used is 220 Hz.

Acoustic Impedance

Recall that the impedance bridge measures acoustic impedance. This means that impedance is expressed in terms of equivalent volumes of air. What does that mean? To understand acoustic impedance, especially in relation to the concept of stiffness, the relation between volumes of air and stiffness must be understood. This is explained through the next example.

Look at the two cylinders in Figure 5.8, which have equal diameters but different volumes. If a piston was inserted into each of these cylinders and used to compress the air inside, which cylinder would provide the greatest opposition to the piston, i.e., which would be "stiffest?" If you guessed the smallest cylinder, you are right. This can be understood intuitively in terms of the air in the smallest cylinder running out of space between particles faster than the large cylinder. Given that the mass and friction differences between the cylinders are negligible (air does not have much mass, and at rest has little friction), which cylinder has the greater impedance? If you guessed the smaller cylinder, you were right again. The greater stiffness of the smaller cylinder gives it the larger impedance because there is little difference between the two cylinders for the other two components of impedance. In fact, the acoustic impedance is inversely proportional to the

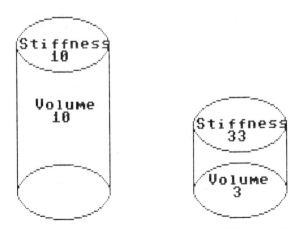

Figure 5.8. Two cylinders of equal diameter but different volumes showing relation between volume of air and stiffness reactance.

volume of air. Thus, since stiffness is the primary component of the impedance of a volume of air, the stiffness of the ear measured with a bridge can be expressed in terms of a volume of air whose mechanical properties are equal to the ear being measured.

If air is kept at a static pressure of 760 mm Hg (the static pressure of air at sea level), 1 cc of air has about 1,100 acoustic ohms of impedance to a 220 Hz signal. It should be noted that an "equivalent volume of air" is subject to changes in atmospheric pressure and temperature. That is, the "normal" impedance of an ear measured at high altitudes, such as at Denver, would appear lower than the impedance measured at Los Angeles because of the lower static pressure (lower stiffness) of air in Denver. Also keep in mind that impedance is frequency dependent, so the static impedance for other stimulus frequencies will be different.

Electroacoustic Impedance Bridges

Previous sections in this chapter have dealt with the theory behind the measurement of acoustic impedance. The instrument used to make the measurement of middle ear impedance is the electroacoustic impedance bridge. This instrument usually consists of six major components: an audio oscillator; a pressure pump; an ear insert containing two microphones, one for producing sound and one for measurement; a voltmeter; a video display; and a recorder. Oscillators and voltmeters have already been discussed along with microphones. Recorders will be discussed in the next chapter, so the present discussion will center around the ear insert, pressure pump, and the video display, which is usually a meter.

The ear insert of the bridge, commonly referred to as the "probe," consists of an acoustic source, a measuring microphone, and an open tube. The ear insert is connected to the bridge by two wires and a plastic tubing that connects the pressure pump to the open tube. The two wires are connected to two microphones in the probe. One microphone serves as a sound source and is connected to a signal generator in the bridge. The other microphone is connected to a voltmeter in the bridge similar to the manner in which a sound level meter is connected. The tip of the insert itself is surrounded by a removable plastic cuff that seals the insert into the auditory meatus.

Several features of the probe are important for the accurate measurement of acoustic impedance. The most important feature of the probe is that it represents a very high impedance relative to the ear. This is necessary for accurate measurement by preventing interactions between the measurement system, in this case the impedance bridge, and the system being measured, in this case the middle ear.

The impedance of the probe is controlled by the volume and cross-sectional area of the probe. As pointed out earlier, the smaller the volume of air, the larger the impedance. It is also the case that the smaller the cross-sectional area, the larger the impedance. A pipe is a good analogy. Imaging pouring a gallon of water into the sink at home, and then pouring the same gallon of water through a sewer pipe. Which would drain faster? The obvious answer is the sewer pipe. The same amount of fluid going through a pipe will encounter less resistance with a larger-diameter pipe than a smaller-diameter pipe.

The ideal middle-ear impedance probe would have three continuous tubes of equal and very small diameter, running from the tip of the probe to the measurement device. The probe for the Madsen Z0-70 bridge is an example of this principle. There are probes made with a cavity between the tubes and the measurement device, i.e., in the probe itself. This results in a complex impedance that will be lower than desired and may cause some nonlinearities in the measurement of impedance, particularly at the extreme ends of the range.

In addition to the characteristics of the probe playing a role in the measurement of impedance, there are two other factors that can affect the measurement: instrument noise and the time constants of the impedance bridge. The way in which they affect the measurement are interrelated. It was observed by early makers of impedance instrumentation that the equipment generated a lot of noise in the measurement. To reduce this problem, a bandpass filter centered on the measurement frequency of 220 Hz was added. While this reduced the noise, it introduced another problem that was of relatively little consequence until recently.

A side effect of adding the filter to the measurement system was that the system now had a time constant on the order of 100 ms. What does this mean? It means that the measurement of rapid temporal changes in the behavior of the middle ear cannot be done by such a system if the changes take place in less than 100 ms. For good accuracy the time window of the measuring instrument has to be considerably shorter than the duration of the dynamic change being measured.

Recently several investigators of middle ear function have noted that the temporal behavior of the middle ear is different for hearing-impaired listeners. If these investigations result in clinical tests, a short, time-constant middle ear measuring instrument will be required. Because of this possibility, a brief discussion of such an instrument follows.

This measuring instrument would still be an electroacoustic impedance bridge, but it would be altered from the standard instrument. The first change would be removal of the filter. The second change would be to average the responses. Response averaging will be discussed later in this book when electrophysiological measurements are described. The same technique can be applied to acoustic impedance measurements. With the advent of computerized measurement instrumentation, this capability can be added quite easily. The removal of the filter reduces the time constant to <5 ms. The addition of averaging permits a more accurate appraisal of the shape of the waveform. This is especially important for very brief signals, which may result in response waveforms significantly different from those for long duration signals.

It should be noted that for most clinical purposes the effects of filtering are not important. The primary effects of the filtering are on the time constant of the system and phase effects on the response waveform. Unless accurate temporal or phase measurement of the middle-ear response is desired, there is no need to worry about filtering. As stated before, it is only discussed here in order to provide for potential future acoustic-impedance measurement requirements.

The pressure pump is just that, a pump for providing control of air pressure in the space between the probe tip and the tympanic membrane. The pump is in the bridge and is connected to the probe through a long tube. The most common cause of difficulty with the pressure system is leaking hoses, especially around joints. The usual symptom is a slow change in meter reading when the manometer is not being adjusted. Unfortunately, this is the same symptom as for an inadequate seal for the probe. If the symptom remains after reinserting the probe, the quickest and easiest way to check is by terminating the probe with the 2-cc coupler used for calibration. If the leak is still there, it is in the instrumentation. If not, the probe was improperly inserted and should be reinserted.

It is surprising how difficult it can be to locate and then fix a leaking hose. One method is to terminate the probe in the standard 2-cc coupler that is used for calibration and to listen for leaks. Another is to take a *very* small amount of water, drip it on the hoses, and look for air bubbles. When the leak is found, any method used to fix it is legal. Glue and tape are the most popular methods. Occasionally it is necessary to replace the entire tube, and it is not a bad practice to do this on a regular basis, depending on usage.

The output of the bridge is via a meter similar to that found on voltmeters and audiometers or via a recorder attached to the bridge. Prior to using the bridge, you should verify the accuracy of the meter. How this is done will be discussed in the calibration section. The meter on an impedance bridge is straightforward and easy to use and is read in the same manner and with the same precautions as other meters.

It should be noted there are also errors associated with meter readout, and that needle meters may not be fast enough; i.e., needle meters have a time constant that is sometimes as long as 200 ms. The manual should be consulted for the exact value. A term sometimes used for the meter characteristics is "meter ballistics." As would be expected, measurements of rapidly changing events such as the temporal waveform measurements described earlier should not be done with the meter, but with a storage oscilloscope. An *x-y* plotter can be used to provide a permanent record. The oscilloscope will be fast enough to store the waveform information, which can then be transferred to the plotter.

All of these pieces together make up the clinical impedance bridge. As with any other instrument, proper care will ensure long life and enhanced reliability. Part of that care is calibration, which is covered next.

Calibration of Acoustic Impedance Bridges

Acoustic impedance and oto-admittance instrumentation should be calibrated instrumentally because biological calibration is unreliable. The parameters that need to be checked are air pressure, sound intensity and frequency for the probe tone, and static volume measurements. If an oscilloscope and/or *x-y* plotter is used, its accuracy should be checked as well.

The air pressure can be measured in two ways. The first and easiest is with a manometer, which is a pressure meter. An example of a manometer is the air pressure gauge that is used to check the air pressure in auto tires. The other method for checking air pressure is to directly connect a U-tube that reads in millimeters of water. The output can then be read directly in millimeters of water pressure. It is recommended that if the pressure differs from the dial reading by more than 5 mm of water pressure or ±5% of the reading, the device should be adjusted. Variations greater than this may affect the absolute acoustic impedance measurements and, to some extent, the tympanometric results as well.

The intensity of the probe tone can be measured by first consulting the specifications section of the manual for the intensity of the probe tone in a 2-cc cavity. The 2-cc cavity is referred to as a "2-cc coupler" (as compared with the 6-cc coupler used for earphone measurements). The procedure is very similar to earphone intensity calibration measurements, which were described in chapter 4.

The probe is inserted into the 2-cc coupler while one makes sure that there is a good seal. The microphone comprising the other end of the 2-cc cavity is then attached to a sound level meter, and the output sound intensity is measured for the probe tone. If there is a balance or compliance control, this will need to be adjusted to the appropriate volume before making the measurement because the bridge will adjust the sound intensity by volume. Some systems have an automatic volume control; for these systems no adjustment will be necessary. If the intensity of the probe tone is in error by more than 3 dB, the intensity should be adjusted.

The frequency of the probe tone can be checked at the same time as the intensity calibration is performed. Attach a frequency counter to the output of the sound level meter or read it directly at the input to the probe. The frequency should be within 5% of the specified probe tone frequency. As with earphone measurements, it is unlikely that the speaker in the probe, which is actually a microphone driven to produce sound rather than measure it, will modify the frequency of the signal. Hence, it is usually easier to make the measurement at the input to the probe rather than from the sound level meter.

Some bridges specify volume measurements, but it is more common to find the output specified in terms of acoustic ohms. In either case, it is a good idea to determine if the bridge is accurately measuring static volumes and hence static impedance. The volume calibration can be done with a variable cavity, of which the best and most readily available is a hypodermic syringe. There are calibrated syringes available that provide cavities from 0.1 to 3 cc. The probe is inserted into the syringe, and one makes sure that there is a good seal. The probe tip should not enter into the cavity; i.e., the tip should be flush with the entrance into the cavity. The syringe should be set to a specified volume, and the volume or impedance should be read from the bridge. Both a singular static impedance and the linearity of the bridge can be calibrated by making this measurement for several cavity sizes over the measurement range of the impedance bridge.

Recall the earlier discussion of the relation between volume and acoustic impedance. Be sure to know the barometric pressure. If the atmospheric pressure is more than 5% different from sea level, you should take the atmospheric pressure into account.

An *x-y* plotter is frequently used for tympanometric measurements. The plotter can be calibrated in much the same manner as the volume measurements for the bridge. Two factors should be in agreement. The dial and the *x-y* plotter should give the same values, and both values should agree with the calibrated volumes. This can be done by using several fixed pressure points and reading the values off the dial and the *x-y* plotter at the same time. The same 5% tolerance should apply. With regard to the ability of the plotter to follow the change in impedance as the pressure is changed by the impedance bridge, most current plotters can easily move fast enough to follow the changes in impedance with pressure that are induced by an impedance bridge.

A final concern is the reflex stimulator, if there is a reflex measurement system built into the bridge. For contralateral measurement systems, the earphone can be calibrated in exactly the same manner as the earphone calibration procedure described in chapter 4. For an ipsilateral system, the measurements can be done in exactly the same way except that a 2-cc coupler must be used instead of the 6 cc-coupler used for the earphone calibration because the effective speaker location is at the probe tip, which faces a much smaller volume than the earphone. The accuracy for intensity, frequency, and rise/fall time should be within ANSI specifications in both cases.

Frequency of calibration for impedance bridges is the same as for other instrumentation. The more heavily the equipment is used, the more frequent the calibration. In no case should the calibration interval be longer than 1 year. It should be noted that many manuals have extensive calibration sections. Both the required equipment (you may have to substitute equivalents) and the procedure will be described. In addition, the procedure for adjusting the parameters of the device will be described.

Chapter Summary

This chapter has described audiometers and impedance bridges. Rather than serve as a substitute for the considerable literature that has been published previously on this issue, the intent of the chapter was to focus upon the basic concepts for measurements made by audiological instrumentation and the fundamental principles of calibrating this equipment.

Audiometers are designed to measure hearing acoustically and to provide the additional capability of limited bone vibration measurements. The calibrations thus involve the acoustic parameters of a signal with some additional measurements for the bone vibration capability. It was pointed out that the acoustic measurements are best made with test instruments, whereas the bone vibrator is best calibrated biologically. Both types of calibration techniques were described.

Impedance bridges are designed to measure the response of the middle ear for both static and dynamic (reflex) conditions. The calibrations thus involve pressure and acoustic parameters, which are best measured with test instruments. The calibration techniques for both pressure and acoustic parameters were described along with a brief discussion of calibrating the most common ancillary piece of equipment, which is an x-y plotter.

Audiometers and impedance bridges are examples of instrumentation that frequently have reasonable documentation, at least from major manufacturers. It is highly advisable not to follow the general rule, "when all else fails, read the manual," which grew out of experiences with poor documentation. The information in the manuals will serve to supplement the materials presented in this chapter, along with the experience gained in the Quiklabs. It was also noted that audiometers are changing rapidly due to the incorporation of computer technology into the instruments. While the basic functions will remain the same as described in this chapter, many additional capabilities will be described in the manufacturers' manuals.

Audiometer Calibration

Introduction

*T*he purpose of this lab is to gain experience calibrating an audiometer. A sound level meter will also be used in this lab. Finally, the lab will provide further experience using test instrumentation introduced in previous labs. The particular audiometer described in this lab is the Grason-Stadler 1701, but the basic principles and procedures used in this lab to calibrate this audiometer for intensity, frequency, and rise/fall time can be applied to any audiometer.

Method

Apparatus

The test instruments for this lab are an oscilloscope, a frequency counter, and a sound level meter (SLM) with the appropriate accessories. The audiometer being calibrated is a Grason-Stadler 1701 clinical audiometer. Information about the use of oscilloscopes and frequency counters has been given in Quiklab 5. Information on the use of an SLM was given in chapter 3. It is assumed that the students for this lab have some experience using an audiometer. If you lack this experience or feel uncomfortable about your level of familiarity, make an appointment with your lab instructor to arrange for some help.

Procedure

Set up the SLM for sound measurement with earphones, using the method given above. Be sure the SLM has been calibrated and that the batteries are good. There will be five phases of calibration that you will follow to check the frequency, intensity, noise floor, linearity, and rise/fall times of the audiometer:

1. To check the frequency, attach the frequency counter to the right ear channel in the test suite using the phone plug output to the headphones. An adapting cable may be required for connection to the frequency counter. Set the audiometer to 90 dB HTL. Starting at 125 Hz,

measure the frequency of the audiometer signal at every audiometric frequency from 125 to 8,000 Hz.

2. To check the intensity, remove the cable from the jack and plug in the earphone. Set the audiometer to 125 Hz, 70 dB HTL. The earphone should be connected to the SLM as shown in Fig. 5.3. Measure the sound intensity at all audiometric frequencies from 125 to 8,000 Hz using the sound level meter. The SLM should be set to "linear". If it is not possible to obtain stable readings with a linear setting, the octave-band filter set should be used. This is done by turning on the octave-band filter accessory (for some sound level meters) and/or setting the dial to the appropriate octave-band center frequency. For test frequencies between the available settings use the octave band just above the signal frequency. Do these measurements for each channel of the audiometer. Be sure that both channels are measured at 70 dB HTL. If the filter set is separate from the sound level meter and is powered by a battery, be sure to turn off the filter set when you are finished.

3. To check the noise floor, measure the intensity for each octave band in the quiet, i.e., with the signal off. Make this measurement using the octave-band filter set. Make sure the earphone is placed properly in the coupler.

4. To check the linearity, set the channel 1 frequency on the audiometer to 500 Hz. Starting at 100 dB HTL, measure the output intensity in 5 dB decrements. Repeat the measurement for channel 2 if this is controlled by a separate attenuator. If in doubt, check both attenuators.

5. Although the rise/fall time measurement is seldom performed, we will do it in this lab. The intent here is to gain experience with this particular measurement. An external filter input or some other way of directly connecting external instrumentation to the sound level meter is required. For a B&K (Bruel & Kjaer) SLM, there is an external filter input setting on the SLM and the silver bar is removed. It will be assumed for the rest of the lab that an external instrumentation connection is available. The oscilloscope is connected to the SLM using the adapter cable included with the SLM. For the B&K SLM, connect the cable to the filter input jack (this is the output from the SLM to an external device). The audiometer is set to 1,000 Hz, 90 dB HTL. Use the single-sweep mode of the oscilloscope, with the storage mode on to capture the beginning and end of the waveform. There are two ways to set up the output of the audiometer for capturing the waveform. You may turn the audiometer to pulsed output and try to time the sweep, or you may manually activate the output with the switch and try to synchronize the triggering of the sweep with the activation of the switch. If you are having difficulty remembering how to do this, reread the

section in the chapter describing rise/fall time measurements. Measure the rise time and then the fall time. Be sure to do this for both switches if the audiometer has two separate channels. Repeat this measure for an 8,000-Hz signal, also at 90 dB HTL.

Results

Three worksheets are required for this laboratory. The first worksheet should have four columns and is for the frequency calibration. The signal frequencies to be tested should be in the first column. The measured frequency corresponding to each test frequency should be in the second column, and the third column should be the absolute difference between measured and test frequency. The absolute difference is the difference between the two frequencies; you can ignore whether the difference is plus or minus. The fourth column should be the percent error (column 3 divided by the test frequency times 100).

The second worksheet, which should be set up with four columns similar to the frequency calibration worksheet, is for the intensity calibration. The first column is the test frequency. The second column is the desired intensity, which is taken from the ANSI standard. The third column is the measured intensity. The fourth column is the difference between the desired intensity and the measured intensity. For the intensity calibration the sign of the difference is retained.

The third worksheet, which has three columns, is for the linearity calibration. The first column is the attenuator setting. The second column is the corresponding measured intensity. The third column is the intensity difference for each successive step, i.e., the difference between the signal intensity at the attenuator setting above the test setting and the intensity at the attenuator setting for the test setting. The absolute difference is used.

Fill these worksheets with the appropriate data. Add whatever tables you think are necessary to adequately present the data, e.g., the rise/fall times. Compute the error from ANSI specifications.

Discussion

Is the audiometer in calibration? If not, how bad is it? Make up a correction factor sheet in order to have the audiometer calibrated to ANSI specifications.

Impedance Bridge Calibration

Introduction

*T*he purpose of this lab is to give experience in the calibration of an impedance bridge. The static impedance and the linearity of the bridge will be calibrated. In addition, the lab will be concerned with measurement of the probe tone's intensity. These are measured because all other impedance measurements are based on these aspects of the bridge's performance. It is recommended that this lab be done after the audiometer calibration lab because this lab assumes familiarity with the measurements made in that lab.

Method

Apparatus

These instruments are required for this lab:

1. Impedance bridge with probe and earphone in headset (if contralateral, if ipsilateral earphone is not required);
2. Sound level meter;
3. A 2-cc coupler;
4. Calibrated syringe with a range of 0.1 to 3 cc in 0.1-cc steps;
5. Barometer;
6. Any cables and/or adapters required to interconnect all this equipment.

Procedure

Probe-Tone Intensity Measurement. The first part of the lab is to measure the intensity of the probe tone when the bridge is balanced. First, connect the 2-cc coupler to the probe by inserting the probe into the coupler. As has been mentioned before, excessive force is not required, but insert firmly. After attaching the coupler to the probe, ensure that there is a tight seal. When satisfied that there are no leaks, attach the sound level meter to the coupler. If the bridge must be balanced manually, do so. Using the sound level meter in the same manner as for the audiometer calibration measurements, measure the

155

intensity of the probe tone. If the manual gives appropriate instructions, this would be a good time to also calibrate the *x-y* plotter, but that is optional for this lab.

Impedance Magnitude and Linearity Measurement.   The second part of the lab is to measure the static acoustic impedance for given volumes of air in a calibrated syringe. The impedance reading on the bridge can then be compared with the known impedance for the calibrated volume of air. Probe-tone intensity must be verified as correct by using the techniques in part 1 of this lab. After this is done, insert the probe into the calibrated syringe. There are several techniques available for setting up the syringe to accept the probe and give a good seal, but the most reliable is to replace the normal needle insert with a rubber grommet. An alternative technique is to use a standard impedance probe cuff that gives an adequate seal. Problems with the cuff are obtaining an adequate seal, differences in insertion depth of the cuff and hence the volume of the syringe between calibrations, and the relation between the probe tip and the opening in the cuff. The exact calibration of the syringe may be thrown off considerably between calibrations because the factors just described make it difficult for the probe to always be the exact same distance into the syringe each time. The rubber grommet solves this problem by being a permanent attachment to the syringe, which permits the same measurement situation each time. It should be mentioned that the syringe will need to be recalibrated after it has been modified to work with the probe. (See the next section for instructions on how to recalibrate the syringe.)

The probe should be inserted into the syringe so that the tip of the probe is level with the inside of the rubber grommet. The seal should then be checked. If the seal is satisfactory, adjust the syringe to a volume of 2 cc and balance the bridge. Repeat this measurement for 0.1, 0.5, 1.0, 1.5, 2.5, and 3.0 cc. Repeat the measurement for two of these volumes. The 2-cc measurement will yield an accuracy calibration, the series of volume measurements will yield the linearity data, and the repeated measurements will yield a reliability measure. Keep in mind the effects of static air pressure on the apparent volume of air. Use the barometer to determine the static air pressure.

These measurements can also be done to calibrate the intensity of the probe tone, but are more complicated and are not described here.

Calibration of the Syringe

The use of a calibrated syringe permits calibration of the syringe with a single volume because the calibration of the change in volume with the movement of the plunger has already been done by the manufacturer. Single-volume calibration is done by putting a given volume of alcohol in an unmodified calibrated syringe that has a needle. Alcohol is used to reduce surface tension effects, which will adversely affect the readings if water is used. The fluid should then be placed in the modified syringe with the plunger in the modified syringe at maximum volume. The plunger of the unmodified syringe should then be slowly turned until the fluid is level with the inside surface of the rubber grommet. The reading should be noted and if there is a constant error, this difference should be added to all volume values. The syringe should then be emptied and cleaned carefully to prevent the alcohol from drying out the rubber grommet. The syringe will remain calibrated until the grommet cracks or wears to the point where it leaks, at which time the grommet can be replaced and the calibration process repeated.

Results

1. Put the expected probe intensity (taken from the manual), the measured intensity, and the difference in absolute and percentage terms into a table. Do the same for the x-y plotter calibration, if this calibration was done.

2. Check the barometer; using the information in the chapter, determine the expected impedance value for the test volumes. Place these values in a table along with the measured values and the difference between predicted and measured values. In addition, plot the measured values with volumes on the abscissa and the impedance values on the ordinate. Finally, note in the table the values and differences between measurements for the repeated measures.

Discussion

Describe the accuracy of the bridge in terms of the intensity of the probe tone and the relation between predicted and measured impedance. Also discuss the plot in terms of implications with regard to linearity of the bridge and any measurements of middle ear function.

6

Audio and Video Tape Recorders

Tape recorders are among the most common instruments employed clinically. Audiologists use audio recorders for presenting speech stimuli for testing, and speech pathologists use audio recorders for recording and analyzing speech stimuli, as well as video recorders for examination of speech and associated behaviors. In addition, researchers in speech and hearing use both video and audio recorders in their experiments. The intent of this chapter is to introduce the basic principles of operation for audio and video recorders. As in previous chapters, the focus is on using, not designing, instrumentation.

Audio and video recorders are currently regarded as a consumer "high-tech" area, and there is considerable discussion of digital and laser technologies being applied to recorders. Therefore, there will be an introduction in this chapter to these technologies because of their potential prevalence in the field. An attempt will be made to provide some perspective for the user of this type of instrumentation in the context of current instrumentation and to indicate when such advanced technology might be useful and when it might be unnecessary.

The area of audio recording will be discussed first for several reasons: (1) this is an area that is used in both speech and hearing and was applied to these fields before video recording; (2) many of the basic principles of recording media are common to both audio and video recording; and (3) most people are more familiar with audio recording and hence will be better able to make generalizations from audio to video than vice versa. After audio recording principles have been discussed, calibration of audio speech tapes and some of the issues with regard to definitions of intensity will be described. The final section in the chapter will describe some basic principles of video recorders, followed by a discussion of their use, including some discussion of calibrating tapes.

Audio Recorders

Audio recorders are intended to record and reproduce audio signals, i.e., signals in the frequency range 20 to 20,000 Hz. Audio recording has been done for a very long time and in many ways. Probably the first major breakthrough in recording audio information for storage and retrieval was Thomas A. Edison's invention of the phonograph and phonograph record. Although the original record was actually a wax cylinder with grooves representing the sound, and the dynamic range was nowhere near 20 Hz to 20 kHz, the basic principles were the same as for today's common stereo phonograph systems.

Phonograph records are actually a good media for storing and reproducing sound. They are especially appropriate when the sound to be reproduced is the same every time and no recording capabilities are required. However, there are some clear disadvantages to the use of a phonograph in a clinical setting. These include the lack of fine control for stopping and starting tests; the inability to reproduce the recording when it wears out, which really translates to the lack of an easy way to make a backup copy; and the difficulty of tailoring recordings so that different subsets of the recordings can be easily generated at different times. While the last factor is not desirable from the standpoint of standardizing test materials, it is done by clinics and so is included as a disadvantage. An instrument that overcomes these disadvantages is the audio tape recorder.

The more proper term for most common audio tape recorders is "recorder/reproducer," although reproduce-only machines are available. The latter are occasionally confusing to the beginning user because such devices are frequently referred to as "tape recorders" although they do not record. The two most common types of tape recorders are reel-to-reel and cassette. The commonalities between the two types outweigh the differences, and there are advantages and disadvantages to each. Since the field is going more and more toward cassette recorders, the discussion of use will concentrate on cassette recorders. This will hardly be a problem for reel-to-reel users, however, because the two types of recorders have so much in common.

Some of the principles of recording on tape will be discussed, before discussing how to use an audio tape recorder. There are two primary methods of recording, both of which will be described: direct and frequency modulation (FM) recordings. How the sound gets on the tape will be briefly described, and then how to take care of tapes and tape recorders as well as how to use them will be discussed. The discussion will begin with a description of magnetic tape and some of its properties.

Magnetic Tape

The medium used to store information for both audio and video recording is magnetic tape. The tape is typically composed of two parts: a backing that provides support and strength to the tape and a recording surface that is made up of materials that hold a magnetic charge.

The backing, or base layer of the tape, is generally composed of a plastic (PVC, or polyvinylchloride) that has been especially designed for good tensile strength. The high tensile strength helps reduce stretching of the tape when it is spun back and forth, which is important for the accurate reproduction of sound. The base materials are also designed to reduce: (*a*) "cupping" which is a tendency of the tape to bend across its width with added tension that causes poor head contact; (*b*) a bias or stretching of the tape more along one side than the other, which can cause poor spooling and potential jamming, as well as eventual damage to the edges of tape; and (*c*) a curl or uneven stretching of the tape from side to side of the tape, which results in pitch distortions because the same relative positions are not maintained across the entire width of the tape.

There are several different types of recording materials used for the recording surface on the tapes, as well as different lengths and widths. The length of the tape can also affect the thickness of the tape. The different widths range from 0.15 inch (3.81 mm) to 2 inches (5.08 cm) and are used for different machines. Wide tape is typically used in commercial machines, ¼-inch tape is standard for most reel-to-reel machines, and 0.15-inch tape is used for cassette recorders.

Tapes have both shiny and matte recording surfaces. The matte surfaces are better for spooling, but are not as smooth and can promote wear on the machine. Tapes that are expected to be subjected to a lot of back-and-forth movement have special lubricants on the recording surface to preserve the media and the machine. However, the most important aspect of tape surfaces from the point of view of speech and hearing is the fidelity of recording, which is related to the oxide used as a magnetic substrate for recording.

All recording surfaces are applied in the same general manner; it is the materials that change. The general technique is to essentially pulverize the material into small particles that can be suspended in an adhesive compound. The adhesive compound with the suspended material is then applied in a thin coat, ranging from 0.05 mm to 0.009 mm in thickness, to the base material. The two materials combined form the magnetic tape. As mentioned before, the thickness of the recording substrate depends on the length of the tape. The longer the tape the thinner the recording substrate.

Ferric oxide is the most common recording surface. It has been around a long time and is very inexpensive. However, ferric oxide has a very limited frequency response, generally about 5 kHz, and a poor signal-to-noise ratio. In the last 10 years, a number of new materials have been developed to improve tape response. The most common of these is chrome dioxide, which is sometimes referred to as "metal tape," and symbolized as CrO_2. It does have a much better high-frequency response, along with a fair degree of high-frequency tape hiss. The hiss can be reduced by appropriate design of recorder amplifiers. This difference between ferric oxide and chrome dioxide in the way the amplifiers are set up means that the two types of tapes cannot be run on the same machine without some modifications. Most current machines provide controls to permit the use of both tapes, but care must be taken to see that the settings are appropriate for the type of tape being used. Unfortunately, chrome dioxide tape is very abrasive and wears out the recording and playback portions of the tape recorder faster than ferric oxide.

A new coating has been developed recently in which ferric oxide is "doped" with cobalt in the same manner as semiconductors (see chapter 1). This produces a tape with the frequency response, dynamic range, and signal-to-noise ratio characteristics of chrome-dioxide tape. Since the surface is composed mostly of ferric oxide, it retains the smoothness of ferric oxide; thus the recording and playback surfaces do not wear as they do with chrome-dioxide tape.

Tape Recording

This section will first describe the general method by which signals are placed on magnetic tape, and then there will be a brief discussion and comparison of the direct and FM recording techniques.

A signal is placed on a tape by altering the magnetic fields on the tape. This is done by increasing or decreasing the strength of the field with a device that can place variable amounts of magnetic charge onto the tape. The device that does this is referred to as the "write head" on a tape recorder. The write head transduces the electrical signal into a magnetic signal that is placed on the tape.

All tape recording begins with a blank tape, which is a tape that has no magnetic charge on it. Zero magnetic charge corresponds to zero signal, and there are devices called "demagnetizers" that will "clean" a tape. What the demagnetizer actually does is pass the tape by a transformer (recall that coils generate magnetic fields) and put a constant charge on the tape. This is not really "demagnetizing" the tape, but works just as well because a constant DC signal is not audible. The same process is performed by rerecording on a tape with no input signal. The write head will place a constant amount of magnetization (the internal noise for the recorder) on the tape, which yields a very low-level random signal. It should be noted that this is actually the second step in "recording a blank tape." Tape recorders have an erase head that precedes the write head, which actually tries to write a very high-frequency (50 kHz to 100 kHz) signal on the tape. Due to the characteristics of tapes and the write heads, this demagnetizes the recording strata on the tape. Incidentally, although x-ray machines can scramble a tape with noise, they do not actually clear the tape in the manner just described.

The signal needs to be read off the tape, which is done, not surprisingly, by the "read head." The read head does the reverse process of the write heads; write heads sense the magnetic signal on the tape and transduce the magnetic signal into an electrical signal. Occasionally, read and write heads are integrated into a single unit, but they are more commonly separate.

Figure 6.1 shows the common arrangement of the erase, write, (or record) and read (or playback) heads on an audio tape recorder. Note that the consecutive arrangement of the heads theoretically permits each of the operations to be performed in order. Many recorder manufacturers can take advantage of this arrangement to permit the user to monitor recordings as they are made because the read head follows the write head. The lag between the two heads is very small because of the short distance between placement of the two heads, and so most people do not notice any lag.

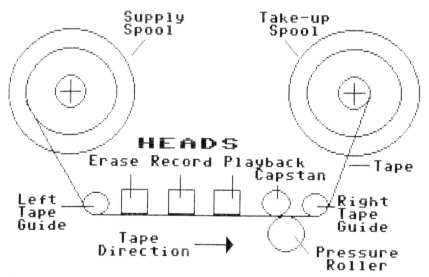

Figure 6.1.   Tape and head arrangement on an audio recorder/reproducer.

Signals are stored on tape in tracks. Figure 6.2 shows the configuration for three types of track arrangements on ¼-inch tape. These examples show that two-track recording and replay can be done in at least two ways: with either half-track or quarter-track recorders. Note that if the quarter-track tape is turned over, it would be possible to record on the other two tracks.

Head alignment is an issue in writing and reading tapes. This involves both proper height and the orientation of the head to the tape. The strength of the magnetic field produced by the write head is in proportion to the orientation of the head to the tape. This orientation is referred to as the "alignment of the head." Manufacturers try to design the recorders for optimum head alignment because it reduces noise and puts the best signal on the tape. Regardless of the actual alignment value, the performance of the recorder is specified assuming a particular alignment, and if this goes awry, the specifications go awry. Since checking and correcting head alignment is not something that can be done without special instrumentation, it is best to have all tape recorders sent to an appropriate facility, usually the firm from whom it was purchased, to have the heads checked out and realigned if necessary.

Another problem with the read and write heads on a tape recorder is that they will obviously not work properly if they are dirty. Unfortunately, tapes are not clean, and although manufacturers have significantly cut down on the friction produced by heads rubbing against tape, tape debris will build up on the heads over time. Therefore, it is necessary to clean the

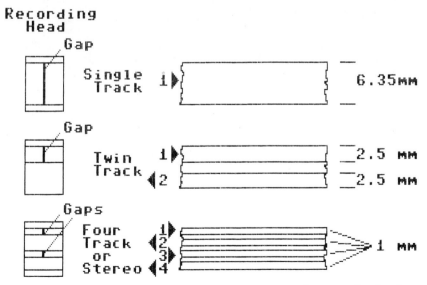

Figure 6.2.   Track arrangement on tapes and corresponding recording heads.

heads of a tape recorder on a regular basis and to do it more often if new tapes are used frequently because new tapes generate more debris than slightly used tapes. Old tapes can also be a problem because the substrate that holds the magnetic charge starts breaking down after a while. The simplest solution to this problem is to replace the tape. The frequency of tape replacement obviously depends on use, with more frequently used tapes being replaced sooner than seldom-used tapes. It should be noted, however, that tapes will deteriorate on their own even if not used, so do not assume that a tape is satisfactory just because it has not been used. A good general rule to follow here is to always have a copy of any tape, thus avoiding being stuck without a tape at a critical time.

A summary of the process of recording on magnetic tape is shown in Figure 6.3. An acoustic (or video, although there are some differences) signal is transduced by a microphone into an electrical signal that is sent through the recorders input circuits into the write head. The write head transduces the electrical signal into a magnetic signal that is stored on the tape. To play back the material on the tape, the playback head reads the magnetic signal and transduces it into an electrical signal that is sent through the output circuits of the recorder and into a speaker or earphones to transduce the signal back into the acoustic domain. This figure makes apparent the number of transformations and potential sources of error impacting the integrity of the signal as it goes from the acoustic domain to the tape and back.

There can be from 1 to as many as 16 channels of information written simultaneously on a single tape. This does not mean that there are 16 write heads on the tape recorder. While there may be multiple heads, a single head can be designed to write several channels simultaneously. If this is done, each channel appears as a striation on the portion of the head that will face the tape. If more than one head is required, the heads will be offset so that the heads will not be writing on the same part of the tape. A

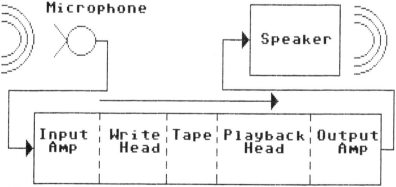

Figure 6.3. Recording and reproduction process for audio tape recorders.

small but sometimes important point concerning multiple-head machines is to know which heads write to which channels. This is important because, unless the machine has a time delay built in to compensate for the difference in time of arrival of the tape at the write heads, or unless the read heads are offset by exactly the same distance as the write heads, there will be a small time difference between channels. Manufacturers are aware of the problem, but because the time differences are so small, manufacturers may not have elected to compensate for it. Therefore, this issue should be checked on a multiple-head machine.

There are two ways that a signal can be coded onto the tape. The first method, *direct recording*, places the signal on the tape by altering the strength or the amplitude of the magnetic field on the tape in direct proportion to the amplitude of the input signal. The other method, *FM recording*, places a constant amplitude signal on the tape whose frequency varies as a function of the amplitude of the input signal. The difference between the two methods is that the direct method has a very good signal-to-noise ratio but not a very broad bandwidth, i.e., it cannot handle very high frequency signals, whereas the FM method has a very broad bandwidth and not as good a signal-to-noise ratio. Video and multichannel recorders use the FM method, whereas audio recorders generally use the direct method.

Tape Editing

It may be necessary from time to time to edit a tape, whether it is to remove a noise section from the tape or to accomplish some research purpose. One of the major advantages of reel-to-reel tape recorders, in addition to their generally higher quality capabilities, is the ease of editing tapes on them. "Ease" here is a relative term; it means editing is easier than on a cassette tape, which is an almost impossible task.

Editing is usually achieved by physically cutting and rejoining the tape although recorders have now been developed which permit sophisticated electronic editing. Such machines are currently very expensive. It is possible, with practice, to edit speech syllables or excerpts of music together without upsetting the rhythm. This method is also used for splicing on leader tape to enable accurate cueing when reproducing several sequences in a row.

The procedure is to play back the tape until the cue is heard. The machine is then stopped, and the two spools are rotated slowly backwards and forwards by hand until the exact point of the cue is established. With practice it becomes possible to recognize cue points even at a very slow speed. A mark is then made on the tape to coincide with the reproducing head (Fig. 6.1) or against a marker post that is fitted to some machines at a measured distance from the reproducing head. The tape is then removed from the head and placed in a special guide, which is usually made of aluminum and has a lip that is slightly narrower than the tape. The guide has a diagonal slit either at a 45- or 60-degree angle to the tape. The mark on the tape is lined up with the slit or with a mark on the guide at the same distance from the slit as the marker post is from the reproduce head. The tape is cut by running a razor blade along the slit. The razor blade should be nonmagnetic.

The recording tape, or leader tape to which it is to be joined, is laid in the guide and cut in a similar manner. The reason for the diagonal cut is to create a smooth transition and prevent a click occurring due to a sudden change in the signal level. Recall that the magnetic charge is across the width of the tape; so if the tape is tapered, the magnetic charge will be tapered likewise.

The two tapes are then butted together, and about 3 cm of special adhesive tape are stuck over the "join" on the back of the tape. Care should be taken to put the adhesive tape on straight and to touch the sticky side as little as possible with the fingers.

A consistent procedure should be followed when editing tape. One convention is to use white leader tape (about 1 m) at the start and to write the title on it, short lengths (about 15 cm or 6 inches) of yellow leader between separate inserts, and red leader tape at the end. It is a good idea to get into a routine of marking the tape for splicing in a particular manner, for example, always along the bottom of the tape. This avoids confusion and reduces the risk of joining the tape on backwards when the splice is made. Also, the frequent statement that these operations are possible with practice should be interpreted to mean "with a *lot* of practice."

Noise Reduction in Tape Recorders

Tape recorders, like all instrumentation, generate noise. Because the human ear is so sensitive to noise, a number of noise-reduction techniques have been employed over the years. To improve the signal-to-noise ratio, a system of "companding" can be used; i.e. the volume range of the signal is compressed to raise the average level before recording and then expanded, depressing the quieter elements of the program (and with it the noise) on reproduction. Unfortunately there are two main problems in designing an effective companding system. One is the difficulty of making the compression and expansion system "track" perfectly over the whole frequency and volume range. The other is preventing the background noise level from going up and down with the signal, which only makes background noise more obvious. Noise reduction methods that have been successful enough to be adopted by the industry are the Dolby and the DBX noise-reduction systems. In both cases the noise being reduced is primarily high-frequency noise.

Dolby Systems

The Dolby process, named in honor of the engineer who discovered the process, has two types of systems: A and B. The Dolby-A system provides the signal with two parallel paths: one via a linear amplifier and the other via a differential network, the output of which is added to the "straight through" signal when recording and subtracted when reproducing. The differential network divides the frequency spectrum into four bands and treats each one separately so that the action is applied only where it is needed. With music, for instance, most of the sound energy tends to be concentrated in the lower middle band, whereas tape hiss is largely in the high-frequency range and too far removed in frequency for "masking" to take effect. This is the effect whereby the ear tends to be less sensitive to sound in the presence of, and for a short time after, hearing louder sounds of similar frequency. The Dolby system exploits this effect by restricting the action to narrow-frequency bands.

The system is adjusted so that with a low-level input (below −40 dB) the output is 10 dB higher than the input for frequencies up to about 5 kHz, above which the output increases progressively to 15 dB gain at 15 kHz. As the input signal rises above +40 dB, the output is progressively less affected. At high levels (where the possible ill effects of companding are most obvious), the compander has less effect and is virtually bypassed. The Dolby-A system is normally used only as an intermediary process, the final product having a straightforward response. This is in contrast to the Dolby B process where the recording is sold with the modified characteristic incorporated, on the assumption that the complimentary characteristic will be applied in the reproducing apparatus.

The Dolby-B process is simpler than Dolby-A and is used mainly in the tape cassette market to reduce the high background level of noise that is inherent in this type of recording due to the low tape speed and narrow track. As in the Dolby-A system, Dolby-B has a main signal path and a side chain. The side chain incorporates a compressor that is preceded by a high pass variable filter covering frequencies from about 500 Hz upwards. In the record mode, signals below a given threshold level are boosted by the compressor and added to the side chain. The increase in level is applied progressively by the variable filter from 0 dB at 500 Hz up to 10 dB at 10 kHz.

Thus low-level, high-frequency signals are recorded up to 10 dB higher than the original. An overshoot suppressor (diode clipper) is provided, following the compressor, to prevent high-level transients that are faster than the time constant of the compressor from being added to the output. Any resultant distortion is masked by the high-level signal and tends to cancel on replay.

The Dolby-B decoder, which is fitted to most high-quality cassette machines, is identical to the coder except that the side chain is fed with a phase-inverted signal so that the output of the compressor is added to the main chain in antiphase and is effectively subtracted from it, thereby producing an exact complement of the coding process. As the low-level, high-frequency response is reduced on playback so is the tape hiss and system noise that has been introduced by the recording, giving an improvement in signal-to-noise ratio of up to 10 dB. The difference between the Dolby system and the simple application of pre-emphasis to the recording and de-emphasis on playback (which is applied anyway) is that the Dolby-B characteristic only affects low level signals.

DBX System

The DBX noise suppression system, like Dolby-A, is a complementary system. The DBX system employs a wide range 2:1 compression ratio to encode and decode. Problems of tracking the compression and expansion are eased by the straightforward ratio and the fact that the level sensing is done on a root-mean-square (RMS) basis, i.e., controlled by the total power of the signal regardless of the phase relationships of the various components. The DBX system exploits the fact that, in most material, the bulk of the power is in the low frequencies and that high power in the high frequencies occurs only when the general volume is large.

The signal fed to the compressor is heavily preemphasized to increase the overall power recorded. The signal is similarly deemphasized to restore it to normal, while at the same time reducing the high-frequency noise when the signal is decoded. To prevent the recording from being overloaded by any powerful preemphasized high-frequency signals, a similar pre-emphasis is applied to the side chain of the compressor so that, in effect, the high-frequency recording level increases as the frequency increases and as the high-frequency level decreases.

The DBX system also takes into account the masking effect of our ears, which makes us relatively insensitive to noise (in this case high-frequency noise), in the presence of loud sound of a similar frequency. The use of DBX can result in an improvement in high-frequency signal-to-noise ratio of up to 30 dB.

How to Use a Tape Recorder

A tape recorder is an extremely simple instrument to use, in part because it is such a large consumer item that the manufacturers have made an effort to make them easy to use. There are systems that will take a reel-to-reel tape and thread the tape automatically, as well as stop it automatically when it comes to the end of the tape. Cassette recorders are even easier to use. As with audiometers and much other instrumentation, tape recorders are incorporating computers into the instrumentation, making them more flexible and easier to use. There are a couple of areas that will be covered here because they cover some of the practical aspects of tape use and because the totally automated recorder is still not generally available. These two topics are covered: starting the record or playback process and using a calibration tone.

Recording and Playing Back on an Audio Tape Recorder

The first step in using a tape recorder is the same as with all instrumentation—make sure the power is on and the tape recorder is connected to the speaker(s) or other transducer that is to receive the output. The second step is to load the tape into the machine. For cassette machines, this means merely inserting the tape, with the proper orientation, into a slotted plastic lid that will open up when the eject button is pressed. The proper orientation can be determined by looking for the location of the writing and reading heads. The open end of the cassette that shows the tape is always inserted so that it faces the heads. After the cassette is firmly in place (do not place your fingers on the tape, always hold the cassette by its edges), simply press down on the lid, and the tape will click into place.

For a reel-to-reel tape recorder, the operation is the same except loading the tape requires threading the tape across the heads and onto the empty reel. If a reel-to-reel recorder is a common piece of instrumentation, it is a good idea to keep one or two spare empty reels. (For some reason, empty reels frequently disappear, and the recorder is useless without them.) Threading a tape is usually very easy to do if it is done gently. Simply take the end of the tape and pull out about 2 feet of tape. Keeping the tape relatively taut without actually pulling hard enough to pull more tape off the reel, slide the tape into the tape slot by the heads. Sometimes this will require *slightly* twisting the tape to go under the shelf of the head cover; remember not to twist the tape too much, or it will snarl or crimp, which can result in permanent damage to the tape. If necessary, you can frequently take the head cover off for easier access, but this is not a recommended procedure as it makes it much easier to damage the heads. After the tape is threaded, the tape needs to be started on the empty reel. Lay the end of the tape flat on the inner part of the reel without twisting the tape, and then by holding the tape onto the reel with a finger through one of the slots in the side of the empty reel, rotate the reel until the tape is covered by the next layer of tape. Provide enough slack to be able to rotate the reel until several turns of tape are on the reel. Make sure that the tape is taut and there is no slack.

There are several tape transport controls for a tape recorder, which generally include forward, fast forward, reverse, record, play, and stop. Some tape recorders have a pause control. The functions of these various controls are self-explanatory. The only confusion may be that many recorders require that the play and record functions be activated simultaneously in order to record.

Recording and playback functions on either a reel-to-reel or a cassette recorder are the same. To record, press both the play and record buttons, or levers, simultaneously until they stay down. Some recorders have a single record button that does the same thing. When done recording, hit the stop button. To play back a fresh tape, just press down on the play button until it stays down. To stop playback, most recorders permit using either a pause button (to stop for a very brief time) or a stop button. As a general rule, do not use the pause button to halt playback for a long period of time because this leaves the heads in position and the tape locked in place. Trying to remove the tape in this situation can damage the tape. Only use pause for brief breaks on playback.

Most tape recorders have tape counters and VU meters. The tape counter counts the footage of the tape as it passes by the heads. It does this by monitoring the tape transport. The readout for the tape counter is either a mechanical rotary counter or a digital display. The VU meter monitors either the input or output of the tape recorders. It is a relative voltmeter; that is, it monitors the voltage relative to some arbitrary value. The readout for the VU meter can be either a needle meter or a bar display. The bar display consists of lighted bars whose length is proportional to the intensity of the signal read by the VU meter.

When recording on a tape recorder, be sure to record at a intensity such that the VU meter on the tape recorder stays around zero. This will ensure that the recording will take full advantage of the signal-to-noise ratio of the recorder. When doing acoustic recording that must be calibrated for level, be sure to provide a calibration signal that has been recorded with the same input parameters as the material of interest. That is, the VU meter should be at zero for the calibration signal and at zero for the recorded material, without changing the record level. This will ensure equivalent record and reproduction levels for the calibration tone and the recorded material.

When you have completed a session with the tape recorder, rewind the tape, hit the stop button, and remove the tape. For cassette recorders, this means hitting the eject button after the tape has been rewound and stopped. After removing the tape, press the lid back into its closed position. This will help keep dust and debris from getting into the recorder. For reel-to-reel recorders, this means removing the tape from the machine and the empty reel, if it is yours, after the tape has been rewound and stopped. Make sure the tape recorder power is off. Then place a dust cover over the recorder to help keep dust and debris from getting into the recorder. If you do not own a dust cover for the tape recorder, it is highly recommended that you get one.

Generating a Calibration Tone

A calibration tone is very important for determining the output intensity of recorded material, which is important for both clinical and research purposes. All tapes should have on the first section of tape a calibration tone that is at the same intensity as the material on the tape. If different sections on the tape are to be played at different levels but were recorded at the same level, then each section should be preceded by a calibration tone. This makes setting the output intensity much easier for variable intensity material such as speech or music.

A single-frequency sinusoid is the best signal to use for a calibration tone. The most common frequency used is 1,000 Hz, because this is within the operating range of most instruments. The signal can be generated either by a function generator or by a sine wave generator. Connect the signal generator to the tape recorder. Set the record level on the tape recorder to the midrange value. For example, if the record level dial runs from 0 to 10, set the dial to 5 and adjust the intensity of the sine wave generator such that the VU meter is at 0. Record the tone for 2 min. After recording the calibration tone, play it back to make sure that it was recorded properly. This procedure is the same for both the reel-to-reel and cassette recorders.

Some Pointers on Audio Recording

There are a few simple rules for audio recording that will help ensure consistently good and reliable recordings. These rules concern the recording level and some of the things that should be known about a recorder before using it.

Speech is the most difficult signal to record well, with a pure tone being the easiest signal to record. For a pure tone, it is simply a matter of adjusting the input level of the recorder so that the VU meter on the recorder is at zero. The steady intensity of the signal will assure that there is little change from this level. A VU meter value of 0 is used to attain the maximum signal-to-noise ratio for the recorder. For speech the situation is more complex because speech does not have a constant intensity over time or frequency. However, the goal is the same, namely, to record at the maximum signal-to-noise ratio. To do so requires some knowledge of the specifications of the tape recorder.

All tape recorders are not equal. In addition to the obvious differences in price, there is considerable variation in capabilities within a given price range. There are a couple of specifications to look for that may help narrow the selection, once an affordable price range has been established. The first is the signal-to-noise ratio of the tape recorder. This value comes from the manufacturer inputting a signal at the maximum nondistorting intensity that the recorder can handle and then measuring the noise level. The ratio between the intensity of the signal and the noise is the signal-to-noise ratio specification that is used for tape recorders. The main point here is that the signal-to-noise ratio is not constant for all input signal intensities. The lower the input signal, the lower the signal-to-noise ratio. The moral in this is to know the intensity of the input signal used by the manufacturer to get the signal-to-noise ratio for the machine of interest.

Another important specification is the peak factor of the instrument. This means how much above VU zero can the signal input into the recorder be without distorting the signal. This value is especially important for constantly varying signals such as speech, which have some average value but may frequently peak above that value for short periods of time. The peak factor is the specification that determines where on the VU meter the input speech signal is maintained. For a tape recorder with a peak factor of <10 dB, the input speech level should be at −3 on the VU meter. For a tape recorder with a peak factor of 10 dB or greater, the input speech level should be at zero on the VU meter.

Another consideration for recording is the use of microphones. When recording speech, one must keep in mind that high frequencies drop off quickly with increasing distance from the source. The microphone must be kept close to the mouth in order to capture high frequencies in a speech recording. A constant microphone-to-mouth distance must be maintained to ensure that the recording has the same frequency emphasis throughout the recording. The same rule has to be applied whenever recording any sound in a free-field situation.

The final aspects of the recorder to examine are the controls and flexibility of the recorder. Keep in mind that the recorder is an instrument that will be used a great deal, and so should be easy to use. Things to look for are the size and placement of the controls. How much pressure is required to actuate any function? Can a catastrophic error, such as recording over a critical tape, be done easily or has it been made difficult to do while still maintaining ease of use? What kind of tape(s) can the machine handle? What functions can be controlled from the front panel, and what from the rear? Look at the placement and labeling of the input and output jacks and controls. Are they clear and easy to read? Are LEDs provided for critical functions such as power and record mode? These are small items that can nevertheless determine satisfaction with an instrument over a long period of time.

There are some other cautions to observe when using tape recorders. One is to handle the tape carefully; avoid touching the tape with your fingers in an area where you will be recording. Another is to keep in mind that when you record, you are erasing the material that was on the tape. In fact, one way to erase a tape is to record with no input. Finally, try to avoid shuttling (going back-and-forth) the tape at high speed any more than is necessary. This will stretch the tape and make the recording inaccurate. Most tape recorders are not built to handle this problem.

Video Recorders

Video recorders are most frequently used by speech and language professionals because of the need to observe and record speech and other behaviors. However, they are also frequently used by audiological researchers investigating lipreading and the relation between sound and sight in speech perception. In addition, video recorders are used in rehabilitation programs and for teaching.

Both reel-to-reel and cassette video recorders will be described and discussed. Just as in the audio world, cassette recorders are becoming more prevalent and their quality is improving. The differences between the two types of recorders relate primarily to ease of use. The laser video machine is a newer video instrument that is not yet a regular item in the field, although potentially this is the best solution of all to the video needs of researchers and clinicians. Laser machines will be discussed briefly for this reason.

A video recording system actually consists of several parts, of which the video recorder/reproducer is just one (Fig. 6.4). The two other primary pieces of instrumentation are the camera and the monitor. The camera is important because the quality of the output can only be as good as the quality of the input. The monitor is important because it is the output channel for the recorder. Using a poor monitor on an expensive video system is the same as putting poor-quality loudspeakers on an expensive stereo system.

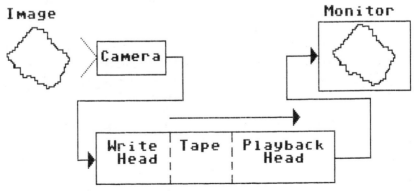

Figure 6.4.   Videotape recording and reproduction process.

Cameras

The camera is the input source for the video tape. Almost all video cameras are color cameras, but for special lighting conditions, a black-and-white camera is sometimes used. Video cameras are benefiting enormously from the advances in digital technology, which is reflected in the growing ease of use and in the fact that almost all video will be done digitally within the next few years. The focus here will be on using the camera rather than on an explanation of its principles of operation.

The most important aspect of camera use is lighting. There are several aspects to consider. The first is amount of lighting. Color photography requires a lot of light. Although new films are constantly being developed that require less light than previous films, the maxim still holds true. In general, black-and-white photography requires less light than color photography to achieve very high resolution. Two other factors to consider are the orientation of the light and the composition of the light source.

The orientation of the light is important because the video camera operates by receiving the light reflected off the object of interest. The camera receives the light, transduces it to an electrical signal and transmits it to the recorder. There it is magnetically transduced onto the tape. Thus the camera can be thought of as a video microphone, and many of the same principles of operation apply. The camera must be properly oriented toward the object, and the light must be appropriately oriented so that the camera can see the object. The light cannot be facing directly toward the camera because that light would mask out the light reflected from any object, and the camera would only be able to record the light facing the camera. There must be sufficient light directed toward the object enabling the camera to clearly "pick up" the object. The orientation must be such that there is no glare, which is essentially a parallel reflection of the light, making the object a source rather than a reflector. If certain features must be examined on a rough surface, it may be necessary to have several light sources in order to avoid shadows.

Avoiding shadows can be extremely important in some situations. For example, some video work is done photographing physiological structures, such as the larynx while a person is speaking. The camera in this case receives its image from a fiberoptic tube. Also, there is not much room for a light source, and the surface being measured is not smooth. This creates a very difficult lighting situation in which both amount and orientation of the light source (which is not fixed) are critical. Most applications do not face this critical situation, but care must be taken, in this situation, or the desired structures may not be visible.

The final lighting concern addressed here is the composition of the light source. This is critical for color photography because any light source, except a laser, has multiple colors in it with various weightings of the different colors. Thus what we might think of as white light from several different lighting sources is not actually white. While this is not too critical for the human eye because the compensation is made automatically unless the lighting is significantly different from "true" white, it is very important for the video camera because it does not have an automatic compensating mechanism. Thus the camera must be preadjusted for the lighting situation. This is very easily done on some cameras by holding up a large white card facing the camera and having the camera automatically calibrate its color balance. On other cameras the adjustment is done manually. The key to remember is to calibrate the color balance before filming, because otherwise the colors will be incorrect.

A word of advice: It is extremely difficult to become an expert in both video and sound. Therefore, it is better to find a person who is knowledgeable and has had experience with the same kind of video work that is needed, and to work with him or her until you are satisfied with the product.

Video Tape Recorders

The video tape recorder is actually a recorder/reproducer, just as for audio recorders. This section will discuss similar topics to those for the audio recorder section. The principles of operation for video recorders and some of the characteristics of the tape are described. In particular, some of the differences between the various types of videocassette machines are highlighted. Some pointers for how to use video recorders are also given.

Videotape

Videotape is very similar to audiotape, and the signal is recorded on the tape using the same magnetic principles described for the audio recorder. However, the mechanical manner in which the signal is placed on the tape and played back is quite different.

The principle of recording a television signal is no different from that used in recording sound. The practical problem arises because of the very high frequencies required to produce a detailed picture on a television set. For a typical modern TV this frequency is around 3.5 MHz.

The highest frequency that can be recorded on a tape depends on two factors: the size of the head gap and the tape speed. The smaller the head gap size and the faster the tape speed, the higher the frequency that can be accurately recorded. Current FM data machines run at a maximum speed of about 120 inches/s. To record a TV signal on one of these machines would require a tape speed of around 500 inches/s, which is an excellent way to use up a lot of tape and is bound to be extremely expensive and difficult to implement.

The solution to this problem involves a couple of factors. First, the speed with which the tape is scanned, which is the key problem, can be increased by moving the heads as well as the tape. The second is to record the information on the tape in such a way that the information on the tape would change fast enough to accommodate the higher speed scanning. Each of these solutions is discussed next.

The most obvious difference between audio and video recorders is the use of the helical scanning technique to record and play back videotapes. The helical scanning technique means a different arrangement between the tape and the heads and a very different loading mechanism from that used for audiotapes. The helical scanning technique is covered very briefly to give an understanding of basic principles. The loading mechanisms and characteristics for U-matic and VHS format tapes will also be described in order to explain some of the differences and to get a feel for what the machine is doing during its automatic loading procedure.

The two key features of helical scanning are the moving tape heads and the fact that the tape is scanned at an angle, unlike audiotape. Figure 6.5 illustrates the basic principle for one type of helical scanning arrangement. Note that the tape leaves the head drum at a different height than it enters. Also note that the drum containing the heads is rotating in a direction opposite to the tape motion.

Imagine a tape wrapped around a cylinder: If the tape is at right angles to the axis of the cylinder, the two ends of the tape will be level with each other. If the angle between the tape and cylinder's axis is adjusted, as in Figure 6.5, the bottom of the tape coming round the cylinder and out can be made to come out at the top of the incoming tape. The tape circling the cylinder is in contact all around, but the circle is slightly askew, forming

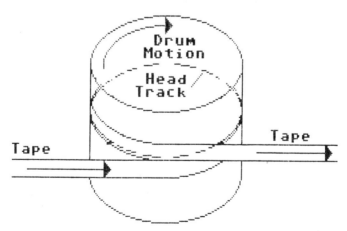

Figure 6.5. Schematic representation of two key features (drum and tape) for helical scanning system.

what is known as a "helix;" hence the name helical scanning. If the cylinder is now rotated, a point *A* on its surface under the top edge of the incoming tape will travel around under the tape, crossing it at an angle until it reaches point *A*, the bottom edge of the outgoing tape, where the latter touches the top edge of the incoming tape. The head will now have traced a path at an angle across the tape for the length of the tape around the cylinder. If the tape was moved forward a little before the cylinder rotated a second time, the next time the cylinder rotated it would trace out a path parallel to the first. By moving the tape steadily, we could scan a series of such parallel diagonal tracks.

Recall that an effective speed of 500 inches/s is required to produce a modern TV signal. To show how this technique achieves this speed, we can calculate the effective speed of this system for some typical parameters. Using a tape speed of 7½ inches/s and a cylinder of 3 inches in diameter, the cylinder would have to rotate at a little over 50 revolutions/s to achieve a head-to-tape speed of 500 inches/s; with a 360-degree helical wrap, only one head would be needed. Each diagonal track would be about 9.6 inches long running from tape edge to tape edge. This is in effect a tape savings of about 70 times and makes the system mechanically practicable.

There are some differences between this system and a broadcast quality system, but the general principles are the same. There is some loss in video quality because the tape is narrower, which means reduced signal strength; also, the scanning speed is about ⅓ that of a broadcast system, which means that there is some loss of definition. However, a very acceptable picture is still produced.

It has already been noted that the track layout on a videotape is very different from that for an audiotape. On an audiotape the tracks are parallel to each other and the edge of the tape. For a videotape, the tracks are at an angle of 3 to 5 degrees relative to the edge of the tape (Fig. 6.6). On a videocassette each track represents one complete "TV field." The concept of a TV field requires some expansion. Therefore, it is discussed next.

The picture on a TV screen is not a single picture but actually represents the drawing of many parallel lines very close together running horizontally

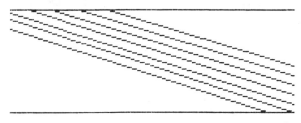

Figure 6.6.   A few sample tracks of a videocassette track format.

across the screen. The TV screens in Europe have 625 lines, and those in the United States have 525 lines. In practice, alternate sets of lines are drawn, with a screen that has one set of alternate lines being referred to as a "field." Two fields, which are interlaced, constitute a frame. These fields are updated 50 times/s in Europe (25 frames/s) and 60 times/s (30 frames/s) in the United States.

The implication of having one field per track is that if the tape transport is stopped but the drum keeps rotating, the result will be a still frame. If the tape speed is adjusted, slow- or fast-motion scan can be effected. Because of overlapping bands and head design, a horizontal band of "noise" will float vertically across the picture, but this is a small price to pay for variable-speed playback. If the picture is stopped, the noise band will freeze also, but this can be adjusted so that it is out of the main viewing area.

U-matic and VHS Formats

Given that helical scanning is the technique employed in all videocassette machines, what is the difference between U-matic and VHS machines? First, what is "U-matic?" The U-matic system refers to the videocassette tape format that was developed by Sony and it was the first widely available cassette format. This format is still very commonly used in clinics and laboratories.

The first thing to note is that the U-matic and VHS machines both use a two-head drum in a helical scanning mechanism for recording and playback. This means that the tape only needs to go halfway around the drum to get the same effect as a single-head drum with a complete wraparound. The main differences are in the size of the tape and the manner in which the tape is loaded by the recorder. The U-matic tape is a ¾-inch tape, whereas the VHS tape is a ½-inch tape. The implication of this difference is that the U-matic will give a stronger signal. Another, perhaps not so obvious implication is that some of the signal will be lost when copying from U-matic to VHS format tapes.

The differences in the manner of the loading mechanism are invisible to the user. For all cassettes the hinged flap is raised when the cassette is inserted into the machine. The U-matic uses a loading arm to pull the tape to the drum and around a little over 180 degrees of the drum. The VHS uses a simpler mechanism that uses two loading pins to press the tape around 180 degrees of the drum. For the U-matic system the tape is actually pulled around the drum, whereas for the VHS system the tape is simply pulled straight out of the cassette and pressed against the drum.

Is there an obvious advantage to using one or the other format? The answer depends on the application. If it is necessary to get a very high-definition picture, this is better done on a U-matic cassette. If the cassette is intended for use by a patient at home, there are two possible choices,

Betamax and VHS. The most common home format is VHS. Neither of these formats is compatible with U-matic machines. Incidentally, the reason that Betamax and VHS tapes cannot use the same machine is the difference in the track layout on the tape, although the tapes and cassettes have the same physical dimensions.

Some Pointers on Video Tape Recording

The preceding discussion of some of the mechanics of video tape recorders will be useful in explaining some of the tips given here for using video tape machines. For example, it is not advisable to leave a tape recorder in pause or still-frame mode for too long because it will wear out the tape much more quickly. Recall that in this mode the heads continue to rotate while the tape stands still. Most current recorders now have an automatic shut-off feature that removes the machine from single-frame mode after a fixed time.

It is also a good idea to work with duplicates of original data tapes if video analysis is being done. While there is some loss in quality when the material is copied, using copies will permit replacement of the videotapes when they wear out, which they will eventually. The tapes will lose video quality even more quickly if frequent stop-frame analysis is required.

Some other recording tips are similar to those for audio recording. Do not shuttle the tape excessively as this will stretch the tape and ruin the picture. Keep the tapes stored in a cool, dry place. The tapes should always be kept in an enclosed package or carrier when not in use to prevent dust and dirt from getting into the cassette. Do not handle the portion of the tape with the video signal with your fingers as this will leave oily deposits on the tape. Do not cover the top of a video recorder when it is on; most recorders have fairly complicated mechanical systems and numerous electronic components inside the case that build up a lot of heat, and venting is necessary for proper operation of the machine.

While videotape can be edited, it is not recommended that you do this yourself. Find an expert who will do it. The principle for videotape editing is very similar to audiotape, but the practice requires it to be done electronically because of the way the tracks are laid out on a videotape.

Various aspects of recording, such as calibration of the tape, are best handled by observing the points made earlier during the discussion on the use of a camera for filming. It is also an excellent practice to monitor the recording while it is taking place. This will help avoid obvious blunders, such as blissfully recording for two hours, only to find out later that the camera was not attached to the tape recorder. This reinforces the point made throughout all of our discussions about the most basic rule of instrumentation: Make sure that the instrumentation is turned on and properly connected.

Laser Systems

Several video systems have recently come into the market that promise to revolutionize the use of video for research, clinical practice, and training. The video disk systems, or "laser disk systems," as these systems are called, offer the potential advantages over video tape machines of virtually unlimited media life and random access of video material.

There are actually two main types of video disk players on the market: the capacitive type and the optical type. Only the optical type will be covered here because the majority of units are of this type.

An interesting aspect of video disc players is that, in a sense they are a return to older instrumentation, namely the phonograph. A video disc looks very similar to a phonograph, and if we think of the laser as a phonograph needle, the principles of operation are very similar also. The basic principle of operation of a laser video disc player is shown in Figure 6.7.

The laser video disk player is strictly a playback system, which is the main drawback of the system. It is currently not possible to record on laser disk in the lab or office. The system operates by shining a laser onto the disk, which is composed of a structural layer that is pitted to various depths and lengths. These pits represent the signal. There is a reflective layer

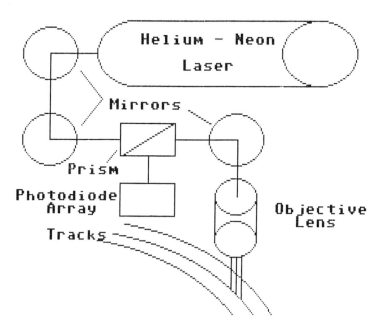

Figure 6.7. Basic operation of a laser videodisk player.

overlaid onto the pits and sandwiched between the structural layers. The laser is focused at the level of the reflective layer, and the amount of reflection is read by a lens and transduced into an FM signal that can be used by the video display portion of the system.

The material is read off the disc by positioning the stylus containing the laser over the track that contains the desired picture. Because the current convention is to store one frame per track, stop-frame work is easy. A single disk can easily store 100,000 frames. The stylus itself is under electronic control and can be positioned at any track on the disk. This makes random access extremely easy and very fast. Some of the current machines permit computer control of the player, and thus some very sophisticated programming and research work is possible, even with very inexpensive computers.

The fact that the laser is focused has a definite advantage. As long as there is nothing opaque between the reflective layer and the laser, the system is unaffected. This means that dust and grime and other particles on the surface of the disk have no effect on performance; the disk can simply be cleaned with a damp cloth whenever necessary. In addition, because there is no physical contact with the disk, it cannot wear out and offers a permanent archive for video information. This also allows unlimited single-frame analysis without having to worry about wearing out the media.

The biggest disadvantages to the video disk player as a useful system for general use are the expense of making a disk and not being able to record on-site. Work is being done to overcome these disadvantages because they are also impeding penetration into the consumer market. It is anticipated that the problems will be solved within the next 3 to 5 years.

Monitors

Monitors are a topic that will be further discussed in the final chapter on computers. This section will focus on a couple of use issues and then defer the rest of the discussion of monitors to the final chapter.

The primary concern for color monitors is clarity. This is especially important because of the amount of time that a clinician or researcher may spend watching the monitor. The monitor should have true color balance and have good enough resolution for easily seeing the structures or behaviors of interest.

Another concern for monitors is lighting. The lighting concerns here are very similar to those for filming. The best environment for viewing film is the dark, because you are viewing reflected light off a screen and too much light will mask out the image on the screen. The situation is different for viewing video images on a monitor. The monitor is actually a light source that fluoresces certain parts of the screen to get the desired output. As a result, the monitor does not need to be viewed in a dark room; however, the masking principle still applies: If there is too much light facing the viewer, the image on the screen will be difficult to see.

An additional concern for monitors is the orientation of the light. The light should be oriented so that it does not fall directly on the monitor screen. Monitor screens, especially older ones, have very smooth surfaces, and the light will cause glare very easily. Viewers should also be oriented such that they are directly facing the screen. Viewing monitors at an angle is very fatiguing, and the images will appear to blur. Another consideration with regard to viewer orientation is distance. Stereopsis is lost if the viewer is too close to the screen. In addition, the actual grain of the monitor becomes visible, which makes viewing of target images more difficult. Ideally the viewer should be close enough to see the images clearly and far enough away that the grain of the image is not visible. This distance will depend on the monitor. Chapter 9 will discuss this topic further in regard to the relation between these rules and the type of monitor.

A final concern is the composition of the light. If the light is dominated too strongly by one color, it will color the images on the screen and throw off the color balance.

Chapter Summary

This chapter has discussed audio and video recorders, with some additional discussion of peripheral equipment used with these devices, such as cameras and monitors. In addition, laser disk players were highlighted as a system with considerable future potential for replacing the current video tape systems. However, at present video tape systems will clearly be the most common type of video system in use in laboratories and clinics. The recent introduction of a hand-held video tape camera that generates VHS tapes is a good example of the robustness of the video tape system.

The laser system was highlighted because of its potential advantages of longevity of media and random access of material. It should be noted that the same concepts are being applied to audio recorders and offer the same advantages. The main disadvantage of the laser system is the lack of a read/write capability.

It was noted that digital electronics is making great strides in this area. It is anticipated that within 3 to 5 years, both video and audio instruments will be entirely digital. Digital systems will have a lot of advantages in terms of interfacing these instruments to computers and for consistency and flexibility of operation. Digital design will also help bring down the cost and provide capabilities such as autocalibration.

Audio Tape Recorders

Introduction

*T*his lab is intended to provide some experience with tape recorders. Tape recorders are a ubiquitous instrument in speech and hearing. Speech clinicians use them to gather speech samples for later analysis, and audiologists use them to present speech for testing of speech perception. Thus, it behooves the speech or hearing clinician to be familiar with tape recorders and how they work. In particular, this lab will contrast cassette and reel-to-reel tape recorders and examine the difference between electronic and acoustic output. With the advent of high-quality cassette tape recorders and the expectation that they will become the instrument of choice in clinics because of ease of use, this lab will use both reel-to-reel and cassette recorders to study the differences and similarities of the reel-to-reel and cassette recorders.

Method

Apparatus

This is the apparatus for this lab:

1. Sine wave generator;
2. Frequency counter;
3. Digital multimeter, or VOM;
4. Sound level meter;
5. Cassette recorder;
6. Reel-to-reel tape recorder;
7. Appropriate tape for each recorder;
8. Appropriate cables and connectors.

The use of the first four instruments has been described in previous labs. This lab will provide instructions for the use of the tape recorders. Both types of recorders run in a similar manner, and the main difference is in the packaging and size of the media and some tape control capabilities. A general description on how to use tape recorders was presented earlier in the chapter ("Recording and Playing Back on an Audio Recorder"). Review that section before beginning the lab.

There are some cautions to observe when using tape recorders. One is to handle the tape carefully. Avoid touching the tape with your fingers in an area where you will be recording. Another is to keep in mind that when you record you are erasing the material that was on the tape. In fact, one way to erase a tape is to record with no input. Finally, try to avoid shuttling the tape at high speed (going back and forth) any more than is necessary. This will stretch the tape and make the recording inaccurate. Most tape recorders are not built to avoid this problem.

Procedure

This lab will have three phases associated with each of two recorders: a reel-to-reel recorder and a cassette recorder. The first phase will involve recording a calibration tone, and the second phase will involve recording and measuring the output of several test tones. This recording will be done electronically and the output measurements will be done electronically and acoustically. In the third phase, the linearity of the output will be examined.

1. *Recording a Calibration Tone.*   Set the sine wave generator to 1,000 Hz and approximately 0.5 volts. Connect the sine wave generator to the tape recorder. Set the record level on the tape recorder to the midrange value. For example, if the record level dial runs from 0 to 10, set the dial to 5 and adjust the sine wave generator such that the VU meter is at 0. Record the tone for 2 min. This tone will serve as your calibration tone. Do this for both the reel-to-reel and cassette recorders. After recording the calibration tone, play it back to make sure that it was recorded properly.

2. *Recording the Frequency Sweep.*   Select between 5 and 10 frequencies within the range of 100–10,000 Hz such that they span the range in a systematic manner. These tones will be used to examine the frequency response of the tape recorders. Ideally, we would like to examine both the input and output stages of the tape recorders. Recall that there are amplifiers for both the input and output of the tape recorder and these may or may not have the same characteristics.

2a. *Recording for the Input Stage Testing.*   Set the amplitude of the sine wave generator (with the frequency equal to 1,000 Hz) such that the VU meter reads 0, with the record level at the same setting as for the calibration tone. Starting with the lowest frequency in the set of frequencies selected earlier, record a 1-min segment on each recorder at each frequency that was selected. *Note: Make all recordings on the reel-to-reel at 3¾ inches/s, if possible.* Do not change the amplitude of the sine wave generator or the record level on the tape recorders. Be sure to note the setting of the tape counter for each segment so that the appropriate segment can be found when testing the output of the tape recorder for that segment. After recording the segments, do the recording portion of phase 2c, then come back to the test section (2b) of this phase.

2b. *Recording from the Output Stage Testing.*   Start with the record level at the midrange value. Record a 1-min segment at each frequency selected earlier, adjusting the record level such that the VU meter always reads zero. Do this for both recorders. Again, be sure to keep track of the tape counter.

2c. *Testing the Input and Output Stages.*   Connect the output of the tape recorder to the digital multimeter. Set the playback level to the middle of the range and play back each segment that you recorded in section (2a), starting with the first segment. Measure the output amplitude of the calibration tone. Measure the amplitude of the output for each segment. Keep the playback level constant during these measurements. Repeat this measurement for the other tape recorder. To acoustically test the output, select one of the tape recorders and connect an earphone to the output of the recorder. Connect the sound level meter to the earphone. (The procedures for doing this were described in Quiklab 7.) Repeat the same output measurements with this test setup as for the electronic testing. Now repeat (2c) for the segments recorded in (2b).

Note: Be prepared to spend at least 30 minutes of recording time for this lab. Do not hesitate to contact the lab instructor if you run into trouble; this will avoid this lab running overly long.

3. *Testing Linearity.*   Use the 1,000-Hz calibration tone for this series of linearity measurements. The output level control on each recorder will have several settings indicated on the dial, which may or may not have numbers associated with them. For each setting on the dial measure the output level. The tape may have to be rewound back to the beginning of the calibration tone in order to test all level settings.

Because of the many recordings and measurements that have to be made in this lab, a suggested order for work is provided to aid in the swift completion of the lab. This work order is *recommended* although not required:

Before lab:
  1. Prepare output level measurement worksheets (two for each recorder).
  2. Prepare linearity worksheets (one for each recorder).

During lab:
  1. Record calibration tone.
  2. Verify calibration tone.

3. Record single-frequency segments on reel-to-reel recorder once for a constant playback.
4. Verify recorded segments.
5. Record single-frequency segments on cassette recorder setting and once for a constant VU reading.
6. Verify recorded segments.
7. Measure electronic output on cassette recorder.
8. Measure electronic output on reel-to-reel recorder.
9. Measure acoustic output on reel-to-reel recorder.
10. Measure acoustic output on cassette recorder.
11. Measure linearity on cassette recorder.
12. Measure linearity on reel-to-reel recorder.

Results

Present your results for each phase using appropriate tables and figures. When analyzing your data, recall that all of your measurements are a combination of the input and output stages of the recorders and that the function of some of these procedures is to factor out as best as possible the contribution of each stage. This means taking the measurements from phases 2*a* and 2*b* and looking at the two of them together. Be sure to describe any manipulations done to the data in order to factor out the contribution of the input or output stage. When presenting the data from the third phase, use your experience with linearity measurements from Quiklab 8 to guide you.

Discussion

Describe the frequency response of each stage of the tape recorder. Is it adequate for any needs that you might envision (e.g., the recording and playing back of speech)? Is there any difference between the electrical and acoustic output? Are these differences, if any, important in terms of your needs? Also discuss the linearity of the volume control.

Discuss the differences between the two tape recorders, if any. Is one of the tape recorders preferable for any needs that you may envision?

7

Physiological Measurement Instrumentation

Physiological measurements are frequently made in speech and hearing. The most common measurements in the clinical area are noninvasive measurements of neuroelectrical activity during particular perceptual or motor behaviors. Such measurements will be the focus of the present chapter. In addition to these types of measurements, researchers in physiology make direct, invasive measurements of neural activity during the same types of behavior. Much of the instrumentation used by physiological researchers is the same as that used clinically, although the location of the measurement differs. Consequently, only brief descriptions of the research instrumentation and measurements are presented.

Neural behavior is not the only type of physiology measured in the field of speech and hearing. Although all physiological measurements are electronically based, measurements of the movement of physical parts of the speech and/or hearing mechanism, such as the larynx or the middle ear bones, are also performed. Some of the instrumentation necessary for these measurements will be described in this chapter. A physiological measurement that will not be covered in this chapter is acoustic impedance or middle ear measurement, as this was already done in chapter 5.

As a result of the extremely large number of possible measurements that can be made in the fields of speech and hearing, not all physiological techniques will be discussed in this chapter, and those that are discussed will not cover all aspects of those measurements (To completely describe each measurement technique would require a separate book). A good example of techniques that will not be discussed are the x-ray based and magnetic resonance techniques for the measurement of physical structures.

The intent of this chapter is to make the reader aware of at least some of the techniques and instrumentation available to make physiological measurements in order to enhance their capabilities as researchers and clinicians.

The first measurement techniques that are discussed, the auditory evoked response (AER) and electronystagmography (ENG), are probably the most ubiquitous physiological measurements made in audiology, next to middle ear measurements. Because of their frequency of use and because many aspects of these measurement techniques generalize to other physiological measures, AER and ENG will be discussed in more detail than other techniques. The measurement of speech physiology will also be described.

Auditory Evoked Response

The intent of this section is not to cover the whole area of auditory evoked response (AER), but rather to focus on the instrumentation used for this type of measurement. In particular, details of the physiology will not be described here. It is recommended that such knowledge be gained, however, before attempting to do these measurements.

There are several pieces of instrumentation involved in making auditory evoked responses. The two most obvious are the electrodes, which are attached to the patient and serve as the input sensors, and the computer or signal averager, which is used to analyze the responses. There are also several other pieces involved, as shown in Figure 7.1.

The AER measurement system involves a signal generator, headphones (or loudspeaker system), an amplifier, an averaging system (which can be a computer), and a plotter (or other graphic output device such as an oscilloscope) (Fig. 7.1). The signal generator and headphones are necessary to deliver the eliciting stimulus to the patient. The amplifier is required because physiological responses, especially those that are measured "far-field," as are most AERs, are extremely small in amplitude and must be amplified somewhere between 100 and 10,000 times to achieve sufficient amplitude to be usable by other instrumentation. The averaging system is required to get a stable and reliable response measure. The plotter or oscilloscope is required to view and/or store the response. Other storage devices such as computer disk drives are also used to store the response.

These components, with the exception of the averaging system, have been described in previous chapters, and their operation will not be detailed here. Therefore, all of the calibration and maintenance requirements that apply to these instrumentation components and described in previous chapters must be kept in mind when using them for this application. The operating principles of the averaging system will be described in this chapter, with a description of computers reserved until chapter 9.

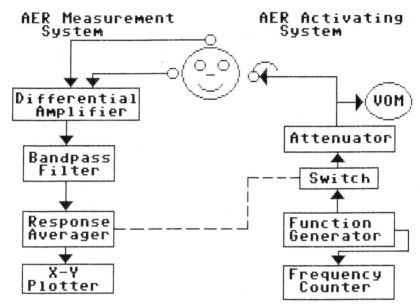

Figure 7.1. Instrumentation setup for creating and measuring an auditory evoked response (AER).

The electrodes and the instrumentation used to capture and analyze the response are two additional aspects of this measurement system that have not been discussed before. Since computers, which are the instrumentation used to capture and analyze the response, will be described in a later chapter, this chapter will focus on the general principles of capturing the response and the methodology used to analyze the response. Electrodes are discussed first.

Electrodes

Measurement of AER is based on the measurement of electrical potentials generated by the nervous system in response to an acoustic stimulus. The potentials are measured "far-field," which means that the site of measurement is distant from the site of generation. The neuroelectrical potential is picked up at the measurement site by a device called an electrode, which is simply a conductive material attached to the input of the measurement instrumentation.

There are many different types of electrodes; these are differentiated by size, shape, and composition. For example, electrodes are always constructed of a highly conductive material such as silver, but this material is not always a metal. A good example of this are glass electrodes, generally referred to as "microelectrodes", that are used by physiologists who measure neural potentials from single cells or nerves. The conductive material for these electrodes is a liquid solution.

Electrodes are generally named according to their size and shape. Electrode size can vary from disks that are several inches in diameter to needle electrodes whose active surface is < 10 μm. Size also influences the composition of the electrode, because materials have limitations as to their viability as size changes. Larger electrodes are generally composed of metallic substances, whereas the very small electrodes are generally composed of a pliable or flexible material such as glass.

The discussion here is restricted to electrodes that are used externally for noninvasive types of measurement. This means that electrodes with metallic composition, in particular, silver-silver chloride electrodes, will be the focus of the following discussion.

Care and Use of Electrodes

The electrodes used for AER are usually small (less than 1 inch diameter), circular, and composed of silver-silver chloride. These electrodes are attached to the skin at the forehead, mastoid, and/or the top of the head. Occasionally other placement locations may be used. To get accurate and usable measurements, you must apply these electrodes using appropriate methodology and maintain them properly.

The key to being able to measure small potentials is the electrode's good electrical contact at the measurement site; two major factors are the site of the measurement and the method of application. Determination of the best site for measuring evoked potentials, which has been the subject of much debate, obviously depends on the type of measurement, for example, brainstem or electrocochleography (ECOG). For brainstem measurements, the best location for at least one of the recording electrodes has generally been considered the mastoid. For ECOG, the greatest sensitivity is in the round window niche which can only be reached by penetrating the eardrum. However, practical concerns will play a role, and other sites may be selected, such as the ear canal for ECOG, if a physician is not available and anesthesia is not to be used.

Regardless of the site of measurement, the electrodes must be properly applied because the amplitude and reliability of the measurement is directly proportional to the care employed in applying the electrodes. First, make sure the electrodes are completely clean. Second, thoroughly clean the area where the electrode is to be placed. Do not just clean a little circle the size of the electrode; clean a *big* circle about twice the size of the electrode. Use a good-quality solvent and a slightly abrasive pad designed for this purpose. With children, the potential for a reaction to the solvent should be checked by cleaning a small area on the arm and seeing if there is a reaction. The medical chart, if available, or the physician, if the chart is not available, should be checked to see if there is any history of skin sensitivity. With older adults there is the problem that the skin may be very thick and not as flexible as in younger adults and children. For this case, more scrubbing may be necessary, but try not to overdo this. Third, the electrode paste should be applied to the surface of the electrode. Try to maintain a balance between the amount necessary for good adhesion and good conduction. The only way to do this is through practice, but in general, a thin coating is sufficient most of the time. Do not prepare the electrodes too far in advance because the electrode paste will dry out and be useless. After the area and electrodes have been prepared, the electrodes are ready to be applied.

The electrodes should be applied as soon as possible after the skin is prepared. For children it may be necessary to have the electrodes ready just before the child is to be tested. It is better to have two testers available, with one to handle the equipment and another to handle the child. After the electrodes are applied, the impedance of the connection should be checked. If the skin and electrodes have been properly prepared, the impedance will be low. The maximum cutoff is 5,000 ohms, with desirable impedances being 1,000–2,000 ohms. It is possible to get impedances <1,000 ohms, but if the impedance is zero, something is wrong, and the instrumentation should be checked. Equally as important as the magnitude of the impedance is the impedance balance among electrodes. All the electrodes should be within a few hundred ohms of each other, or you will get an imbalance that will affect the readings.

Capturing the Response

Auditory evoked responses are elicited by a stimulus, and the nature of the response depends a great deal on the nature of the stimulus. For purposes of discussing the hardware, a lot of detail about stimulus-response relations is not necessary, but a brief description is required. How the response is captured and analyzed by the instrumentation is described next.

The most simple and commonly used stimulus is the pulse. The pulse is used because it elicits a response from the whole cochlea and hence yields the largest response, although it must be kept in mind that the largest contribution to the response is from the basal end of the cochlea. For frequency-specific responses, either a pulsed sinusoid is used or a broadband pulse in combination with a selective masking technique, which involves a high-pass noise with the cutoff frequency decreasing for each measurement of the response.

The measurements of interest in AERs are the amplitude of the response and the latency of the response. The most commonly used clinical measure is the latency of the response to a particular aspect of the waveform, such as wave V of the brainstem evoked response (BSER). This latency measurement implies that there is a time-locking between the stimulus and response. This assumption is the basis for capturing the response for auditory evoked response, as well as for other physiological measures.

There are two types of response measurements, single and multiple, and the techniques and circumstances for doing each are slightly different. In both cases the basic instrumentation is the same as that shown in Figure 7.1. The response comes from the electrode into a storage area inside the instrument. At the same time it is displayed on a screen that operates just like an oscilloscope. In fact, in some clinical installations and in many research installations where the response is captured by a computer, an oscilloscope is actually used as the display device. If an oscilloscope is used, it must be a storage scope.

The single-response measurement, as the name implies, involves displaying the response to a single stimulus. This means that just one trace is stored and displayed. For single-trace measurement it is essential that there be an excellent signal-to-noise ratio and that the response be a large response (in physiological terms). There must also be the capability to do artifact rejection, that is, reject spurious responses. For a certain class of artifact, this can be done either by not displaying responses that are too large, which is done by monitoring responses in a frequency region around 75 Hz and rejecting responses in this region, or by not measuring responses past a certain latency. The large signal-to-noise ratio is required because the physiological responses are generally very small (microvolts or even nanovolts in amplitude) and there is a fair amount of general physiological noise that can mask the response.

The single-trace measurement is not used much for the early responses to auditory stimuli because large signal-to-noise ratios are difficult to obtain and there can be considerable uncertainty about the response waveform. Since most clinical measures require an interpretable waveform, this makes the single-trace measure unsuitable. However, for some of the late potentials the single-trace technique can be used effectively because the potentials are much larger than the early responses and fine details of the waveform are not as crucial to the clinical interpretation.

The most common type of measurement technique involves using multiple responses, each of which is elicited by a single stimulus. These responses are averaged to get the final response waveform that will be used by the clinician or researcher. Some newer techniques attempt to apply rules for objective determination of the response; one of these will be described briefly after the description of the standard averaging technique.

The standard clinical measurement involves the storage and averaging of multiple responses. The averaging is done to improve the accuracy of the waveform measurement. How averaging results in an improved waveform is based on some assumptions about the nature of the background noise and signal itself. These assumptions are that the noise is random and not time-locked to the signal, that the response to the signal is time-locked to the stimulus that elicits the response, and that the response has a constant waveform shape.

If noise is random and fluctuates about a signal with a particular amplitude, then adding together a lot of noise waveforms and taking the average will eventually result in a signal with that amplitude. This will not work if the noise is the same each time it is sampled. In addition, the signal that provides the base amplitude for the noise must be constant and time-locked to the same external referent that is being used to scan the noise. Averaging does not make the noise disappear immediately. The improvement in providing a true measure of the signal amplitude, that is, the improvement in signal-to-noise ratio, is inversely related to the number of signals that are used for the average. The number required to achieve a given improvement in signal-to-noise ratio is given in the equation below. It is important to note that this equation gives the improvement in signal-to-noise ratio and that the final signal-to-noise ratio for a given number of averages will depend on the signal-to-noise ratio in the original.

$$S/N = (S/N) \times (\text{number in average})^{1/2}$$

The improvement in signal-to-noise ratio with averaging not only makes it easier to detect whether a response occurred, but also smooths out the shape of the waveform. Furthermore, the waveform becomes more uniform from trial to trial, which enables the observer of the waveform to analyze aspects of its shape, as well as to determine the presence or absence of a waveform.

The effectiveness of the averaging, in terms of the assumption about time-locking, depends on the stimulus used to elicit the response. In general, the best stimulus to use is a stimulus that turns on very abruptly because the nervous system responds best to rapid changes in the environment. For an acoustic stimulus, this means that the best stimulus for eliciting a response is a rectangular pulse, which sounds to the listener like a click. Such a stimulus provides a very clear onset signal to the auditory system and ensures the highest probability of getting all the nerves to fire at the same time, which is referred to as "synchronous firing." It is synchronous firing that is responsible for the constancy of the waveform shape, as well as the time-locking of the response to the eliciting stimulus. The disadvantage of a click is that all parts of the cochlea are stimulated at once, and hence there is no way to tell what happened in a specific region. To do so requires either a special stimulus, a shaped sinusoidal pulse, or a special procedure, which requires successive measures using high-pass masking noise.

All of the assumptions listed previously are important for the signal averaging technique, but the major contributions of instrumentation have been to facilitate the generation of a stimulus and response averaging. Current instrumentation incorporates signal averaging in order to provide the clinician or researcher with the aforementioned advantages. The instrument also provides a suitable click stimulus to elicit the response. Since the instrument is both generating the stimulus and measuring the response, it is easy for it to do the time-locked averaging required.

Instrumentation for measuring AER is generally very easy to use and focuses on providing the user with a clear display of the waveform and controls that permit adjusting both the number of averages and the amount of time over which the response is sampled. The systems also permit adjusting the amplitude of the display by multiplying the waveform amplitude by some factor. Usually some factor of 2; such as 2, 4, 8, or 16; is used.

Some systems provide cursor controls that permit placing the cursor at a particular point on the waveform. As the cursor is moved, there is a readout that gives the time delay between the point on the waveform pointed to by the cursor and onset of the stimulus. This measurement, referred to as "response latency," is one of the most common measurements made from an AER waveform. Detecting a response is usually done visually. The observer looks for a particular waveform shape occurring in a specific latency range. The presence of a particular peak in the waveform or the latency to a particular peak in the waveform are the measures used to assess the waveform.

Recently, methods have been developed that may permit automatic threshold measurement from the brainstem evoked response (BSER). Although current instrumentation does not incorporate such capabilities, there are active efforts to implement such schemes. A representative scheme is covered briefly in the next section.

Automatic Threshold Detection of the AER

Methods for automatic detection of AER threshold fall into two categories: pattern-recognition schemes and statistical-decision-theory schemes. Both of these methods require the same instrumentation as a standard AER measurement, except that an additional computer system may be required unless the computer itself has been set up to acquire the response, as well as perform the calculations necessary for implementing the automatic detection scheme. Both methods also do averaging as part of their methodology and require multiple responses.

The pattern-recognition schemes generally use a template that represents the "ideal" response and matches, within some limits, the observed response to the ideal response. It does this by storing the averaged response and matching it on a point-by-point basis with the template. The amount of deviation from the template is computed, and if it is less than some criterion value, the response is accepted as a valid response. This can sometimes be done as the average is built up, with the evoking stimulus terminated when the response meets the criterion. More often, a fixed number of stimuli are presented, and the analysis is done afterwards.

Statistical-decision-theory methodologies generally use some form of maximum likelihood estimation. The probability for a particular point on the waveform to exceed a specified criterion value with a specified standard deviation is determined. When that probability exceeds a specified value, such as 95%, the response is said to have been detected. As with the pattern-recognition method, the calculations can be done after a specified number of responses have been averaged. However, ideally the calculation is done after each response beyond some minimum number. This permits the implementation of a "stopping rule," which states that stimuli will no longer be presented when the response is verified.

Calibrating the System

Regardless of whether a visual recognition or automatic detection method is employed, the accuracy of the response measurement still depends on having calibrated equipment. The calibration procedures for most of the various components have been described in previous chapters, and reference should be made to those chapters when necessary. Only one aspect of the instrumentation calibration has not been discussed before, and that is the calibration of the input to the averaging system.

The input to the averaging system must accurately track the amplitude of the response in order for the averaging to work properly. Thus, the input acts as a very accurate voltmeter and the calibration technique is very similar to that used for a voltmeter. The input amplitude is converted to a number inside the machine. The calibration setup is shown in Figure 7.2.

Calibration of the input to the averaging system requires a signal generator, a voltmeter, and a way of reading the number generated at the input. The signal generator is set to output a DC voltage at a particular value according to the voltmeter. The signal generator is then input to the machine, and the number generated for that input voltage is determined. This number is compared to the desired number, and the input is adjusted until they match. The typical requirement is to set the maximum, the minimum, and zero, which represents the midpoint. Thus it is frequently necessary to go back and forth among the three settings until all are appropriate.

Output of the system is calibrated in a similar manner. In this case the number in the machine should generate a specific voltage. This is checked by doing the above operation in reverse, that is, setting the number and looking at the output voltage. Again, minimum, maximum, and midpoint are tested until correct. When the input and output have been calibrated

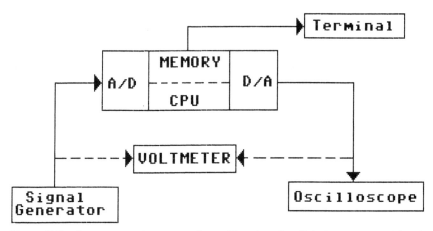

Figure 7.2. Instrumentation setup for calibrating the digital averager, which is used to analyze AER.

and the other instrumentation calibrated, the averaging system is ready. Some systems have internal calibration procedures that make the job much easier. Do not forget that the ancillary instrumentation, such as the amplifiers, oscilloscopes, and plotters, must be calibrated as well.

Originally, dedicated instruments were used to make AER measurements, but those instruments are now giving way to general-purpose computers that can perform the same measurements, which has been the case in laboratories for years. A future use of general-purpose computers might be to serve as workstations for a large computer, which would permit access to the data by a large number of users and easier formation of a patient database by an active clinical or research center. Another use might be to have multiple personal computer workstations linked either to a large computer or via a network.

Vestibular Evoked Response

Caloric stimulation and physical positioning movement techniques are the two main techniques for measuring vestibular evoked response. Electronystagmography (ENG) is the basis for both types of measurement.

Electrodes

The electrodes used to measure vestibular evoked response are identical to the electrodes used for measuring AER. The only difference is in the positioning and the extra care required for these electrodes because of their proximity to the eyes. The electrodes are generally positioned next to the corner of each eye on each side of the head. Occasionally four electrodes are employed. In this case, the second pair of electrodes are positioned on the forehead above the middle of each eye.

Capturing the Response

Measurement of eye movement due to stimulation of the vestibular nervous system is the basis for electronystagmography. The vestibular system is activated by movement of the body or by direct stimulation of the vestibular system. When the vestibular system is activated there is reaction by the visual system through the vestibulo-ocular reflex. The parameters of this reflex are used to test the integrity of the vestibular system.

The instrumentation configuration for ENG is shown in Figure 7.3. The electrodes are attached to the patient, and the electrical signal is amplified and then recorded. The display for the waveform is usually either an x-y plotter or strip chart recorder. In research situations, the signal may be recorded either on a tape recorder or with a computer.

The vestibular system can be stimulated through abrupt temperature changes in the ear canal because of its proximity to the cochlea. In fact, the fluid spaces of the cochlea and the vestibular system are connected. This technique of stimulating the vestibular system is referred to as "caloric stimulation." Caloric stimulation is used so often for ENG measurement that ENG and the measurement of eye movement in response to caloric stimulation have become synonymous.

The system can also be activated by abrupt changes in body position, for example, by quickly turning the head. This technique is referred to as

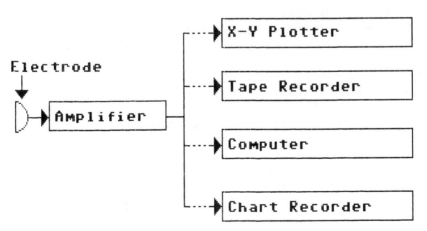

Figure 7.3. Instrumentation setup for electronystagmography (ENG), which is used to measure vestibular evoked response.

"positional nystagmus." When the vestibular system is activated by either movement or temperature changes, the eyes will turn rapidly back and forth in a systematic manner.

The eyes themselves have an electrical polarity; that is, the cornea is positive and the retina is negative. Owing to the placement of the electrodes on the outside edge of the eyes, the movement of the eyes can be sensed. As the eyes move back and forth, the cornea will move relative to the electrode and the amount of positive charge sensed through the electrodes will change.

The eyes move in a systematic way and so the waveform depicting the movement should be regular and have certain characteristics in a normally functioning system. The basic parameters are these: both eyes should give the same results, and the waveform should follow the normal pattern. The normal pattern is that of a slow phase followed by a rapid phase. The first phase is away from the midline, and the second phase is back toward the midline. The presence of tumors or other abnormalities will affect the amplitude and shape of the waveform. Electronystagmography should be done by an expert. There are currently no automatic measurement techniques for ENG, and it takes experience to analyze the recording.

There are some cautions to be observed when making these measurements (just as with AER) that will improve the accuracy and reliability of using this instrumentation. The electrodes and the mounting surface should be clean to ensure good contact. Keep in mind that these measurements are far-field measurements, just as for AER. There may be artifacts as a result of extraneous electrical activity. Furthermore, in the two-electrode configuration there are several eye movements that cannot be sensed. Both vertical and rotational nystagmus cannot be measured using a two-electrode configuration; therefore, the eyes should be observed during the measurement in order to see if these occur.

The restriction of measurement to the horizontal dimension has generated a search for instrumentation that can measure all the components of nystagmus, namely, horizontal, vertical, or rotational. The four-electrode configuration mentioned earlier is one technique. Another technique is to rapidly take several photographs of the eye during stimulation or movement. While this can be done with high-speed photography, it is expensive and time consuming because the results are not available until the film is developed. In addition, the photography requires a lot of light, and nystagmus is reduced in the presence of a focused light source.

Computer imaging systems that use infrared light to photograph the eye have been developed recently; since the eye cannot see infrared rays, the light does not impact nystagmus. While these systems are also expensive, the results are available immediately, and all the analyzing power of the computer is available to extract the desired information. Such systems are still restricted to laboratories, but if they prove clinically useful, in combination with the decreasing price of computer graphics hardware, it may be possible to produce a reasonably priced system capable of measuring all three aspects of nystagmus.

Electromyography

This section will focus on instrumentation for electromyographic (EMG) measurements, i.e., the measurement of muscle activity through measurement of the electrical activity associated with it. The focus will be on surface measurements and will highlight some of the issues that must be dealt with when making such measurements.

Electrodes

Most of the pertinent information was covered in the earlier sections. The electrodes used for AER and EMG measurements are very similar. The only differences are in the placement of the electrodes and in what is being measured by the electrodes.

The EMG electrodes sense the excitation of motor neurons. Electromyography is used by muscle physiologists in many disciplines, but in the speech and hearing field the users are speech physiologists. Hence, the placements are in areas of muscles important for speech, such as the lips and jaw. There are other muscles that are clearly important for speech, such as the tongue muscles, but the activity of this articulator is monitored with other techniques. The main difficulty in this area is the specificity of the measurement. This is because of the multiplicity and small size of muscles.

One attempt to increase the specificity of the response is to use needle electrodes. The concept here is the same as for the AER measurements. The needle is closer to the nerve, and in some cases is embedded in the muscle tissue, so the electrode is less sensitive to extraneous sources and more sensitive to the activity of that particular muscle. However, the problem then is to find the correct muscle. Since the muscles for the lips and jaw are small and not easily separated, this is very difficult and hence surface measurements are generally used.

Capturing the Response

Some of the concerns for EMG measurement are the same as for AER measurements. In particular, the signal-to-noise ratio is critical here. The EMG measurement is generally a far-field measurement. The muscles of the body are never still and are present in the same area as sensory nerves. The electrode will sense all electrical activity in a region rather than just activity associated with a particular muscle response.

An additional complication with muscle activity is the antagonistic action of groups of muscles that can seriously complicate waveform interpretation. That is, groups of muscles will have a time-locked response to a stimulus. Within the group, the polarity of the response may differ, which will result in a summed response rather than separate responses. Matching a response to a group of muscles under these circumstances can be a thankless task.

The instrumentation used for EMG measurement is essentially the same as that used for AER measurements, with some changes due to the characteristics of the waveforms being measured (Fig. 7.4). To reduce noise in the signal, just as for AER, EMG is measured with some frequencies excluded. For EMG the frequency range is up to 5,000 Hz.

As noted before, placement of the electrodes is critical to obtaining good measurements. This is especially true when using surface electrodes because of the loss of specificity. Fortunately, many muscle responses have a distinctive waveform shape when a particular movement is made that have been determined by needle electrode measurements. On-line waveform measurement combined with a good procedure for generating appropriate muscle activity can be extremely useful for accurate placement of electrodes. This can be done by sending the output of an amplifier to an oscilloscope, as shown in Figure 7.4, and having the patient make the desired movement. This can be done relatively quickly while the electrode paste is curing. When the waveform approximates the expected response, the electrode should be fixed in place.

Muscles frequently operate as groups, with different muscles having a different response pattern. To facilitate measurement of these patterns, you must use a multichannel recorder. Multichannel FM tape recorders, which were described in a previous chapter, are good for this application. These recorders permit off-line analysis of the responses of each muscle to see how they interrelate. These recorders also give a permanent recording,

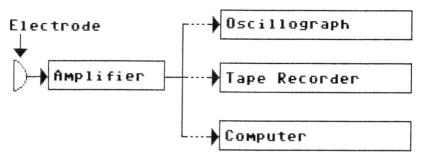

Figure 7.4.   Instrumentation setup for electromyography (EMG), which is used to measure muscle activity.

which can be useful when trying to determine progress of a particular therapy procedure.

Articulatory Measurement

Lip movement can be measured indirectly with EMG, but direct measurement is also possible. This can be done with instruments that use strain gages, which are primarily laboratory tools at the present time. Strain gages are also used to measure other movements associated with speech production. The discussion here will be general, with a couple of references to particular applications.

The resistance of a wire is directly proportional to its length and resistivity and indirectly proportional to its cross-sectional area. If we stretch a wire, its resistance will change. This simple theory is used as the basis for transducers called "strain gages."

If we stretch or compress a wire from its length at rest, we get a resistance change similar to that shown in Figure 7.5, which illustrates some important points about strain gages: First, there is a region where the change in length leads to a linear change in resistance. The slope, extent, and location of the linear region differs depending upon the length, thickness, and the elasticity of the strain gage material. Second, there are regions where the behavior clearly becomes nonlinear. These nonlinear regions generally

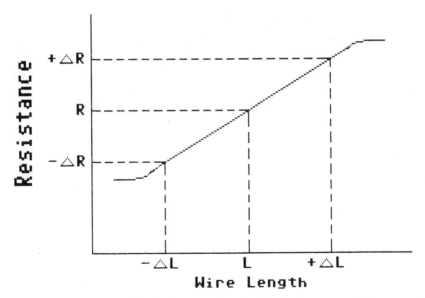

Figure 7.5. Length (tension)-resistance function for strain gages, which are used for measurement of articulatory motion.

occur at the limits of compression and stretching, but may also occur due to the frequency of variation in length of the strain gage. Again, the slope, extent, and location of the linear region differs depending upon the length, thickness, and the elasticity of the strain gage material.

The dependence of the linear and nonlinear strain versus resistance function on frequency is especially important for speech measurements because of the requirement that the strain gage not impact the speech production behavior itself. That is, the strain gage must be light and flexible enough to move with the articulator or structure being measured without being a load on the structure, and therefore altering the movement itself. This requirement results in materials that must be carefully measured to determine their linear performance region in order to ensure accurate results.

Strain gages are based on the same general principles just given but are implemented in various forms. These include unbonded, metallic filament; bonded, metallic foil; and bonded piezoresistive or semiconductor gages. The type of gage chosen depends on the application.

Semiconductor (piezoresistive) strain gages are the most common because of their greater sensitivity, small size, and long life. This type of gage exhibits more than 100 times the resistance change for a given strain. This means that, if semiconductor gages are connected in a manner that forms the arms of a Wheatstone bridge (recall our impedance bridge discussion in an earlier chapter), a very large output voltage can be generated. Unfortunately, such large resistance changes result in nonlinear behavior from the bridge with a constant-voltage power supply. This problem can be solved using a constant-current power supply. The key here is to be aware of potential nonlinearities that can impact your measurements.

Strain gages have been used most extensively in speech research into respiration and articulator movement, especially the lips. For example, there is a certain lip movement measurement system that was developed, which uses strain gages that are attached to the lips with an adhesive collar. The gages are anchored by a headband that attaches firmly to the head, so that the gages have a stable platform from which to measure movement. Without this stability, the reading would reflect not only the movement of the lips but the movement of other structures such as the jaw muscles.

This lip movement measuring system serves as a good illustration of a potential problem with interpreting strain gage measurements. Strain gages are sensitive to any deflection of the gage. This deflection may not be all in one direction (up and down), but is more properly regarded as a vector sum of movement in three dimensions (up and down, in and out, and side to side). If the subject being measured can move in more than one dimension, then strain gages should be positioned such that the various dimensional factors can be measured and utilized in an analysis of the motion, In fact, the lip movement measuring system does attempt to do this with a strain gage measuring the thrusting motion of the jaw as well as the up-and-down motion of the jaw. There are other complications as well, and the reader is encouraged to refer to other sources for further information.

There is another system that has been developed to deal with the issue of three-dimensional motion movement. This system uses infrared LEDs that are attached to the structures of interest. Infrared sensors relay the position of these LEDs over time to a computer. The computer generates a series of coordinate positions in three-dimension space from the information provided by the sensors, which are each oriented in one of the three dimensions. Again, users of this system are still mainly laboratories.

Laryngeal Measurement

The larynx is another moving structure of interest to speech scientists. Measurement of laryngeal movement has been accomplished in a variety of ways, including EMG. The two systems described here are only two of several systems that could be used.

Fiberoptic System

The recent development of fiber optics in the communication industry has resulted in a boon for medical researchers. Fiber optics, which refers to the channeling of light by fibers of glass or plastic, were originally developed for telephone systems and data transmission lines. An important advantage of the fiber optics system is its immunity to outside electromagnetic interference. The fiber optic bundle looks like a long, thin tube. This tube is actually composed of many, very small, hollow fibers that are bound together. The center fibers transmit a strong light source toward the area at the tip of the bundle. The surrounding fibers transmit reflected light from the imaged surface back toward a camera. The images are put on film or videotape for later analysis, or they can also be viewed on-line by the physician.

Medical applications of fiber optics include motion sensing and imaging of hard-to-reach structures. The general configuration of a fiber optic system for imaging is shown in Figure 7.6. A good example of this technique in the medical diagnostic field is gastrointestinal endoscopy, which is used to search for cancer in the intestinal tract.

Research into the operation of the larynx can also be done using a fiber optic system. The fiber optic tube is small enough to be pushed through the nasal cavity and into the nasopharynx. The tip is then pointing down toward the larynx, but is not resting on it and is interfering minimally with the production of speech. Despite these advantages, there are two major

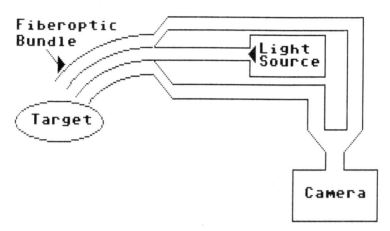

Figure 7.6. Fiberoptic camera system used in medical and research applications for imaging physiological structures.

issues that must be addressed with this system. These are absolute versus relative measurement of glottal movement and aspects of properly viewing the image. The difficulty with regard to absolute measurement of glottal movement with this technique is that the glottal structures are not stable in the field of view. Since the distance from the tip of the fiber optic bundle to the surface being imaged is not constant, absolute measurements of distance are not possible. The other issue is that the fiber optic light source is not always powerful enough to provide sufficient light for viewing the structure with as much detail as desired. Due to the constant movement of the vocal folds and associated structure there are interposing structures that can limit viewing of desired landmarks. Furthermore, the image is being sampled 60 times/s and this is not fast enough to really follow the fine or higher-frequency movements of the laryngeal structures. More light and a higher-speed camera are required to solve this problem. Some researchers have tried to resolve this by using high-speed photography and a different type of imaging system, which is not discussed here.

A computer-assisted technique for making measurements of the relative displacement of videotaped glottal structures has been developed. This system uses a computer interfaced to a video mixer that overlays a cursor onto the display. Through appropriate calibration of the cursor position, relative distance between points on the screen, and hence between landmarks on displayed structures, can be measured. A computer program provides for calibration of the cursor and for making the measurements. It must be emphasized that this system makes *relative* measurements and that the time resolution between successive measurements is limited by the rate at which the screen display is updated, namely, 30 times/s or 33 ms.

Electroglottograph or Laryngograph

Activity of the vocal folds can also be measured with an instrument called a "laryngograph." This device was developed to measure vocal fold activity using a noninvasive procedure. Noninvasive procedures are those that do not require inserting probes into the patient or subject. This is in contrast to the fiber optic procedure, which actually requires a physician to place the fiberscope and to administer any necessary anesthesia. Therefore, the fiberoptic technique would be classified as an "invasive procedure." The advantage of noninvasive procedures is that they are less risky medically and are generally easier to implement clinically. The advantage of invasive procedures is that they generally provide greater accuracy.

Electrodes.   The electrodes for the electroglottograph (EGG) are different than the electrodes described earlier. The EGG electrodes are larger than EMG and AER electrodes, approximately 1¼ inches in diameter as opposed to <½ inch, and are made of lightweight gold-plated aluminum rather than silver-silver chloride. All of the comments made earlier about electrode care also apply to these electrodes.

The electrodes are placed on the subject's neck at the level of the vocal folds, one on each side of the thyroid notch ("Adam's apple"). The electrodes must be applied with a firm pressure to assure good contact, but electrode paste is not used. For adults, a Velcro band is used to secure the electrodes; for children the best results are obtained by having the experimenter or clinician hold the electrodes in place. On-line monitoring of the response on an oscilloscope is helpful here to assure that the electrodoes are properly placed, just as for the EMG measurements. In this case, the patient does a continuous phonation of a vowel, and the electrode placement is adjusted to obtain the maximal amplitude response.

Capturing the Response.   The EGG measures the opening and closing and, to some extent, the motion of the vocal folds. The basic principle in capturing the response is that a small current is passed between two electrodes that are placed on either side of the vocal folds. One of the electrodes serves as the source, and the other serves as the "sensor." The relative impedance is derived from the amount of current passing between the electrodes at any given time. The impedance is determined by the amount of vocal fold contact. When the folds are open, the impedance will be highest and the current lowest because of the open space that the current has to cross or go around. When the folds are closed the situation is just the opposite. Thus, changes in current flow correspond to changes in the transverse electrical impedance or changes in vocal fold contact area.

There are several measurement issues that relate to the impedance change, which is small, and the absolute degree of closure, which is impossible to ascertain for small amounts of opening because of the manner in which the vocal folds open and close. That is, the folds do not open and close with nice clean edges like a sliding glass door, but rather with rounded edges and varying amounts of contact along the depth dimension of the contact surface. Hence, exact measurements of the motion of the vocal folds is precluded. The extent to which motion can be deduced from the waveform coming from the EGG is a theoretical matter, which will not be discussed in this book because the intent of this book is to discuss instrumentation and not the motion of vocal folds.

There is another measurement issue that is amenable to instrumentation: improving the accuracy and viewability of the waveform. This involves two factors: (*a*) random noise that is either generated in the electronics or that results from radio frequency energy picked up by the electrodes; and (*b*) variations in electrical conductance between the electrodes due to movements of structures other than the vocals folds, such as the tongue, velum, or laryngeal musculature. These factors generate a low-frequency component in the output that makes analysis of the waveform very difficult.

A potential solution to this issue is to high-pass filter the output of the EGG to reduce the low-frequency information. However, the analysis of the waveform is based on its temporal properties, and these can be altered by a standard high-pass filter. Thus, it is necessary to use a special filter, such as a linear phase high-pass filter, that will not alter the temporal characteristics of the waveform. Details of this special filter will not be discussed, but the basic point is that this filter permits high-frequency information to pass through without altering the time relations among the frequencies. Thus, the temporal aspects of the waveform are preserved accurately. The waveform itself is usually stored either on a strip chart recorder or on a tape recorder. The latter is recommended as this will permit repeated viewing and more flexibility for off-line analysis.

Respiratory Measurement

Respiration can be measured in a number of ways, but this section will focus on techniques using a *spirometer*. A spirometer is an instrument that directly measures airflow and volume. The common name for the device is a *respirometer*. There is also a technique using *magnetometers* (small magnetic disks for sensing the movement of the chest wall), but this technique will not be discussed here. The technique that is described here involves two types of spirometers: the *static respirometer* and the *ambulatory respirometer*.

Static respirometer measurements are made to determine lung capacity. An example of this instrument is the Collin's respirometer. This measurement can be made by requiring the subject to fully exhale into a variable-volume container after inhaling several times to ensure that the lungs are completely full. The inhalations should be slow with the subject being asked to take deep breaths, not quick breaths that tend to fill only the upper part of the lungs. The exhalation should also be slow. Care should be taken that no air escapes through the nose.

The exhaled air goes into a variable volume with an indicator that varies as the volume varies. The volume itself looks like a large can with a sliding end. As the cavity is filled, the top will slowly rise along with the indicator. The variable volume is calibrated with a known volume of air prior to the measurement. This can be done for everyday purposes by having an experienced user exhale completely, breathe a known volume of air from a calibrated volume, and then exhale into the respirometer. Quick checks can be made by making the measurement on a person whose lung volume is known, in much the same way as quick checks are made on audiometers.

A static respirometer is useful for making measurements of lung capacity, but it is not appropriate for making measurements while the subject is speaking. This is because the user must be blowing into a tube to make the measurement. There are other ways to measure respiration during speech behavior, such as wearing a mask with a pressure transducer that measures airflow as the user speaks; however, these are cumbersome and not very suitable for clinical application. A method that may be useful for clinical application is the ambulatory respirometer (plethysmograph) or "Respitrace."

Respitrace is a brand name for a system that consists of a vest with zig-zag coils of wire (transducers), one of which is centered on the rib cage and the other on the abdomen, and a sensor that translates the output of the two transducers into voltages. There is a constant, very-low-amperage current passing through the wires. As the chest or abdomen changes its circumference, the coil wires will either straighten out more or become more compressed. The wires operate in a manner similar to a strain gage, with the impedance of the wires varying with the amount of coil compression or expansion. As the impedance changes, the current changes, and the amount of movement of the rib cage or abdomen is reflected in the amplitude of the current. The output of the wires is fed into a small box that contains instrumentation to provide rib cage, abdominal, and summed displacements associated with speech and nonspeech breathing.

An important factor in the accuracy of the measurements is the correct placement and anchoring of the vest. This can be critical when using this instrument with children, for whom this instrument is especially applicable. If the vest is positioned improperly, the movements being transduced will not be those associated with the desired structure. Vests come in several sizes to accommodate different patients, but adjustments of the vests is still required to ensure accurate placement of the wire coils. The coils should be level and in the upper region of the rib cage without turning over the top part of the vest; the same is true for the abdomen placement. In addition, the vests should be well anchored in front and back so that they do not slip. The vests are made of a stretch fabric, but they will slip if care is not taken to anchor them properly or to select the right size.

The Respitrace is calibrated using isovolume maneuvers and a "spiro-bag," which is a bag with a calibrated volume. While this works fine with most adults, most young children cannot perform such maneuvers. The device is most suitable for measuring gross aspects of respiratory behavior and for examining the timing aspects of respiration associated with speech. Data are recorded either on a strip chart recorder or on a tape recorder. The latter is recommended as this will permit repeated viewing and more flexibility for off-line analysis.

Chapter Summary

This chapter provided an overview of several types of instruments that measure physiological aspects of speech and hearing behavior. There was no attempt to be comprehensive, and several instruments were mentioned but not described. The focus was physiological measurements in humans. Therefore, physiological measurements in animals were not addressed.

Some general principles were elucidated throughout the chapter. Electrodes for all types of measurements tend to be very similar. The placement technique is critical for all measurements, as is the ability to identify a valid response. Because instrumentation has to be designed and utilized in a way that will not alter the phenomenon being measured, there must be an appropriate way to handle artifacts as these are especially common in physiological measurements. New instrumentation has many more features for making measurements easier and more reliable and for expanding the potential arena of measurements, for example, making physiological measurements in children.

10

Measuring an Auditory Evoked Response

Introduction

*T*he purpose of this laboratory is to measure an auditory evoked response. Either BSER or the late response can be measured; the choice is up to the instructor.

Because Quiklab 10 depends greatly on the availability of special instrumentation that may be especially hard for some readers to acquire, only an outline of the lab is given here.

Method

Apparatus

1. Electrodes;
2. Some means of averaging or measuring responses. This can be a hard-wired signal averager, a computer, or a physiological amplifier connected to an oscilloscope.

Procedure

The electrodes should be attached as described in the chapter. The measurements made will depend on the instrumentation available, but they should include at least a single waveform. The waveform should be repeated in order to assess reliability of the measurement. Preferably, an averaged waveform should be obtained at several signal intensities.

Results

A plot of the waveforms and a tabulation of factors such as reliability and skin resistance should be done. If plots of the amplitude of the waveform are done, these should be made as a function of the signal amplitude.

Discussion

What conclusions did the measurements reveal to the experimenter? Were there any problems that may have affected the measurements?

Measuring Lung Capacity

Introduction

*T*his lab is different in that it may permit some ingenuity by the student and/or instructor. The basic problem is to measure lung capacity.

Because Quiklab 11 depends greatly on the availability of special instrumentation that may be especially hard for some readers to acquire, only an outline of the lab is given here.

Apparatus and Method

If a respirometer is available, use that; if it is not available, use the variable-bag-size technique. If a respirometer is going to be used, refer to the chapter for the respirometer technique. Otherwise, (and this is a *lot* more fun!) figure out how lung capacity could be measured using variable-size bags. How would these be constructed? What is the best procedure? It is up to the students and instructor to come up with the appropriate materials. Be ingenious!

Results and Discussion

These sections should be a straightforward tabulation of the results and a discussion of the strengths and weaknesses of the chosen technique.

8

Instrumentation for Signal Acquisition, Generation, and Analysis

P revious chapters have discussed analog methods of signal generation. This chapter will focus on the use of instruments which use a digital representation for the acquisition, storage, and generation of acoustic signals and electrical signals which are based on acoustic events. The waveform analysis portion of this chapter will discuss both analog and digital techniques.

Waveform Acquisition and Generation

There are two methods for representing real-world signals:

1. An analog representation, in which the three domains of signal representation are continuous, that is, they can be any number, fractional or otherwise;
2. A digital representation, in which the three domains of signal representation are discrete, that is, they are restricted to a specific set of numbers.

The first method will be discussed very briefly, with the rest of the discussion of signal acquisition and generation focusing on the digital method.

Analog and Digital Signal Representation

An analog representation of a signal is a continuous version of the signal; that is, there are no discontinuities or breaks in the waveform. The digital waveform is a discontinuous version of the signal; that is, the signal is represented as a series of steps, with the amplitude at the beginning of the step representing the amplitude at that moment in time. This basic difference in representation of a signal has many implications. For example, each step in a digital waveform has some finite duration; therefore, by the end of the step there will be a difference between the original waveform and the digital waveform if the amplitude has changed during that time. This will not be true for the analog waveform. How to make digital signals accurately represent analog signals and how to go back and forth between the two domains will be one of the major topics of this chapter.

Figure 8.1 shows an original signal waveform and the corresponding analog and digital waveforms, if we assume no distortion in the representation. Note that the analog representation is a copy of the original. The typical pictorial representations of waveforms are analog; that is, the waveforms are continuous and smooth. What is meant by continuous and smooth?

The terms *continuous* and *smooth* actually have mathematical connotations, but for our purposes it is simpler to think of continuous and smooth as meaning that there are no breaks in the waveform. That is, no matter how small the difference between the numbers representing adjacent points in an analog waveform, there is theoretically always a number between them for a continuous waveform. The importance of this concept and how well it applies in the real world will be seen later when analog and digital methods are contrasted.

Figure 8.1 shows that the digital waveform is very different from the analog and original waveform. It is composed of a series of steps. Actually

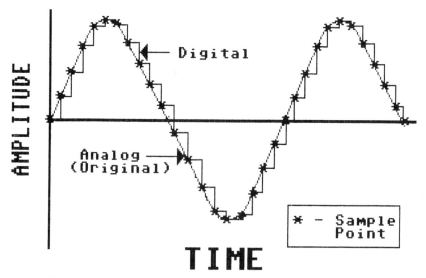

Figure 8.1. Analog (original) versus digital sinusoidal waveform.

this is just a plot of what happens when a signal is converted to digital form. The actual transformation is from a smooth, continuous situation to a series of numbers representing instantaneous amplitudes of the waveform at particular points in time. Until the next sample is taken, the digital representation stays at a constant value. The degree of correspondence between the original waveform and the digital representation of it depends primarily on two factors: the range of numbers available (Fig. 8.2), and how often the numbers are derived from the waveform or sample rate.

Figure 8.2 shows two levels of digital representation: One level that has only four amplitude values available to match to the waveform, and another level with many amplitude values available. It is obvious that the grain is determined by the number of numbers available. Figure 8.3 illustrates the effect of sample rate.

Figure 8.3 displays three waveforms. The two digital waveforms represent different sample rates. The figure shows that as the sample rate is increased the digital waveform more closely approximates the original waveform. In fact, if too few samples are taken (<2/cycle) the original waveform cannot be reconstructed from the digital waveform. There will be further discussion of these two factors later in the chapter.

Analog and digital waveforms require different types of storage and generation instrumentation. The next section describes some of the necessary instrumentation.

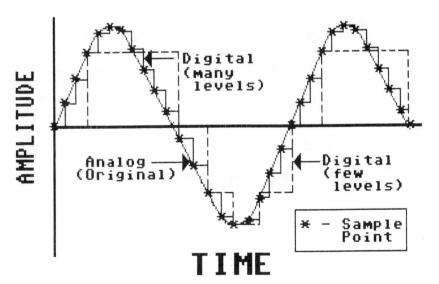

Figure 8.2. Effects of number of levels on digital waveform representation.

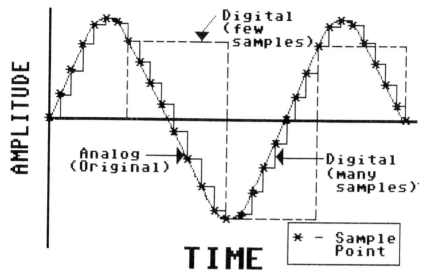

Figure 8.3. Effects of number of samples on digital waveform representation.

Analog Recording and Generation

Previous chapters have covered instrumentation which does analog signal acquisition, namely, various types of tape recorders. Since they and the necessary transducers were discussed earlier in chapter 6, they will only be mentioned here as examples of analog signal-acquisition instrumentation. Two additional methods of recording are oscilloscopes (storage and nonstorage, with storage scopes permitting permanent storage through pictures) and various forms of *x-y* recorders, including oscillographs. Oscillographs, which were mentioned in the previous chapter, are simply very-high-speed strip chart recorders that use a "light pen" to burn a trace on photographic paper rather than an ink pen. Their advantage is their ability to record higher-frequency waveforms than the standard strip chart recorder. Their disadvantage is the amount and expense of the paper required to do the storage.

The signal generators discussed in earlier chapters were all analog signal generators. That is, the signals were generated by circuitry that operated with voltage levels. As a foundation for later contrasting of analog and digital techniques, specifications and the generally expected levels of accuracy (as shown by distortion), signal-to-noise ratio, and absolute noise level from analog recorders and signal generators will be briefly described.

A standard function generator will produce a sine wave signal with harmonic distortion of 0.5% or about −46 dB relative to the peak amplitude of the signal. Signal-to-noise ratios will be about 60–80 dB. The absolute noise level can range from 100 μV to 5 mV which may or may not be a problem, depending on the transducer and the environment for the signal. Similar specifications exist for most analog recorders. If dedicated or special instrumentation is used, then these specifications can be improved. For example, a sine wave generator capable of 0.03% (−70 dB) harmonic distortion is available, as are recorders with this amount of distortion and signal-to-noise ratios of 90 dB.

Digital Recording and Generation

Digital recording and generating instrumentation operates with voltage levels at the input and output, but all internal circuitry operates with numbers. This means that the voltage levels being input and output from the instrumentation must be converted from voltages to numbers and vice versa. The hardware devices that perform the conversion are called "analog-to-digital" (A/D, voltage to numbers) and "digital-to-analog" (D/A, numbers to voltages) converters.

Digital-to-Analog Converters

The digital-to-analog (D/A) converters will be covered first because they are frequently used as part of an analog-to-digital (A/D) converter. Most D/A converters use a current summation technique. The D/A is based on a set of switches, in combination with a reference voltage. The switches are actually part of a resistor ladder coming from the reference. Recall the discussion of how an attenuator works and the earlier discussion in chapter 2 of a voltage divider. For our discussion here the implementation of the voltage ladder is not critical. Figure 8.4 illustrates one implementation of a D/A using an R-2R resistor ladder. The number representing the desired output voltage is sent to the D/A with some resolution; for example, the number is accurate to 1 part in 256. To represent this resolution in terms of on/off switches would require eight switches. (For now, take this on faith. The binary number system will be explained in the next chapter.) The amount of voltage represented by each switch is some multiple of 1/256 times 2. The number is converted to a binary number, a set of ones and zeros, to turn each switch on or off. An example of how this works will be described.

For our example, we want to output a voltage of 1 volt. The reference voltage for our D/A is 5.12 volts. The resolution of the D/A is one part in 256. Equation 1 gives the general equation for voltage (V out and V ref) and number (N) relations in a D/A. Equation 2 shows the algebraic representation of what has been described so far.

$$V \text{ out} = \text{sum}(V \text{ switches})/\text{resolution} \times V \text{ ref} \qquad (1)$$

$$1V = \text{sum}(V \text{ switches})/256 \times 5.12 \qquad (2)$$

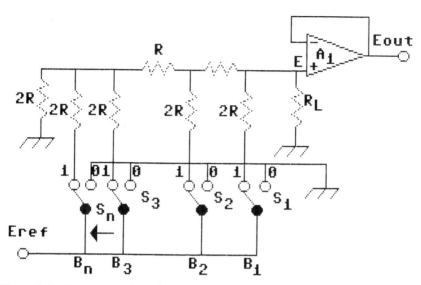

Figure 8.4. Implementation of a digital-to-analog (D/A) converter using an R-2R resistor ladder.

The number to be sent to the D/A is represented by the sum(V switches), and in this case the sum of the switches has to equal 50, as shown by Equation 3. Similar calculations can be done for any set of parameters described by Equation 1, namely, output voltage, number, resolution, and reference voltage.

$$\text{sum } (V \text{ switches}) = 256 \times 1V/5.12 = 50 \qquad (3)$$

Analog-to-Digital Converters

There are several types of methods used to perform analog-to-digital (A/D) conversion. Some of these are *integration, voltage-to-frequency, parallel, binary counter* (also called "servo" or "ramp") and the *successive-approximation* methods. The voltage-to-frequency and binary counter methods will not be described, although it should be noted that the binary counter and successive approximation methods are very similar in concept.

Integration Converters

The integration converter method is described here so that the reader is aware of the technique. Because of its slower speed, it is not a recommended technique for audio work. The integration converter method (Fig. 8.5) consists of an input control switch, an operational amplifier integrator (voltage summer), a comparator (compares two voltages and outputs a signal when they are equal), a clock-driven binary counter, and a control-logic section that "ties the whole thing together."

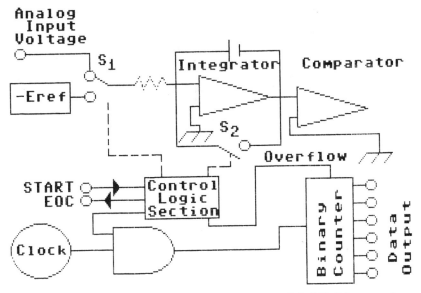

Figure 8.5. Dual-slope integrator used for analog-to-digital (A/D) conversions

A signal at the start input clears everything and connects the analog input to the integrator. The output of the integrator will start rising, and the counter will start counting. The comparator is connected to ground. When the counter overflows, the reference voltage is connected to the integrator input. At this time the counter is back to zero. Since the reference has a polarity opposite that of the analog input, the integrator will start discharging and the counter will start counting again. When the integrator output has discharged all the way back to zero, the comparator will send out a signal to the control logic to stop the counter and send an end-of-conversion signal. The number in the counter (data output) will be proportional to the analog input voltage applied to the input.

The integrating type of converter is too slow to follow high-frequency signals, but is considered very good for low-frequency signals because of its inherently good noise rejection. An integrator is a form of low-pass filter, so noise artifacts are reduced. This type of converter is often used in digital multimeters because of this feature.

Parallel Converters

The parallel (or "flash") converter method is used in our field for some video applications. The key factor for this type of A/D (Fig. 8.6) is that the voltage at the input is routed to a parallel set of comparators. Thus all comparators compare the reference voltage, stepped down by the appro-

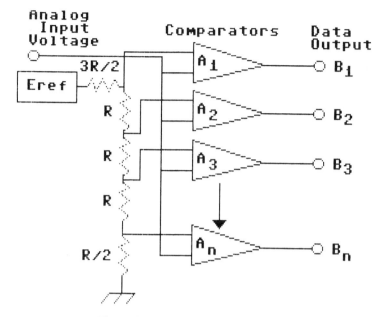

Figure 8.6.   Parallel A/D converter.

priate factor for that comparator, and the input voltage at the same time. This results in the fastest type of converter.

In addition to the fact that there must be sufficient comparator circuits for the resolution of the A/D, the outputs of the comparators must be encoded into a number, which requires additional control logic. These converters are very fast (in the billionths-of-a-second range), but because of the amount of circuitry required, they are very expensive. The cost, combined with the fact that such high speeds are seldom required in audio work, means that "flash" converters are restricted to the video field.

Successive-Approximation Converters

The type of converter that is most common in the audio field is the successive-approximation converter (Fig. 8.7). The main components of this type of converter are a D/A, a comparator, a shift register, register output latches, a clock, and a logic control section. The parallel output lines from the shift register are connected to the digital input lines of the D/A, with the output of the D/A connected to the negative input of the comparator. The positive input of the comparator is connected to the analog input voltage. Thus the comparator will send a positive or high signal to the control logic, which activates the current-latched line, whenever the analog input voltage is higher than the D/A voltage.

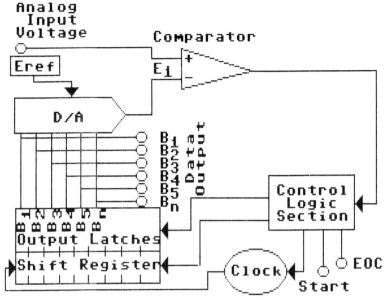

Figure 8.7.   Successive-approximation A/D converter.

Basic operation of this A/D involves setting the D/A 1 bit at a time and testing with the comparator to see if the bit should remain set or be reset. Testing begins with the start signal, which clears the latches and the shift register. At each clock tick, a line in the shift register is set and the corresponding output latch is set also. This causes the D/A to output a voltage corresponding to the binary sum of the bits that have been set to that point. The comparator sends a positive or negative output depending on whether the analog input signal is greater or less than the D/A output voltage, respectively. If the signal is positive, the latched line is left set; otherwise the line is cleared. This is done until all lines have been tested. The end-of-conversion signal is then sent. The resulting value now sits in the output latches and is available to be read as data. The number of lines represents the resolution of the A/D, and although eight lines are shown in Figure 8.7, the operation is the same regardless of the number of lines.

The successive-approximation converter is popular because it is fast, although not as fast as the parallel converter, and relatively cheap. The accuracy and stability are good, and the converter is easy to implement and drive from software. As with all instrumentation, there is the requirement for regular checks to ensure proper performance within specifications.

Two notes regarding this type of A/D converter: First, the speed of conversion will be the same for each conversion and will be a function of the speed of the D/A and the number of lines. Thus, an 8-bit successive-approximation converter will be faster than a 12-bit successive-approximation converter, all other things being equal. Second, there is a built-in error of one-half the size of the smallest step. Recall that the comparison is driven by the D/A output voltage and the D/A output voltage is driven by the shift register. The value of the smallest voltage change that can be produced in the D/A by the least significant line of the shift register represents limits of resolution for the A/D. The comparator can only sense voltage shifts that vary more than one-half this value because there is no next step to provide the comparator with a close-enough voltage.

Factors Affecting Accuracy of Signal Acquisition and Generation

It must be emphasized that A/Ds provide an *estimate* of the waveform. As with all estimates, there will always be errors in the estimated waveform. There are two major sources of error in the acquisition and generation of signals using digital processing techniques. These are quantization error and sampling error, which were illustrated by Figures 8.1 and 8.2, respectively and are now treated more extensively.

Quantization Error

Quantization relates to the range of the number system or level-of-information representation used in the conversion. Interestingly, there is no one-to-one correspondence between a computer's level-of-information representation and that of the A/D. Most current microcomputers use 8 and/or 16 bits to represent information internally, with 32-bit representations becoming more common. However, all of these machines use A/Ds that gather data in chunks ranging from 4 to 16 bits. Just because a computer may use a certain number of bits to represent information internally does not mean that A/Ds with greater or lesser resolution cannot be used with that machine.

Quantization error refers to the noise introduced into the signal-representation process by the size of the steps between adjacent points in the waveform. Understanding of this concept requires that a couple of factors be discussed here. First is the error of estimation of amplitude. The fewer the numbers available to represent the waveform, the larger the steps between adjacent points. This results in a larger difference between the actual and estimated waveform amplitude, with a correspondingly larger error. The second factor is the shape of the estimated waveform itself. Figure 8.1 shows that the estimated waveform looks like a series of pulses on pedestals of varying height. The pulses are not the same as the waveform and will generate sound based on their amplitude and pulse width. It turns out that pulses have a very broad spectrum, and so the pulses create a broadband sound. The fewer the numbers available to estimate the waveform, the greater will be the amplitude of the pulses and the greater the noise. Conversely, the greater the range of numbers, the smaller the errors and the smaller the noise.

An A/Ds resolution in the amplitude domain is described in terms of the number of bits. The system used is a binary system just as for computers. Thus, an 8-bit system has a resolution of 256 steps, a 12-bit system has a resolution of 4,096 steps. Keep in mind that the number of bits refers only to the resolution of the D/A or A/D, not the absolute value of each step. This is determined by the range of the A/D or D/A. To get the step size in absolute units, divide the voltage range by the number of steps for the A/D or D/A as determined by the number of bits.

The number of bits in the A/D or D/A also has implications for the noise floor of the converter. This is because the resolution of the converter also determines the imprecision of the converter. (This is another case of viewing a glass as half-full or half-empty: When it is half-full we are talking about resolution, when it is half-empty we are talking about error.) The relation between number of steps available for representing the waveform and the accuracy of the waveform was shown graphically. The fewer the number of steps, the greater the error. Since this error varies randomly, due to variations in the converter's error, the error results in a noisy waveform overlaying the actual waveform. The greater the error, the greater the amplitude of the noise relative to the estimated waveform. The noise relative to the signal amplitude can be calculated based on the number of bits. The noise level in a converter is calculated as shown in Equation 4, where A is the maximum amplitude of the converter and N is the number of bits.

$$\text{Noise in dB} = 20 \log (A/2N) \tag{4}$$

It can be seen from Equation 4 that as the number of bits increases, the noise amplitude decreases. However, if the maximum amplitude of the converter increases, the noise increases as long as the number of bits stays constant. Thus the noise level in a converter is always relative to the signal amplitude and the number of bits. For acoustic work, a 12-bit converter with a range of ±5 volts is usually sufficient, although the audible range is approximately 23 bits for a normal listener. Beyond a certain point, limitations in other equipment are more of a restriction than the converter's limitations.

Sampling Error

Estimation of a waveform by a converter involves estimation of amplitude at specific times. Sampling error is based on the time interval between estimated points on the waveform. Continuous waveforms are continuous in both amplitude and time. Recall the earlier discussion of the term *continuous.* The digital conversion process is discrete in both time and amplitude. Thus just as there are errors related to the magnitude of the step size in amplitude, there are errors related to the magnitude of the step size in time. This translates to sampling rate, with the higher sampling rates having smaller time step sizes. Figure 8.3 shows the relation between the original waveform, digital representation, and error of estimation.

As is the case with the error in amplitude estimation, the error in sampling results in noise. The error in this case is not amplitude noise, but an error in the estimation of frequency. There is a rule, referred to as the *Nyquist sampling frequency*, which specifies the minimum sampling rate necessary in order for the sampled waveform to have the same frequencies as the original waveform. The Nyquist sampling frequency is twice the highest frequency in the waveform.

Violation of the Nyquist sampling frequency rule results in a particular error in conversion. This error is called "aliasing," which is the appearance in the estimated waveforms of frequencies which were not in the original. These frequencies occur at multiples of the original waveform frequencies. This error can be avoided by filtering the waveform prior to conversion for A/Ds and after conversion for D/As. These filters, referred to as "anti-aliasing" filters, are low-pass filters set at a frequency that is one-half or less of the sampling frequency of the converter. In practice, the filters should be set at 40% of the sampling frequency. This is recommended because almost all filters have some roll-off and do not exclude all frequencies above the cutoff frequency. By setting the filters at 40% of the sampling frequency, we can ensure that all of the frequencies above the cutoff frequency are rejected and all aliased frequencies are eliminated.

Another potential source for error that should be noted is that the analog input voltage has to be within the dynamic range of the A/D. This may seem like a trivial comment, but most A/Ds are protected from overvoltage conditions and hence will yield a value for voltages that are above the upper limit for the A/D. This clearly results in an erroneous value. With a fluctuating signal the peaks of the signal should be carefully controlled to be within the maximum input range of the A/D.

These sections have described a number of aspects of digital signal acquisition and conversion; however, there are also analog signal generators and analyzers. The focus here has been digital because this is the newer technology and it is generally displacing analog instrumentation. Analog instrumentation is still very common, however; the next section describes both analog and digital instrumentation used for signal generation and analysis.

Signal Acquisition and Generation Instrumentation

Analog and digital instrumentation, which is designed to acquire, record, and/or generate signals, is an integral part of any laboratory or clinical program. A brief overview of analog and digital instrumentation is given first; this is followed by a description of instrumentation and techniques for signal analysis. It should be noted that much of the existing instrumentation for signal acquisition, presentation, and analysis uses analog technology, digital technology, or some combination of the two. The next description of digital instrumentation will build on the techniques and concepts described so far; therefore, be sure that the first part of this chapter is understood before proceeding.

Analog Instrumentation

Most of the equipment described to this point is analog instrumentation, so the principles of operation will not need to be discussed here. In fact, almost all the instrumentation discussed in chapter 3, which covered test instrumentation, was analog instrumentation. Examples of this type of instrumentation are oscilloscopes, tape recorders, x-y plotters, and signal generators. There are also analog devices for signal analysis such as spectrum and distortion analyzers.

It should be pointed out that just because an instrument uses integrated circuits it is not necessarily digital; it could be a solid-state instrument. There are many analog devices that come on a *chip*. The chip represents a miniaturized form of the analog components. This is similar to the confusion generated by the term "digital" meters, which implies digital technology but in fact simply means that the meter displays numbers rather than using a needle display. There may be cases in which digital instrumentation will be solid state, but this does not always have to be the case. Recall that the first digital computers were mechanical devices, not electronic.

Digital Instrumentation

It is becoming increasingly more routine to use digital techniques in common instrumentation such as the oscilloscope and signal generators. In fact, most digital instrumentation represents the application of digital technology to analog instrumentation. Some instruments, such as spectrum and distortion analyzers, use largely digital components due to some inherent advantages of digital technology in this area, but other instruments, such as tape recorders, still use a lot of analog technology. Many instruments, such as plotters, are hybrids of analog and digital instrumentation, with the interface and control logic in the plotter being digital and the mechanical plotter drivers being analog. Also keep in mind that all digital instrumentation that generates or analyzes analog signals needs a portion of the circuitry devoted to analog instrumentation (amplifiers on the input side to make sure the signal is at an optimal amplitude for conversion, and amplifiers on the output side for volume control).

Digital technology is applied to analysis instrumentation in two ways.

The first is for control logic; the example given above was the plotter. Control logic is generally the first step in the application of digital technology because it is the easiest and least expensive to implement, since the control logic is generally much cheaper than converters. Digital control logic is commonly referred to as "intelligence" and usually takes the form of an added microprocessor and some supporting circuitry. The microprocessor permits programmability to be added to the instrument and enhances its flexibility, as well as adding additional functionality. The microprocessor also helps prevent obsolescence because the instrument can be upgraded by new programming rather than having to rebuild whole sections of circuitry. Of course, the circuitry that is available in the instrument still limits what can be programmed, but the range of choices increases.

The second way digital technology is applied to instrumentation is in the signal path. That is, once the signal enters the instrument, it is treated as a digital signal. This requires the addition of A/D and D/A converters and is usually the second step in the conversion of analog instrumentation into digital instrumentation. The normal setup is to have matched pairs of A/D and D/A converters "multiplexed" according to the number of channels in the devices. A *multiplexer* is a device that switches rapidly between channels so that a single device can service several channels. This keeps the cost down, and the increasing availability of cheap multiplexers and converters has resulted in an increase in completely digitized instruments (with the caveat noted above for input and output amplifiers).

The computer is the most widely known digital instrument. The computer is a general-purpose tool, but has been used for the specific applications of signal generation and analysis. The general-purpose nature of the computer is very useful for handling a variety of tasks associated with signal analysis, such as database management and human interface. It should also be noted that computers are frequently built into other special-purpose instrumentation, such as sound level meters, in order to control added functions.

Waveform Analysis

The preceding overview of analog and digital instrumentation shows that the instrumentation is very similar, and it is primarily the means of implementing control or the signal paths that differ. Thus the most important aspect of signal analysis is not necessarily whether the instrument is analog or digital but rather how to use the instrumentation to do the waveform analysis. The next section discusses some of those applications.

Waveform Sources

Signals that would be analyzed by digital and analog instruments, as well as some additional instruments to be described next, can come from a variety of sources. Examples are rotary engines, such as propellers, the ear, the voice, and laboratory and clinical instrumentation. Each of these presents special problems because of their form of vibration, frequency characteristics, accessibility, and temporal characteristics. In order to do signal analysis for this variety of signals a variety of techniques are required. Availability of equipment sometimes may constrain the types of analyses that can be done. Techniques run the gamut from quick and easy to difficult (and usually expensive); some of these techniques are discussed next.

Visual Analysis

Visual analysis is the most common and usually the first level of analysis. Sometimes the analysis cannot be done any other way with available instrumentation because of the judgmental nature of the analysis. Two examples of visual analysis are presented: analysis of a waveform with an oscilloscope and analysis of a video image. The instrumentation will not be described in detail here, the focus will be on the nature of the analysis.

Most laboratories and clinics have an oscilloscope, which is probably the most common type of analysis instrumentation. It has the advantage of being easy to use, and the output is in a form that is fairly easy to understand. The user should be aware that it does lack precision, but for many analyses it is just fine.

Commonly, there is some question about a signal generated by a particular piece of instrumentation such as an audiometer. An oscilloscope is attached to the output of the device under test. For visual analysis it is almost essential to use a storage scope. The first task is to adjust the oscilloscope to show the waveform. (This was discussed in chapter 3, and that section should be reread if there are uncertainties about how to use an oscilloscope.)

After the waveform is displayed properly there are several aspects of the waveform that can be analyzed visually. First, the frequency can be estimated. Second, the waveform shape can be examined. The expected waveform shape should be known and compared to the actual. If distortion is suspected, look for small ripples along the waveform. Most distortion is at higher frequencies than the signal frequency and so will show up as higher-frequency ripples along the signal waveform. Third, the duration of the signal can be checked. Finally, the amplitude of the signal can be checked. The caveat for all of these analyses is the degree of accuracy. For example, as the signal duration increases, the time per division on the oscilloscope will increase and the absolute error will increase. However, the preceding discussion shows that for a first-level look at a signal, a visual analysis using an oscilloscope provides quite a bit of information.

Another example of visual analysis is video image analysis of speech physiology. This analysis usually results in a categorical analysis. This is because of the lack of easily standardized measures for video images of physiological speech structures. This is a good example of an area where the experience of the viewer is essential to the analysis. The only way to get such experience is to do it and have the analysis supervised by an experienced person. There are some things that can make such an analysis easier. First, use as high a resolution monitor as can be afforded. This investment will not only reduce eye strain but will permit more accurate visualization and measurement of the video image. Second, pick easily visualized landmarks for orientation. For moving and changing images, it is especially important to have more than one landmark, as landmarks may get obscured by other structures. Finally, try to pick at least a relative measuring system and apply it across images of the same type. This will permit comparison across images and also permit others to have a rigorous procedure for analysis. It is best to start with relative measures because many video images do not permit absolute measurement schemes. It is also important to know the limitations of the video image in terms of resolution and timing. This was discussed in the chapter on physiological measurements.

Visual analysis is especially useful for spotting gross errors or suggesting further analyses. If a particular potential problem shows up, then a single instrument focusing on that aspect of the waveform can be used. The next section briefly discusses the use of single instruments.

Single-Instrument Analysis

The use of single instruments was discussed in the chapter on test instrumentation, so this treatment will be very brief. Single instruments that could be used are any of the instruments described in chapter 3, such as a frequency counter or voltmeter, that analyze a single aspect of the waveform. The primary advantage of single instruments over visual analysis is greater accuracy.

The sophistication of more advanced analyzers has increased to the point that they can be used as well as single instruments, but the cost is considerably more so single instruments are still very useful. In addition, there are many cases when there is only one measurement parameter of interest; for example, when there is a need to monitor only the amplitude of a signal. For this application, it is much more cost effective to dedicate a voltmeter to the task rather than a more sophisticated device such as a spectrum analyzer. There are other cases where a more sophisticated analysis is required, and such instruments will now be described.

Spectrum Analysis

Spectrum analysis is employed to get more accurate information about several aspects of the signal. In some ways it is a more powerful form of visual analysis because it evaluates all the same aspects of the waveform. This is always an instrumentation-based analysis, but the intent of this section is to describe some of the principles behind spectrum analysis and to show the applicability of spectrum analysis techniques to speech and hearing.

Spectrum analysis is a fine-grained look at the content of a signal, and it is implicit in the description of signals used for hearing and of the spectrographs of speech. The intent of this section is to describe some of the theory behind spectrum analysis using an intuitive approach dealing with the relation between the shape of a waveform and its spectral content rather than a heavy mathematical treatment of spectral analysis. The examples used will be a sine wave and a pulse, which have very different waveform shapes and spectral content. The next section will describe various signal analysis instrumentation, along with application examples.

A theory by Fourier is the basis for spectral analysis. In this theory the sine wave is the simplest waveform from a spectral point of view, although the waveform shape is anything but simple. Figure 8.8 shows a sine wave and the associated spectrum. As has been noted before, the sine wave shape can be derived from a point on a rotating circle. This analogy of a rotating circle is apt because it points out the three aspects of the sinusoidal waveform: the amplitude, which is equal to the radius of the circle; the frequency, which is the rotation rate of the point on the circle; and the

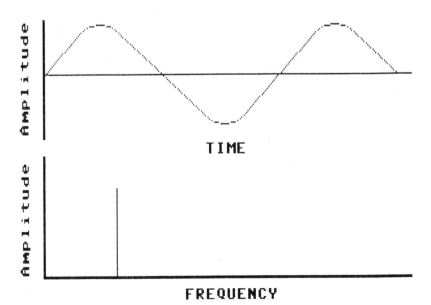

Figure 8.8.   Time waveform and spectrum for sine wave.

phase, which is the location of the point when the circle starts rotating. (Phase was discussed extensively in the treatment of impedance in chapter 2, and that discussion should be reviewed if necessary.) All three aspects of the waveform can be described in spectral analysis, although most analyses focus on the amplitude and frequency aspects. Phase is not a focus because it is not clear what the ear does with phase information, and so this information has been de-emphasized for most speech and hearing applications. However, in other areas such as radio electronics, phase information is extremely important; phase information in speech will probably become more important as more is learned about speech perception.

Figure 8.8 shows that the spectrum associated with a sine wave that starts at zero is a single line on a spectral plot. Fourier's theory maintains that all waveforms consist of a sum of sine waves. To describe the waveforms, the instrument user must know the frequency, amplitude, and phase of the sine waves comprising the waveform. Spectrum analysis is the process of determining those components. To get some idea of how the theory works we will use a pulse train as an example. In order to simplify the analysis as much as possible, we will assume the frequency of the pulse train to be the same as the sine wave shown in Figure 8.8. Figure 8.9 shows the pulse train overlaying the sine wave.

Figure 8.9 shows the pulse train that will be used for the analysis. To derive the spectrum, we must break the pulse train into its component

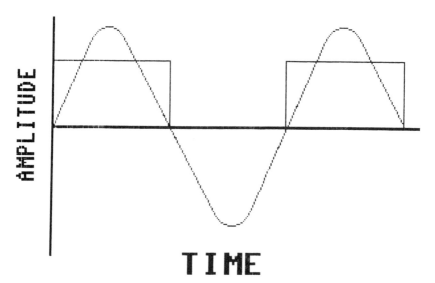

Figure 8.9.   Sine wave and pulse train of the same frequency.

aspects of amplitude, frequency, and phase. The amplitude has been chosen such that the energy in each pulse is equal to one-half the energy in the sine wave. The frequency of the pulse train is the same as the sine wave. (Note: When talking about pulse train "frequency", the term "repetition rate" is frequently employed. Both terms mean the same thing.) The pulse train is starting at zero at the same time as the sine wave (although this is not obvious from the figure because of the zero rise time of the first pulse). Do all these similarities mean that the pulse train has the same spectrum as the sine wave? Figure 8.10 shows the spectra for the sine wave and the pulse train. What concept is being shown in this figure?

The key to the difference in spectra between the sine wave and the pulse train is the difference in waveform shape. Note that each pulse in the pulse train goes immediately to full amplitude, whereas the sine wave gradually approaches full amplitude. If a series of sine waves of increasing frequency were shown, we could see that as the frequency increases, the waveform approaches full amplitude more quickly. This implies that high frequencies are required to generate each pulse. Further examination of the pulse shows that it also remains at a single amplitude for much longer than the sine wave, which is a constantly changing amplitude. These slowly varying portions of the waveform, as well as the time separation between, would require frequencies at least as low as the frequency of the sine wave. There are also the square corners that are sharper than the corners of the sine

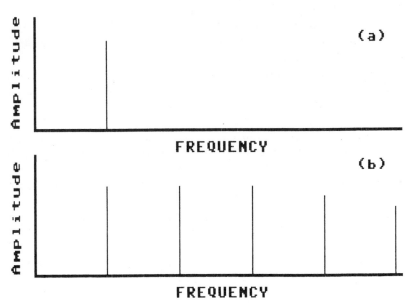

Figure 8.10.   Spectra for sine wave (*a*) and pulse train (*b*) from Fig. 8.9.

wave and would require a combination of low and high frequencies to get the square corner and the flat parts on each side of the corner. Thus, this intuitive analysis shows that both high and low frequencies are needed to generate the pulse train; this is shown in Figure 8.10.

What about the phase and amplitude aspects of the pulse train? The amplitude of the pulse train is more complicated to figure out because it depends on the pulse width, with a longer pulse width emphasizing the lower frequencies (it is staying at a particular amplitude longer and at zero for less time) and a short pulse width emphasizing the higher frequencies (it is staying at a particular amplitude for less time and at zero longer). The result is that pulse trains with very brief pulses have flatter spectra than pulse trains with longer pulses. Review of the effects of rise/fall time in chapter 5 may help to understand this aspect because it is based on the same principles, although it is explained differently.

The phase aspect of the pulse train is relatively simple to figure out. To keep the square corners in synchrony throughout the pulse train, along with the fact that the first pulse in the pulse train began at zero, all the frequencies that make up the square corners have to start at the same phase. In this case the phase is 90 degrees. The phase response would be shown as a series of dots with a value of +90 at the frequencies of the harmonics of the frequency of the pulse train.

Analog Spectrum Analysis

How does signal analysis instrumentation do the same type of analysis that was required to extract the components of a sine wave or pulse train? There are two primary methods employed by spectrum analyzers. The first method, which is primarily associated with analog instrumentation, is to use a scanning filter to find the frequencies in the waveform and to output the amplitude of each component (Fig. 8.11). For example, with the sine wave such an instrument would place a very high resolution filter at a low frequency and progressively increase the center frequency of the filter until it had scanned some preset range of frequencies. The sine wave would be input continuously into the instrument, and when the frequency of the filter equaled the frequency of the sine wave, the sine wave would come through the filter and the voltmeter would read the amplitude of the sine wave.

Several points must be considered when using this type of spectrum analyzer. The first consideration is the bandwidth of the filter, which affects the output of the device. The key point is the relationship between changes as a function of frequency in the signal being analyzed and the bandwidth of the analyzer. For example, if the bandwidth of the scanning filter is 50 Hz, then the signal energy will be summed within the filter for 25 Hz on each side of the center frequency of the filter, giving a flat output over a

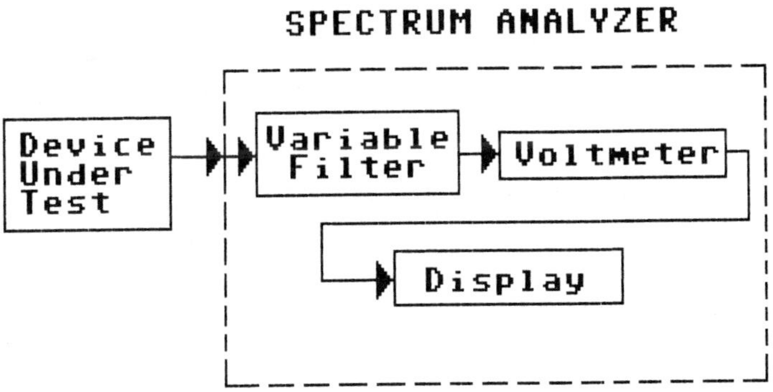

SPECTRUM ANALYZER

Figure 8.11.   Scanning filter spectrum analyzer.

50 Hz range. To examine how the filter bandwidth is interacting with the output, change the bandwidth to a smaller value and see if the same output occurs. In general, if it is suspected that the signal consists of discrete frequency components, the smallest available bandwidth should be used.

A second consideration with a scanning filter analyzer is the scanning rate. Most analyzers permit setting the scanning rate. However, as the filter bandwidth becomes narrower, the analysis time necessary for a valid output becomes longer. This reciprocity between time and frequency has been encountered before, and the same general principle applies here. Some analyzers will report when the scanning rate is too high for a particular bandwidth. (There is no such thing as "too long" an analysis time. It is just an inconvenience.) Other analyzers will not report this, and some caution should be applied. If very narrow bandwidths are employed, just be sure to have the filter scan slowly enough for valid data.

A final consideration is that the analog analyzer is not capturing the signal, and so must have the signal continuously present in order to do the analysis. For continuous signals this is not a problem, but for transient signals it is necessary to repeatedly pulse the signal in order for the signal to be present as the filter scans the frequency range. The problem with this is that pulsing a signal results in the same kind of spectral spread that was discussed earlier for the pulse train. This can lead to an erroneous estimate of the frequency spectrum of the signal because the effects of the pulsing get added to the spectrum of the signal itself. When analyzing transient signals with a spectrum analyzer that uses filter scanning technology, be aware of this problem and compensate for it by eliminating the spectral spreading due to the pulsing from the analysis. The effects will be the same as for the pulse width of pulses in a pulse train; that is, the duration of the transient signal and the presentation rate will interact. The longer the duration of the transient signal, the narrower the spectral spread due to the signal itself. The slower the presentation rate, the better the spectrum as long as the scan rate is kept very slow. This difficulty with handling transient signals is probably the major drawback to analog spectrum analyzers.

Digital Spectrum Analysis

In digital spectrum analysis (Fig. 8.12) the signal is first converted to digital form. The spectrum is computed using a fast Fourier transform (FFT), which is a mathematical method for extracting the spectral components based on Fourier's theory, and then the resulting spectrum is displayed or sent to storage media.

This method is not without its own problems. First, all of the issues dealing with A/D conversion, such as sample rate, amplitude range, and number of bits, apply to these devices. Second, there is usually a limited storage capability, which must be kept in mind when doing an analysis of long-duration signals such as speech signals. Finally, these analyzers do not have unlimited resolution. When a spectrum is computed, the analysis is limited by the number of points analyzed. The greater the number of points analyzed and the longer the time window, which are closely related, the greater the resolution. However, the calculation time is not a linear function of the number of points, but is closer to a power function. Thus, twice the resolution can take four times as long, three times the resolution will take nine times as long, etc. Infinite resolution thus requires infinite time, which is not a design goal for most analyzers. The tradeoff is determined by the speed of calculations and available memory.

The resolution of digital spectrum analyzers is rated in terms of the number of components calculated for a spectrum. The frequencies at which the component values are calculated is based on the frequency range selected. However, the number of components is fixed. Thus a 1,024-line

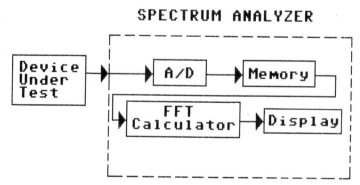

Figure 8.12.   Fast Fourier transform (FFT) digital spectrum analyzer.

analyzer (the number of lines is almost always a power of 2 because of the binary character of digital calculations) will always calculate 1,024 components that are equally spaced within the frequency range selected. The greater the number of components, the better the resolution, but the cost will be proportionally greater.

The real power of digital spectrum analyzers is shown with transient signals. The signal can be captured in memory, and the spectrum can be computed without the confusing effects of pulsing the signal. In addition, many of these analyzers are real time; that is, the spectrum is displayed as the signal is being presented. Actually there is a time lag of up to 20–40 ms, but it is so close that the eye and ear perceive it as simultaneous. Thus, the spectrum of a transient signal can be quickly and easily determined.

Signal Analysis Instrumentation

Several instruments used for signal analysis will now be described. This list is not intended to be exhaustive, but rather to be illustrative so that the student will be able to generalize to new instrumentation that might be best applied for a particular type of analysis.

Oscilloscope.   This device was discussed earlier because of its ability to do visual analysis of waveforms. It is extremely flexible for this application as long as reasonable care is taken to recognize the limitations on accuracy (do not try to analyze voltages to the third decimal place). The primary application of the oscilloscope is as a diagnostic tool and for some quick analysis work such as checking calibrations.

Sound Level Meter.   This device is very useful for amplitude or rough spectral analysis. This example will be described at two levels. The first, an amplitude analysis, should be familiar because it is the way sound level meters are generally applied in the field. To use the sound level meter for this, place the sound level meter close to the sound source with the microphone diaphragm parallel to the direction of sound propagation and record the value. The second, a new sound level meter that includes many of the functions that are commonly used in the field, will be described to show how digital techniques have expanded the capabilities of current instruments. This sound level meter can perform octave band analysis and also compute various sound measures based on the incoming sound. The device has a memory and can be linked to a computer to do further analysis of the sound measured by the device. This is also an example of using a computer-instrumentation partnership to provide more general-purpose instrumentation.

Spectrum Analyzer.   This instrument is almost always required for analysis of complex waveforms and is very useful for noise analysis. It is frequently necessary to check systems for noise, and a spectrum analyzer will not only describe what frequencies are present but also yield the relative amplitudes of the various components. Spectrum analysis is used to measure distortion for particular components and for analyses when there are a lot of unknown factors, but a complex sound is involved. Thus this instrument is useful for diagnostic and calibration purposes.

Distortion Analyzer.   This instrument is a more specialized form of spectrum analyzer that is used to do harmonic and intermodulation distortion analysis. Its use was described in chapter 5 because it is commonly used to check the distortion of audiometers. While it could also be used to examine system performance for a laboratory environment, a spectrum analyzer is a more general tool and would be preferred if the choice was to purchase only one instrument.

Spectrograph.   This instrument is similar to a spectrum analyzer, but is slightly different because of its application as a speech analysis tool. The spectrograph determines the amplitude over time in specific frequency bands of a speech signal. There are two forms of spectrograph:

1. The original spectrograph uses photosensitive paper wrapped around a rotating drum with a stylus that burns the paper according to the intensity of the signal. The stylus is synchronized with a scanning filter with a bandwidth of 300 or 600 Hz. The signal is recorded on a tape loop inside the spectrograph and is played back once for each rotation of the drum, which equates to one setting of the filter. As the drum rotates, the output of the filter at that point in time is burned onto the paper, with the intensity of the burn proportional to the output of the filter. The center frequency of the filter is incremented with each rotation, yielding an intensity-by-time-by-frequency plot. The plots are excellent for determining the frequency-over-time characteristics of a speech signal, but to get accurate assessment of the intensity parameter is much more difficult because it requires a lot of work with contour plots, which display the intensity across frequency for a particular point in time.

2. The new spectrographic analyzers employ digital techniques to do parallel spectral analysis and obtain real-time displays. How this is done was described earlier and has been adapted to generate spectrographic displays. The major difference between digital spectrographs and digital spectrum analyzers is that generally the digital spectrograph has more memory and does the calculations over time slices out of the signal. It is still difficult to determine the relative intensity values from the display, but because all of the component values are stored, offset time-slice frequency spectrum displays can be used to get this information (Fig. 8.13).

Figure 8.13 shows a series of frequency spectra averaged over 5 ms slices out of a speech signal. New analyzers permit adjustment of the duration of each time slice and of analysis bandwidth and frequency range. These parameter changes can even be done without rerecording the signal because the signal is kept in memory. Keep in mind the earlier discussion of the

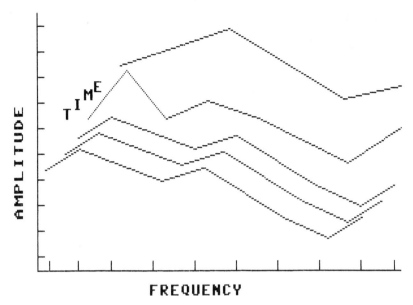

Figure 8.13.   Time-slice frequency spectrum.

strengths and weakness of FFT spectrum analyzers, because the digital spectrographic analyzer is essentially an FFT analyzer that does the calculations on a limited time slice of the signal rather than over the whole signal.

Computer.   The computer is the most general-purpose analysis tool available. It can be used to control other signal analysis instrumentation. With the addition of appropriate hardware and software the computer can function as a signal analyzer itself. The required hardware is an A/D that can sample at a sufficiently high rate to accurately acquire a sufficiently broad frequency range for the desired analysis (remember Nyquist). The computer must have enough memory to hold the desired signals, which primarily becomes a problem with speech analysis. The greater memory requirement and the greater computational requirements mean that this type of analysis (and synthesis) is generally done on super microcomputers and minicomputers. Because of their flexibility, computers are heavily involved in the synthesis of signals as well as experimental control. Any type of signal that can be held in memory can be generated by a computer with a D/A, within the constraints of the D/A as discussed earlier. The same is true of experimental control, which is discussed in the computer chapter (chapter 9). This flexibility is also shown in the variety of analyses that can be done by a computer; for example, the computer-assisted analysis of a video image described in the chapter on physiological instrumentation. A similar system has been used to analyze temporal aspects of speech spectrograms by using temporally calibrated cursors to calculate the time between different parts of the speech as displayed on the screen of a real-time spectrograph. This last example brings us full cycle from a simple visual analysis to a complex computer analysis.

Chapter Summary

This chapter described signal acquisition, presentation, and analysis principles and instrumentation. Applications ranging from the analysis of video images to the analysis of the speech signal were described, along with an introduction to the theoretical basis for such analyses. Specific examples were used with the intent of providing students with a sufficiently broad exposure to the variety of techniques available, which will enable them to generalize to new situations and instrumentation.

12

Signal Analysis

Introduction

*T*here are many different acoustic signals in the area of speech and hearing. A frequent requirement is that these signals be produced with high fidelity. However, the various recording/reproduction instruments and media record and reproduce these signals with varying degrees of fidelity. In order to examine the input and output of these instruments, we must analyze the acoustic content of the signal. This is done through the use of signal analysis techniques.

Virtually all instruments that record and reproduce information can be viewed as *transmission links*. This is true regardless of the type of information that is being transmitted through the instrument. The concept of the transmission link permits the application of communications theory to the analysis of instrumentation. Communications analysis has proved to be a very powerful and useful tool and has resulted in the development of specific instrumentation to do some of this type of analysis. It has also allowed the specification of signals in terms of their fidelity, i.e., the accuracy of the reproduction relative to the original. Since many acoustic signals are specified in this manner in the field of speech and hearing, and since these specifications are important for common tests and examinations, a lab is devoted to an introduction to signal analysis instrumentation.

The purpose of this lab is to introduce the student to the use of signal analysis instrumentation. In addition, the student will gain exposure to the practical application of some communications theory concepts, especially the concept of distortion.

Method

Apparatus

This is the apparatus used in this experiment:

1. Two sine wave oscillators or function generators;
2. Sound level meter with accessories;
3. Multimeter or VOM;

4. Frequency counter;
5. Spectrum or wave analyzer;
6. TDH-39 Earphones;

Instruments 2, 3, 4, and 6 have been used in previous labs. The oscillators are very similar to the function generators used in previous labs, and so their use will not be described here. (Wave analyzer and spectrum analyzer are synonomous terms.) The wave analyzer is being introduced in this lab and it is described thoroughly because it represents the major focus of the lab.

Use of the Wave Analyzer

A wave analyzer is an instrument that examines the frequency content of a waveform. A signal is input to the wave analyzer, and the output is a representation of the frequency spectrum of the signal. That is, the wave analyzer takes the input signal and breaks it down into its constituent sine waves. As is the case for instruments covered in previous labs, wave analyzers come in many shapes, sizes, and capabilities. Hence the description for the use of the wave analyzer will be fairly general.

The typical wave analyzer has an input and three outputs. The input is for the signal to be analyzed. As with VOMs, the input impedance for a wave analyzer is very high to avoid loading (drawing a lot of current from) the system under test. These are the outputs from a wave analyzer:

1. The signal after it has been processed by the analyzer;
2. A pair of outputs to drive an *x-y* plotters;
3. A sine wave output corresponding to the current examination frequency of the wave analyzer.

To understand the sets of outputs, it is necessary to explain some of the theory of operation of a wave analyzer: The purpose of a wave analyzer is to break up the signal into its constituent sine waves. However, until very recently it was not reasonable to do the calculations necessary to determine the amplitude and frequency of the waveform components. There are wave analyzers that do compute the spectrum using a technique referred to as the *fast Fourier transform* (FFT). Other wave analyzers use some form of filtering technique to examine the frequency domain. There is a very narrow and very selective filter in the wave analyzer that has an adjustable center frequency. The output of this filter represents the energy due to the signal at the center frequency of the filter. Thus, the wave analyzer is filtering the signal prior to providing, by way of a meter or CRT display, the amplitude of the waveform component at a particular frequency. Some wave analyzers, for example the GR 1900-A, provide the filtered signal as well as the amplitude information. This dual capability permits the use of the wave analyzer as a filter for those cases where there is a need for very precise filtering of the signal. The amplitude information is sent to the x-y recorder outputs.

The x-y recorder outputs are intended to provide a hard-copy plot of the frequency spectrum of the signal under test. As mentioned before, the output amplitude of the filter is sent to the x-y recorder outputs. In particular it is sent to the y output. However, for the plot to be useful, frequency information must also be provided. The GR 1900-A provides a chain drive that is locked to the frequency control of the wave analyzer to provide this information to the recorder, but most current recorders use an electrical signal sent to the x output that represents the current center frequency of the filter.

The wave analyzer may output the frequency of the filter by means of a sine wave. By attaching a frequency counter to this output, one can determine the current frequency of the filter. This output can be used simultaneously with the amplitude outputs.

Although the calibration procedure for a wave analyzer can be somewhat complicated and time consuming, the operation of a wave analyzer is relatively straightforward. For this lab, we are going to assume that the wave analyzer is calibrated, and so we will get to do the easy part. The wave analyzer, for our purposes, has four parts (aside from the outputs): the signal input, the frequency control, the amplitude dial, and the voltmeter. Operation of the signal input and frequency controls needs no explanation, other than to make sure that the correct connectors are used for the signal input. The voltmeter has a decibel scale and is read in the same manner as the sound level meter.

The amplitude dial is similar to that on the sound level meter. There are usually two controls: one sets the maximum amplitude permitted at that setting, and the other sets the scale for reading the amplitude. It should be noted that the maximum amplitude referred to here is the maximum amplitude of the waveform at any frequency, not just the frequency being examined. Before inputting any signal, always start at the maximum setting in order to avoid damaging the instrument.

To get a spectrum, after connecting the signal to the wave analyzer, set the frequency dial to the frequency of the signal, or in the case of a complex signal, the frequency where the maximum amplitude is expected. When in doubt, use a voltmeter to determine the overall amplitude of the waveform and set the maximum appropriately. Now go to the lowest frequency in the frequency range over which the analysis is being done and start slowly increasing the frequency with the frequency control. Set the scale control to maximum sensitivity (lowest amplitude setting) and watch the meter. When a significant deflection is seen, investigate that frequency to determine the amplitude at that point and then resume scanning. Record the amplitude. Continue this procedure until the top of the frequency range of interest has been reached. If the data collected are plotted (amplitude times frequency), the frequency spectrum for that signal will be displayed.

Procedure

There are three phases to this laboratory. Phase 1 will examine the electronic output of a single oscillator. Phase 2 will examine the electronic output of two sine waves after they have been mixed. Phase 3 will examine the acoustic output for a single sine wave and for two sine waves after they have been mixed.

1. Electronic output of single sine wave.   To measure the spectrum for a single oscillator providing the signal, set the amplitude of the oscillator to 0.5 volt and the frequency to 1,000 Hz. Use the multimeter and frequency counter to do this. Using the block diagram in Figure 8.14, set up the equipment to do the wave analysis. Using the instructions given above, determine the frequency spectrum of the signal from 400 Hz to 6,000 Hz with an analysis filter of 50 Hz.

2. Electronic output of mixed sine waves.   To meaure the frequency spectrum for two sine waves after mixing (which contrasts with the single oscillator signal in phase 1), set both oscillators to 0.5 volt. Set one oscillator to 1,000 Hz and the other oscillator to 1,400 Hz. Use the block diagram in Figure 8.15 to set up the apparatus. Determine the frequency spectrum for the mixed sine waves from 400 Hz to 6,000 Hz with an analysis filter of 50 Hz.

3. Acoustic output of mixed sine waves.   The previous phase determined the frequency spectrum of the signal going into the earphone. Now, to examine the frequency spectrum after it is transduced by the earphone, leave the oscillators at their present settings. Using the block diagram in Figure 8.16, determine the frequency spectrum at the earphone for two sine waves after mixing. Now remove one of the oscillators and determine the spectrum for a single oscillator. Use the same frequency range and filter setting as before.

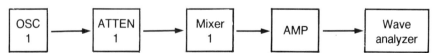

Figure 8.14.   Apparatus for wave analysis of electronic output for a single sine wave.

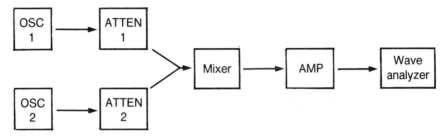

Figure 8.15.   Apparatus for wave analysis of electronic output for two sine waves after mixing.

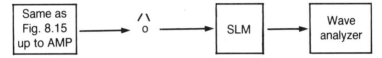

Figure 8.16.   Apparatus for wave analysis of an acoustic signal.

Results

Plot the electrical and acoustic frequency spectra for each stimulus configuration. Plot the electrical and acoustic spectra for the single sine wave signal on one graph and the electrical and acoustic spectra for the complex signal on another graph. Compute the distortion in decibels for all distortion products for all frequency spectra.

Discussion

Describe and compare the performance of each system (electronic vs. earphone) as it is reflected in the spectral measurements, especially with regard to harmonic and intermodulation distortion. For the purposes of discussion, assume that any distortion in the systems is a result of the systems and not of the signal source.

Discuss the performance of the systems with regard to the intended use of the systems, namely, for psychoacoustic investigations. Also discuss the system in terms of any needs that you may have for the system, such as the presentation of speech or other recorded material or for audiometric measurement.

Modular Programming Equipment and Computers

The first computer was built in the 1800s, but computers became common in large institutions in the 1960s. These large computers, called *mainframe computers*, were responsible for computing bank balances, and large corporations were the primary users of such machines. The computers filled whole rooms and required large, sophisticated staffs to maintain and program the computers. On the other hand, laboratories in the fields of speech and hearing and other behavioral disciplines, as well as physiology, used small computers called *minicomputers* to control experiments and store data. Recently, smaller computers, or *microcomputers*, have become ubiquitous. They are found in the home, at school, and at work. For persons in the field of hearing and speech, the microcomputer is becoming a normal adjunct to their work.

Development of the computer as a workplace tool has come about because of the miniaturization referred to in earlier chapters. This miniaturization has been particularly important for computers because of their complexity. The typical microcomputer comprises millions of transistors. These transistors are contained in a console that is smaller than a typewriter. Microminiaturization techniques can now place almost one million transistors in a package less than 1 square inch. The trade publication *Infoworld* (January 1984) estimated that by the year 2000 over one billion transistors will be placed on such a chip.

The small size and growing power of microcomputers has increased the sophistication of the possible user applications for such computers. Examples of applications are word processing, office management, data management, report preparation, mailing lists, and laboratory control.

This is only a partial list; other applications will also be described in this chapter. The only real limits to the applicability of the computer are imagination and money.

While computers are very useful tools, they are also complex and frequently intimidating. Fortunately, this no longer needs to be the case. With some basic understanding of how computers operate and some first-hand experience, one can easily understand computers. The analogy used in the first chapter with regard to the first client and how experience helps applies here as well.

This chapter will describe some of the basic aspects of computers. The terminology and information presented in the chapter is not intended to make the reader an expert in computers but rather an informed user. After studying this chapter it should be possible to make intelligent decisions about hardware and software to suit many clinical and research needs. This does not mean that all types or brands of computer equipment will be reviewed, but rather that understanding the general principles and capabilities of computers will permit appropriate analysis of the situation in order to decide if and how a computer would be used.

In addition to discussing computers, this chapter will describe modular programming equipment. This equipment is frequently used by experimenters, and much of the logic used to program the modules is applicable to computers. In fact, these modules will be described first in order to introduce some of the logic associated with digital computers.

Modular Programming Equipment

Modular programming equipment refers to an instrument environment comprised of combinations of modules. Each of the modules implements a specific function or decision rule. For example, one module might switch signals on and off and another might serve to combine events and make a decision based on the combination or sequence of events. By combining the functions of several modules, the programmer can control a complex series of events. So that the reader can understand how this can be done, the basic logic of module programming is described next.

Modular Programming Logic

The basic logic associated with modules is not restricted to programming modules but is more general and can be applied to other areas as well. In fact, the rules for logic programming come from Philosophy.

The basic rules of logic are simple and have a great deal of generality because of this simplicity. The apparent complexity comes from the combination of the basic rules. When analyzing any type of programming, whether it be for computers or modular programming equipment, keep in mind the basic simplicity of the rules. Tasks should be broken down into their simplest components, and complexity should be created by the combination of tasks rather than by making each task complex and adding together complex parts. This style of programming, referred to as *modular programming*, makes not only the writing and creation of programs easier but also the inevitable changes and additions that will be required later. The best place to start is with the basic rules of logic.

The basic logic rules are *OR*, *AND*, and *NOT*. There is also a special case of *OR* called the *XOR* function. Each of these rules is especially useful for combining certain events. (To simplify the description of these rules, I will refer to events by capital letters.) The logic rules also have certain symbols (Fig. 9.1) and will be used in all logic diagrams. In addition to these conventions, there is also an explanatory vehicle called a *truth table*. Truth tables are very useful for learning the function and for ascertaining the outcomes of chains of events using the rules. When the rules are used in the text, they will be presented as equations and the rules will be enclosed in dots, e.g., .AND.

The first rule to describe is the AND rule. A two-event (*A* AND *B*) truth table is given in Figure 9.2, which shows how logic rules are derived. Each event is assigned one of two states: *true* or *false*. It is important to point out that these are arbitrary assignments and could mean anything in the real world. Modular programming equipment frequently assigns voltage levels to logic states. For example, true could mean that the voltage level is 1 volt, and false could mean that the voltage level is 0 volt. As long as these are the only two voltages in the environment then it is possible to apply logic rules. How to describe multiple alternatives with logic rules will be discussed later in the chapter.

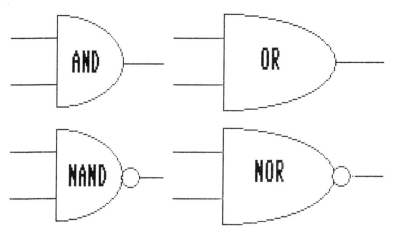

Figure 9.1.   AND, OR, NAND, and NOR symbols.

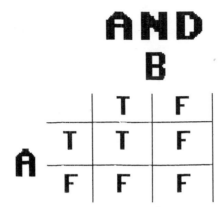

Figure 9.2. AND truth table for two events.

The AND rule is that if both of two events are true, then the outcome is true. In all other cases, the outcome is false. Figure 9.2 shows this in truth table form. Each of the two possible states of events A and B, as represented by true (T) or false (F), are shown at the left side and top of the table, respectively. The outcome for each combination of events is shown in the table and is also represented by T or F. To find the outcome for any combination of events, look for the intersection of the two states of interest. The outcome is given in the cell at this intersection. For example, examine the case of A-true AND B-false. By drawing a line from A-true across the table until it meets with a line drawn down from B-false, you can find the cell representing the combination of these events. Since the rule states that "the outcome can be true only when both events are true," this cell is false because one of the events (B) is false. A similar analysis can be done for all combinations, which results in the truth table shown in Figure 9.2. The other rules can be examined in a similar manner.

Another rule is the OR rule. This rule states that if either event is true, the outcome is true. The XOR rule, which is a special case of the OR rule, states that the outcome is only true if one of the events is true, but not if both events are true. The truth tables for these two rules are shown in Figure 9.3. If the appropriate rule is applied to each cell in the truth tables, in a manner similar to that described for the AND rule, you can see how the truth tables were derived.

The final rule is the simplest rule. The NOT rule is that the state of the outcome is the reverse of the state of the event. The NOT rule is frequently used in combination with the other rules to achieve outcomes that would not be possible otherwise. Examples of NOT combined with OR and AND, which are referred to as the *NOR* and *NAND* rules, respectively. The NOR rule is shown in Figure 9.4. Do you notice any correspondences?

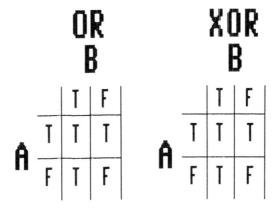

Figure 9.3.   OR and XOR truth tables for two events.

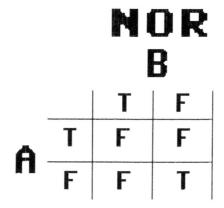

Figure 9.4.   NOR truth table for two events.

The preceding logic rules can also be described using the notation of logic diagrams. How this is done and how logic diagrams can assist in the development of programs to control modular equipment can best be illustrated through a simple example. Assume that there are three events: *A*, *B*, and *C*. Furthermore, assume the three events must occur in a particular sequence: *A* starts first, and B starts halfway through *A*; *C* starts as soon as *A* and *B* end; the cycle starts again when *C* ends. This cycle of events is illustrated in the timing diagram in Figure 9.5.

Figure 9.5 shows that in addition to knowing the logic of the sequence, it is necessary to know the duration of each event. Durations are implemented in modular programming logic through devices called *timers*. As the name implies, these devices remain in a specific state for a fixed period of time. By using timers in conjunction with the logic rules given before, it is possible to generate the sequence shown in Figure 9.5. The logic diagram to do this is shown in Figure 9.6. Three timers, one for each event, an AND logic module, and a NOR logic module are used. The first timer is started independently, and the cycle will continue forever unless it is halted externally. This continual cycling through a particular sequence is

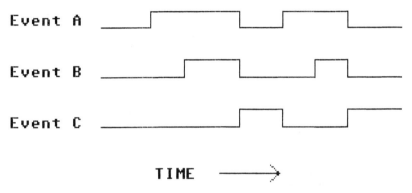

Figure 9.5. Sample timing diagram for three-event sequence.

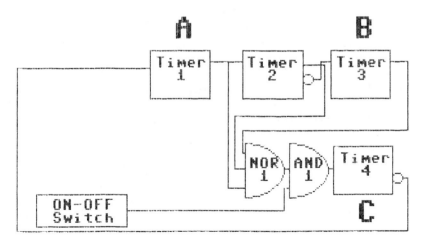

Figure 9.6. Logic diagram to implement Fig. 9.5.

called an *endless loop*, because the looping through events never ends. Such loops should be assiduously avoided. To stop the loop in the present program, a switch has been added that will stop the loop when it is opened.

So that you understand how the program works, I will describe the logic diagram in Figure 9.6 step-by-step. Refer to the figure as often as necessary in order to follow the description. After going through the description and the diagram *slowly*, you will understand why programmers of modular systems use logic diagrams rather than words to describe the programs.

The timers are labelled *A* and *B*, to conform to the event that is being timed by that timer. Timer *A* is started by closing the on-off switch when all events are stopped. Think of the switch as true when closed and false when open. The actual logic sequence that triggers the start of the cycle is having the AND module become true. This will happen when the output of the AND module combining the outputs of the NOR logic module and the switch is true. Note that the timers have both true and inverted outputs, which is symbolized by the *small circle* on the inverted output. This permits the logic state to be sensed both for when the timer is on and when it is off. The true outputs from all timers are input into the NOR module. Thus when all timers are off, the output of this module is true.

An alternative way to get the same effect might be to input the inverted outputs from all timers to an AND module. However, there are some problems with this alternative. These are left as an exercise for the reader (the switch is the key). Timer 2 is used to delay event *B* until halfway through event *A*. This means that when timers 1, 2, and 3 are off, the output of the NOR module will be true. When this module becomes true, event *C*, (timer 4) is started. When timer 4 turns off, and the switch is on, the cycle begins again until the switch is turned off.

Note the frequent references to "when *X* becomes true." This statement refers to a *change* in logic state from false to true. The *change in state* is usually the key event in a logic sequence. As mentioned earlier, logic states are frequently coded as voltage levels in modular programming equipment. Since the key event is the transition between these voltage levels, a brief discussion of these transitions is necessary.

Logic is frequently classified as either *positive logic* or *negative logic*. This refers to whether true is positive or negative. Regardless of whether the logic is positive or negative, the transition from false to true is called the "leading edge of the logic transition," and the transition from true to false is called the "trailing edge of the logic transition." These transitions are not instantaneous, and the time between states may not be the same for both leading and trailing edges. Manufacturers should provide this information in their documentation. Availability of such information is most important when one is programming sequences of events with close timing tolerances and where logic events may be happening together.

Several times I have had a program apparently fail because of this problem even though the logic diagram was accurate and correct. This can be checked out by looking for places in the logical flow where such conflicts in logic state can occur and then observing the logic flow as the program is run. This is called *debugging* the program and will be described more fully when discussing software development, but it is also a necessary process in modular programming.

Programs almost never work properly the first time, and it is dangerous to assume that a program will run perfectly the first time especially when one is pressed for time. Further examples of programming will be given in the rest of the chapter and in the Quiklabs at the end of the chapter to reinforce these concepts of logic and programming.

Up to this point the discussion has been somewhat abstract. Describing logic programming in terms of real-world events may make the concepts more concrete. The first step is to assign meanings to A, B, and C. The presentation of a sine wave will be event A and the presentation of noise will be event B. The sine wave will have a probability of occurrence of 50%. Event C will be the subject's response. We will also want to adjust the intensity of the signal after two consecutive correct responses or two consecutive errors. These additional requirements will need other modules to implement the program. In particular, we will need some kind of counters and analog modules. The logic aspect of the program will be covered first, and then analog modules will be discussed.

The sine wave and noise will have a fixed duration, which will be controlled with timers. The probability of the signal being presented can be controlled in a couple of ways depending upon the module manufacturer, but let us assume that there is a probability module that can be tested and that will respond with a logic true state at a specified percentage of the time. The presence or absence of the signal needs to be indicated; whether two of the same type of response, either correct or incorrect, have occurred consecutively also needs to be indicated. Both of these program requirements can be implemented using a *flip-flop*, which is a module that is discussed next. A summary of correct and incorrect responses would be useful, and these would be implemented with *counters*, which function exactly as their name implies. The logic diagram depicting the signal presentation portion of the program is shown in Figure 9.7. Before the logic diagram is reviewed, flip-flops and counters will be briefly described.

Flip-flops serve two purposes: as memory or as binary counters. The logic modules discussed up to this point implement what is referred to as *momentary logic*. That is, they change as the logic state changes. Flip-flops, on the other hand, reflect the last state presented to the flip-flop and only change state if forced. Thus there are always two inputs to a flip-flop: a true input (usually referred to as the "set input") and a false input (usually

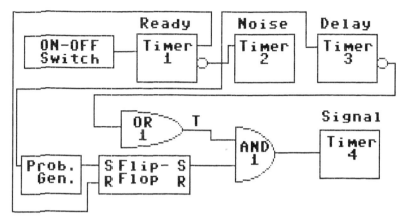

Figure 9.7.   Logic diagram for program described in text.

referred to as the "reset input"). The flip-flop also has two outputs, which correspond to the inputs and reflect which of the inputs last received a true input. What this means is that flip-flops have memory, i.e., they "remember" the last state that was input into the flip-flop. As will be seen when computers are discussed later in the chapter, flip-flops represent the main building block in computers. Many flip-flops also have a *clear* capability that permits making all outputs false regardless of the current state of the flip-flop. Flip-flops are used in the current program to store the state of the last response and the presence of the signal.

The binary counter function of flip-flops is also shown in the program. Recall that flip-flops change state whenever a different input changes state and only reflect the last change. So what happens if the set and reset inputs are pulsed simultaneously? Let us assume that the flip-flop starts in the reset condition. The first time both inputs go true, only the set input will recognize the true condition because reset was the last condition. Hence the set output will become true and the reset output will become false. The second time both inputs go true, only the reset input will recognize the true condition because the flip-flop is in a set condition. Hence the outputs will reverse states. If we do it again, the outputs will reverse again. Note that every second time the inputs are pulsed in this manner, the outputs repeat their state. In effect, the flip-flop is capable of counting events up to two. The number system that has a base of 2 is the binary number system and hence the flip-flop is referred to as a binary counter.

In addition to the flip-flop, counters come in a large number of varieties. This module also provides a type of memory in that the counter is not a momentary logic state module. Probably the most common type of counter is the *cumulative counter*, which accumulates a count of the number of times it has been triggered. Another commonly used counter is the *up-down counter*, so called because the counter can count in either direction. This counter is extremely useful for program control. Both types of counters would be used in the current program, though they are not shown in Figure 9.7. Although there are other classifications of counters, most will fit into one of these two types, as a quick examination of a counter's capabilities will show.

Now that all of the logic modules needed for the program have been discussed, it is time to briefly describe the logic diagram depicted in Figure 9.7. Some of the details will be left to the reader as an exercise. As in the previous program, there needs to be a way to start and stop the program, and the same device is used, a start-stop switch. Examining the program shows that certain parameters have to be specified before the logic can be finalized. In Figure 9.7 it was assumed that the noise burst was longer than the sinewave signal and the sine wave signal would be placed in the temporal center of the noise burst. Thus the noise starts first. This does not mean that the first event after the program is started is turning on the noise as represented by timer 2. There is a timer, timer 1, that represents a "ready" interval that is turned on first. This timer provides a brief period between the subject's button press and the beginning of the next trial for the subject to get ready, hence its name. Another timer, timer 3, representing the delay between the start of the noise and start of the signal, is started at the same time as timer 2. When timer 3 turns off, it starts the signal timer (timer 4). However, note that there is an AND module between the delay and signal timers, and this AND module has a flip-flop as one of its inputs. The input to the flip-flop is from the probability generator and represents whether or not there will be a signal. Also note that there is an OR module between the delay timer and the AND module, with an input only from timer 3. Why is the OR module there? The answer shows how there can be "hidden" problems in programming.

Recall that the "off" output of a timer will be true whenever the timer is off. The state of the flip-flop representing signal presence is determined at the beginning of every trial and hence can become true at the beginning of the trial. Since the timer will also be off at the beginning of the trial (the noise has not started yet), the signal will begin at the beginning of the trial, which is not the desired situation. There are a number of ways to "fix" this problem, but a momentary OR module (an OR module that outputs a single pulse whenever the output becomes true) has been used here. An alternative, and more common method, might be to use a flip-flop. Try to figure out how this would be done. The signal presentation portion of the program is now complete.

The next portion is the response portion. It is assumed that there is an interface to the subject and that the button response becomes true when the subject presses the button. After the signal and/or noise goes off, the subject will respond whether or not the signal occurred. To determine if the response is correct, the programmer must compare it to the signal presence flip-flop. This is done with AND modules and is fairly straight-forward, so it is left as an exercise for the reader to figure out the logic diagram. The outcome of the comparison is recorded on one of four counters, each representing one of the four possible outcomes. These counters are only for checking subject-response bias. That is, these counters are to check whether the subject has a bias toward responding in a set manner regardless of the order of signal presentation.

Based on whether the subject was correct, the program needs to determine the intensity of the signal for the next trial. This is done through another flip-flop, which is used as a simply binary counter, and through an up-down counter, which is connected to a *programmable attenuator*. A programmable attenuator is an attenuator whose amount of attenuation can be controlled remotely. By connecting the counter to the program-mable attenuator in a one-to-one manner, the programmer can directly tie the attenuation to the counter value. Thus changing the counter will change the amount of attenuation. In this case, whenever the "correct" flip-flop becomes false, the counter will count up one, and whenever there is an error, the counter will count down by one. In this manner, the attenuation will change in accordance with the rule given here. This completes the program.

Before leaving the logic section of the program I must emphasize that the logic diagram, although written for a modular system, is equally applicable to any manner of implementing the above program. One reason for using a logic diagram as the basis for describing programs is the generality of the logic. The logic describes a way to implement a particular procedure. It does not specify what equipment must be used to implement the program.

Up to this point the actual instrumentation used to generate the stimuli controlled by the program have been ignored, with the exception of the programmable attenuator. The next set of modules to be discussed are the analog modules. These are the modules that handle the electrical signal that represents the stimulus of interest.

Analog Modules

Analog modules provide many of the functions of the signal generator described in the test instrumentation chapter. Other analog devices pro-vided in modular form are amplifiers, filters, attenuators, and switches. All of these types of instrumentation should be familiar with the exception of switches, which were described only briefly in the chapter on audiological instrumentation. In addition, analog-to-digital and digital-to-analog modules are available, which were described in chapter 8. The only analog module that will be described here is the electronic switch, because all of the other modules perform in the same manner as described in earlier chapters.

The electronic switch is a device that performs two functions: It turns the signal on and off, and it controls the envelope of the signal. It does this by controlling the rate of onset and termination (rise/fall time). Some switches also provide some control of the shape of the onset and termination portions of the envelope. In order to implement the on-off capability, the switch has a logic input that functions in much the same manner as a light switch. As long as the logic is in a true state, the switch is on. As long as the logic is in a false state, the switch is off. By controlling the duration of the true state, the duration of the stimulus passing through the switch can be controlled. Conversely, by controlling the duration of a false state, the time period during which the stimulus is off can be controlled. Both of these situations occur frequently, for example, in psychoacoustic research.

The rate of onset and termination (they are symmetrical on most module switches) is controlled by a knob on the front of the switch. Be sure to read the documentation describing the switch to determine the units for the knob, as it is very easy to make a mistake. In addition, the actual rise/fall time should be verified using the procedure used to check the rise/fall time for an audiometer described in the audiological instrumentation chapter. Do not trust the setting to be accurate.

Just as with logic modules, analog modules need to be arranged in specific ways to generate specific kinds of stimuli and to interface with the logic of the program. This organization of the modules is described, in the same manner as for the logic modules in Figure 9.7, with a block diagram (Fig. 9.8). It is left as an exercise for the reader to examine and understand the block diagram in Figure 9.8, which should be easy because similar block diagrams have been shown in earlier chapters. For any program to be complete, both the logic and analog diagrams must be present. In addition, many of the analog modules are controlled by logic modules. Hence there are interconnections between the logic and analog portions of the programs. These must also be made clear, and this can be done in a number of ways including notations on either the logic or analog block diagrams.

Modular programming is perfectly adequate for single experiments. In fact, if a dedicated setup that can be used to quickly implement simple experiments is desired, modular programming equipment is an excellent choice. However, it should be clear from the preceding discussion that while complex experiments can be executed using such instrumentation, there are many limitations.

Two of the more obvious limitations are with regard to the variety of

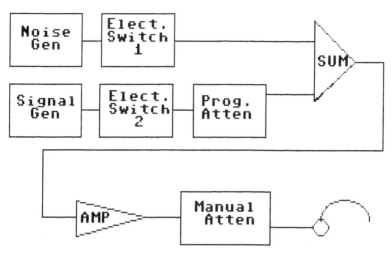

Figure 9.8.   Analog block diagram for program in Fig. 9.7.

signals that can be generated and the ease of doing multiple studies concurrently on the same equipment. In addition, signals with complex time waveforms cannot be generated by modular programming equipment. Through judicious use of external signal generators, one can somewhat overcome this limitation but the result is an increasing complexity of ancillary instrumentation. A less obvious limitation is that only a certain number of modules can fit into a modular equipment cabinet, and there is a limit of four to five modular equipment cabinets per power supply. Complex experiments can require a large number of modules, and thus the modular equipment approach can get very expensive beyond a certain level of complexity due to the requirements for modules, cabinets, and power supplies.

Remote Modular Programming

The multiple-experiment limitation can be overcome to a limited degree by a *patch panel*. Patch panel is a generic term referring to a panel that provides a flexible, remote, physical interface between equipment and the user. A patch panel for modular programming equipment consists of two pieces: a plastic board with rows of small holes and a holder, into which the plastic board is inserted. The back of the holder has holes into which are inserted connectors from the various modules in the programming system. The connectors consists of a multipin connector that slips onto the back of the modules and has several wires with pins on the end. These pins are inserted into the holes on the back of the holder. The front of the holder has rows of pins corresponding to the holes in the plastic board. To use this system, which is sometimes referred to as a *remote programming panel*, the user connects the programming leads between holes on the plastic panel that represent the desired locations on the modules. When the board with the leads is inserted into the panel, the pins contact the leads and provide a connection between the two modules represented by the holes on the panel. By programming individual experiments on separate panels, the remote programming system provides a way to quickly change between different experiments.

Helpful Hints

Several pointers to the user of such panels may be helpful at this point:

1. Be aware that setting up a patch panel is time consuming. Each wire has to be inserted into the panel using a special tool. If there are 20 modules with an average of 8–12 wires each, this means the insertion of between 160 and 240 wires. Added to this is the time to insure that it is done properly, i.e., the time to fix the mistakes that will inevitably occur.

2. Spend some time laying out the panel prior to doing step 1. For example, do you want all the OR modules to be in a single section on the panel, or do your want them scattered throughout the panel in order to reduce lead lengths? The time spent planning the organization of the panel represents one of the main benefits of a panel system, which is that, regardless of where the modules are in the equipment rack, the panel will be laid out in the logical order that is best for you. It should be noted, however, that laying out the panel and modules in the equipment rack in the same fashion will be helpful in troubleshooting the system. After laying out the panel, commit the layout to paper and make many copies.

3. Be sure to have plenty of programming leads and panels. Calculate how many you think you want and then double that amount. The same can apply to modules, although the ratio here is more 1.5 to 1.

4. There will always be some front panel (module) connections. This may be due to various reasons, such as equipment breakdown, a pin in the panel breaks, or insufficient panel programming leads (which will not happen if step 3 is followed, right?). The same rule applies as to step 2, namely, put the front panel connections on paper and make many copies.

5. The analog connections should not go through the panel, as this exposes the pins and is an open invitation to noise. Thus, the remote panel does not remove the need to handle the analog connections for each experiment.

6. The lead connections must be diagrammed as well as any front panel connections for each experiment. This is in addition to the logic and analog diagrams discussed earlier. All this documentation may seem like a lot of work, that is, until something goes wrong and you are in need of that documentation. Then the work will pay off tenfold.

If these steps sound somewhat cumbersome to follow, it is because they are. Experiments can be changed within minutes, but if the changes are extensive, considerable manipulation of instrumentation is necessary to implement this system for complex experiments or a series of complex experiments. Luckily, a tool has come along to make much of this manipulation a lot easier—the computer.

Computers

There are many different kinds of computers made today, but one of the main sources of fascination with the computer is their general-purpose nature. While special-purpose equipment definitely is appropriate for certain needs, the types of computers most useful to the person working in a scientific or clinical environment share the common strength that a variety of tasks can be handled by the computer system. This generality usually means that referring to a computer as if it were a single entity is frequently a mistake. Most current computers actually consist of a central computer to which are attached a collection of additional devices to perform various functions. Thus to understand current computers really requires some discussion of hardware. As is the case with most other sections of this text, the intent is not to teach hardware design but to familiarize the reader with a variety of hardware in order to help him or her make informed decisions about classes of hardware required for certain needs.

Computer Hardware

Computer hardware is a complex topic, but within the limited purview that has been chosen here it is not as complex as is frequently implied by "computer mystics." The key is to be able to specify clearly the function of a particular piece of hardware and to understand enough jargon to be able to communicate with the technical person responsible for installing and/or maintaining the system. Therefore, this section will describe classes of hardware, with the focus being on the application for the hardware. The progression will be from the center outward, which means that the "brains" or core of the system will be described first, followed by devices that are usually inside the main case, or cabinet, of the computer system, and finally the devices that are usually attached external to the central cabinet, or case, of the system. The class of computers implicitly assumed during this discussion will be microcomputers, but the principles described in these sections can generally be applied to minicomputer and mainframe computer systems.

Core Hardware

Core hardware includes the system components generally regarded as central to any computer: a processor, memory, and some communications link between the two (Fig. 9.9). It should be noted that this diagram in Figure 9.9 assumes a particular type of computer architecture (i.e., how the basic components of the computer are organized) called "Von Neumann architecture."

Figure 9.9 shows that all instructions are decoded by the processor, but that both instructions and data are stored in memory. In fact, in a computer all information is treated as a data stream. It is the content of the data or the intent of the processor in manipulating the data that determines the classification of the data. Physically, it is not required that data and instructions be retrieved from memory over separate data lines; to save space many computers do not separate these lines. The paths indicated in Figure 9.9, when implemented in hardware, are referred to as *busses*.

Computer Architecture

Computer architecture is a very exotic and esoteric field but is very important in terms of computer performance. The only architectural topic that will be lightly touched upon now is the difference between serial and parallel architecture because the field is moving from serial to parallel

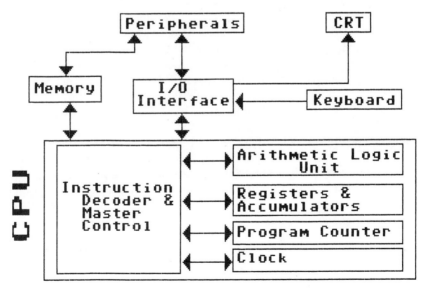

Figure 9.9. Simple computer architecture.

architectures and some understanding of these issues will be helpful when selecting computer systems.

As mentioned previously, present computers are Von Neumann machines. This means that instructions are executed and memory accessed serially in the time domain, i.e., one operation is done at a time. In a parallel architecture, instructions are executed and memory is accessed simultaneously, i.e., several operations are done at the same time. The serial method has obvious advantages from a design viewpoint. The design is simpler conceptually and requires much simpler schemes for handling data streams that may represent either memory, data, or instructions because all processing is done in a single channel. The main advantage of a parallel design is a clear edge in speed of processing. This edge has to be qualified, however, because parallel processing does not provide clear advantages for all types of processing. A simple example is text entry, where the speed of the operator is so slow that parallel processing does not speed up the task noticeably, if at all. In other contexts, for example, calculations requiring matrix mathematics such as fast Fourier transforms, parallel processing provides dramatic improvements in performance.

There are many different types of parallel architecture; two concepts that are used in current machines are shown in Figure 9.10. The architecture in panel *A* is referred to as a *data-driven architecture* and essentially involves routing the data through the processors so that computations are performed in parallel. Due to the parallel nature of the structure, if many operations need to be performed simultaneously on different data, this machine would be much faster than the Von Neumann machines described earlier.

The concept in Figure 9.10*B* is interesting because it is an attempt to represent software concepts in hardware. It is called a *reduction machine* and is a *demand-driven architecture*; that is, a computation or task is done as needed. As can be seen from the figure, this means that a large number of parallel processors will usually be required at the beginning of a problem, but as the solution is approached, the number of processes will shrink. Of course, as the processors are freed up under this scheme, they can be applied to other tasks that the computer is processing. This type of parallel processing is very similar to both an operating system (the software that controls the flow of information in a computer) called UNIX, which we will discuss in more detail later, and some software languages, most notably LISP. This reduction machine will be extremely well-adapted to the types of problems that such software was developed to solve, namely, artificial intelligence, which is also going to become more important in the future and will be discussed later in the chapter.

Parallel processing is a fascinating topic and is most likely the machine

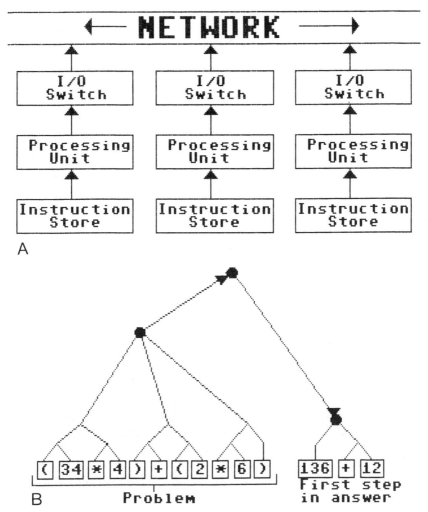

Figure 9.10.   *A*, Data-driven computer architecture; *B*,Reduction computer architecture.

of the future. However, for the next several years the Von Neumann architecture machine will be utilized. The rest of this chapter will discuss computers without much regard to their serial or parallel nature.

Processors and Memory

So far, the discussion of computers has been on the organization of core hardware, namely processors, memory and the connections between them, which are referred to as "busses." Now it is time to discuss the components. The story of processors and memory has been the same as the story of integrated chips. The capabilities have increased, the size has decreased, and the cost has gone down. As mentioned in the introduction to this chapter, along with the shrinkage of the parts has come the shrinkage of the whole machine. This has led to a succession of terms that refer to computer size and can be very confusing.

The original computers were huge beasts and took up whole rooms. The Electronic Numerical Integrator and Calculator (ENIAC) is a famous vacuum tube computer, which was followed by more powerful machines of similar size. The rooms had special environments for these machines. There were raised floors for the cables, and large air-conditioning units to remove the heat dissipated by the components. These machines were (are) called "mainframes." The large computers used by universities and large institutions are mainframe computers. As the size decreased, new terms such as "minicomputer" and "microcomputer" came to be used. In fact, the latest term was threatening to be "nanocomputer" (used to refer to handheld-size computers), instead "lap" and "portable" are used to describe the smallest current computers. (As an aside, I assume that if the size-term correspondence continues, a computer that fits on a finger will be called a picocomputer.) The only useful aspect of all this jargon is to refer to the size of the computer because the manner of operation for these machines is almost identical. (This is from the viewpoint of the user. Obviously, many aspects of the design are different for the different machines.) As a result, the rest of the discussion in this chapter can be taken as applying to all sizes of computers, although details may differ slightly for the different sizes of machines. For example, the larger computers use larger processors.

It was mentioned before that processors have become more powerful during the course of their evolution. Power in a computer is usually quantified as being able to do a given number of tasks in a given time. There are two ways that processors have been involved in increasing computer power.

The first power increase is because processors have become faster. Recall that the processor has to decode instructions. The rate at which the processor can decode and execute instructions is the *processor speed*. The first processor operated at a rate of about 100–200 instructions/s. Current state-of-the-art processors operate in the range of one billion instructions/s. In fact, this speed increase has generated its own jargon. Millions of instructions/s are referred to as "MIPS". The superseded processors are rated in terms of the number of millions of floating point operations/s or "megaflops" and billions of floating point operations/s or "gigaflops."

The second power increase is the result of an increase in the size of the data that the processor can handle in one "chunk." To visualize this requires some understanding of how data are stored in a computer.

Data Storage in a Computer

There are several aspects to data storage in a computer. One is how the data are physically stored in the machine. Another is the representation of the physical data, and still another is the number system used for the representation. Each of these will be discussed in turn.

It was mentioned earlier in this chapter that flip-flops play an important role in computers. The role they play is in the memory of the computer. All data in a computer are stored in memory. While this memory can take many forms, the discussion in this section will be restricted to *core memory*. Core memory is the memory that is inside the computer and represents, for most computers, the memory containing current data. Recall that there is no differentiation to the computer as to whether information is program code or program data and there is no difference in the way the information is stored in the machine. The information in physical memory is contained in groups of flip-flops. Within the groups, each flip-flop is in either the set or reset state.

Representing information stored by the computer means coding the state of the flip-flops in computer memory. This is done by having each set flip-flop coded as a 1 and each reset flip-flop as a 0. Since there are only two possible states for a flip-flop, this is a binary situation, and each flip-flop is referred to as a *bit*. Think of it as a *bi*nary *t*oggle switch. The flip-flops are generally represented as being in groups of eight, which are referred to as *bytes*, although this is not how physical memory is constructed. In physical memory the flip-flops are organized in large matrices. Large-scale integration has made possible matrices on the order of 256,000 or even one million bits on a chip. Incidentally, memory-chip size is given in terms of the number of bits on the chip, not the number of bytes, and appropriate abbreviations are employed. For example, a 64K chip is a memory chip that contains 64,000 bits of memory. Current core memory is constructed as a given number of memory chips, while other chips, called *support chips*, which do things such as handle information routing, are placed on a circuit board. Boards can contain millions of bytes of memory.

The difficulty of using number systems to represent data in memory has two facets. One is representing the data itself. The other is representing its location in memory, which is most important to programmers. That is, programmers not only are concerned with the data, but also its location (called "address" in computer jargon). Although the intent of this chapter is not to train programmers, a brief explanation of number systems is included to aid in communication between programmers and nonprogrammers when discussing applications.

Number Systems

Representation of the data itself when it is output by the computer is determined by the application, not by the manner in which that data is stored in memory. The decimal number system is usually used for output because that is the number system in most common use. The only limitation is the size of the number that can be represented on the particular computer. For the programmer, however, the details of how the data are represented in memory can be very important, and primarily three number systems have been employed for these representations: the *binary, octal,* and *hexadecimal* (frequently abbreviated "hex") number systems. Because most people are trained in the decimal system, this can be confusing to the nonprogrammer, but these other number systems are actually straightforward and use all the same rules as the decimal system. The only difference is in the base of the system.

The binary system has a base of 2 and each number can be one of 2 numbers. Since all number systems start at 0, the two numbers in the binary system are 0 and 1. Just as in any number system, a number can be an arbitrary number of digits long.

The octal system has a base of 8 and each number can be any one of the 8 digits from 0 to 7. The hex system has a base of 16 and so each number can be any of the 16 numbers between 0 and F. Where did the "F" come from? The F came from the fact mentioned earlier that people are trained in the decimal number system and it is easier to learn a number system if it can be represented in a decimal-like manner. Since a number system with a base of 16 would require numbers such as 15,15129, which is a four-digit number in such a system, it was decided to use the letters from A to F to represent the numbers from 10 to 15 in the hex system. Thus the above number in the hex notation would be FFC9. Much clearer, right?

A difficulty that obviously arises is the translation of numbers from these number systems into the decimal number system because the decimal system is most common. Fortunately, the user does not have to do this very often. What is important to realize, however, is that these strange number systems are not designed to obfuscate, but rather to help the individual who has to program the computer on a very detailed level. Why are these number systems so helpful to the programmer?

Interestingly enough, the basis for the answer lies not in hardware, but in the way computers are programmed. Although to a computer the bits in memory are just a long string of binary digits, it is not easy for the programmer to think of them in that manner and it is also very cumbersome. For example, the hex number given as a previous example would be 1111111111001001 in binary. However, hardware now reflects the bias of programmers and is organized in bytes. As the size of memory and processor capacity increased, data came to be represented as "words" with 2–8 bytes per word, and there came a need for number systems capable of handling large numbers to describe both the numbers themselves and the addresses where the data were located. For now at least, the hex number system seems to be satisfactory.

One of the main purposes of a computer is to handle data. However, even with boards constructed to hold megabytes of data there are many cases in which computers have to handle 10s of megabytes of information and information from many users simultaneously. In addition, there is a need for permanently storing information. To satisfy all these requirements, different types of memory have been designed. Although the preceding discussion has been restricted to core memory, these other types of memory will be discussed a little later in the chapter. At this point we return to discussing processor power in terms of size.

Data Transfer and Handling

As discussed previously, data in the computer are stored in bytes. However, this is not necessarily how the data are processed. Two factors need to be considered here. One is the data size that the processor can handle in one chunk and the other is data size that the memory can send to and receive from the processor. It was mentioned before that one reason for the increase in the power of computers was the increase in the size of the chunk. The first microprocessors handled data in 4-bit chunks. Current processors in laboratories and industry handle data in 32-bit chunks. Even some home computers operate on 16-bit chunks. State-of-the-art processors use larger chunks and some of the special architectures described earlier.

Memory originally was set up to send data to the processor in the same size as the processor typically handled. However, as processors were able to handle larger chunks of data, this rule of thumb was not maintained. Ideally, the data transfer size from the memory matches the data-handling capabilities of the processor, but it may not be economical. For example, some machines advertised as 16-bit computers transfer the data in 8-bit chunks. This actually means that the processor can handle 16-bit data, but is using an 8-bit data transfer. Why is this important? It turns out that the speed of a computer is actually determined more by the speed of its data transfer than by the speed of its processor. Hence, the main bottleneck in computer power is not the processor, but the memory and the data transfer between processor and memory. Since we have returned to the topic of memory and have added the issue of data transfer, the topic of the different types of memory will now be discussed.

Types of Memory

Memory in computers fulfills the same needs as memory in the everyday world. Our brains store and change information constantly, but when we want to remember something for a long time, we generally write it down. We also use video and audio tape recorders, to store information of that type. These examples should make clear that there are many types of memory in the everyday world that fulfill different needs. How computers use different types of memory to fulfill various needs will now be discussed.

Random Access Memory

In previous discussions on core memory, it has been implicit that this memory could be changed at will by the programmer, i.e., that it was read/write memory. Core memory is referred to as *random access memory* (RAM) because any location in memory is immediately available. The first personal microcomputer had 1,024 bytes of RAM.

The size of computer memory is currently measured in kilobytes (usually abbreviated as Ks), i.e., the first personal computer had 1K of memory. Each K is worth 2^{10} bytes, or 1,024 bytes. Thus a 64K RAM computer has $64 \times 1,024$ bytes of RAM or 65,536 bytes of RAM, not 64,000 bytes of RAM. With the increase in RAM size, memory is starting to be measured in Ms (megabytes). The tradition started with Ks has continued so each M equals 1,000 Ks or 1,024,000 bytes, not 1,000,000 bytes. This lack of correspondence between English and computer jargon is sometimes confusing, but can generally be ignored because, in spite of the maxim that programs expand to overflow available memory, the differences in size implied by the jargon are usually not great enough to make a difference.

Random access memory is the workhorse memory for a system. It is where data for calculations are stored and accessed and has the great advantage of being fast. It is similar to our brain. Another type of memory that is fast, but does not permit easy changing of its contents is read-only memory (ROM).

Read-Only Memory

Read-only memory is constructed in much the same manner as RAM, but in such a way that once a program or data have been written in the memory they cannot be removed or changed. At one time, ROMs were permanent in the sense that they could only be written into once. but newer models permit changing the data in ROMs. An example is an Electrically Erasable Programmable Read-Only Memory (EEPROM), which is usually abbreviated to PROM. A PROM can be erased with an appropriate electrical current and then written to again. It should be pointed out that this process of erasure and writing is much slower than erasing and writing in RAM. Probably the closest analogy is writing on a piece of paper. The usual technique is to have RAM of equal or greater size than the PROM, and after the desired information has been written into RAM and verified, the PROM is erased and the RAM transferred to the PROM.

Why use ROMs if they are so slow? While ROM is slower than RAM, it has the advantage that it is permanent. That is, when the power goes off, the ROM retains its contents, whereas RAM is erased or garbled. In addition, while ROM is slower than RAM, the difference is not noticeable by a user. Thus ROM is very useful for programs that should be run when the computer is turned on or for programs that will seldom change; a common example is game programs. Another application for ROM is to store data that seldom change or that must be retained when the power is removed. Current computer terminals are examples of this.

All of these memories are typically semiconductor memories. RAM and ROM are available on circuit boards, and thus memory can be expanded to the extent that the machine has space and the microprocessor can access the memory. However, there are other types of memory designed to satisfy some of the needs mentioned earlier, namely, permanent storage of work in progress and storage of amounts of data exceeding the RAM space of the computer. Another need, which may not be so apparent, is the requirement for portability. This need is also being addressed in another way through advances in data communications and will be discussed later. These needs have been addressed through several devices, most notably magnetic tape and various disk media. These devices are attached peripherally to the central core of the computer, and thus are referred to as *peripherals*. Hence the discussion of peripherals will begin with a description of memory peripherals.

Manufacturers are increasingly trying to make their machines more portable, and so the line between peripherals and core is becoming blurred just as the lines between mainframe, minicomputer, and microcomputer have become blurred. This should be kept in mind because you should not expect to find these peripherals necessarily separated from the computer. The division is based on function rather than location.

Magnetic Tape

Magnetic tape was (and still is) used a lot on larger computer systems. Most systems use seven to nine track tapes (seven to nine rows of data are written simultaneously) as permanent data storage devices. The data storage technique is very similar to that of multichannel FM tape described in chapter 6. A lot of data can be stored on a single tape. For example, a 2400-foot tape can store 35–100 million bytes of data. This means that it does not take a large number of tapes to store all the data that might exist on a computer system, which is the purpose for the tapes. They are also useful because they are relatively compact and very portable. Hence tapes can be used to transfer data or programs between machines.

As in other areas, cassette tapes have become popular as tape storage media and are frequently used for microcomputers. They are used for the same purposes and in the manner as reel-to-reel tapes.

A disadvantage to the use of tape is that randomly accessing data on tape can be very slow. Data on a tape must be accessed sequentially, that is, the tape must be read until the point that contains the data of interest is found. Although this can be overcome to a certain extent by the use of directories (which are effectively a table of contents) at the front of the tape, the additional factor of speed must be overcome. Tape drives neither read nor write rapidly. A typical speed for a tape drive on a personal computer might be 1200 bits/s, approximately 120 characters/s. At that rate it would take about 40 min to transfer 300,000 bytes. Tape drives on larger computers operate considerably faster, but you get the idea. Imagine the time it would require to find and read two pieces of data, one at the beginning of the tape and the other at the end. Due to this speed of access difficulty and the need to access large amounts of data rapidly, disk drives were developed.

Disk-Drive Storage

The common usage of disk storage is a relatively recent phenomenon and is due to the incredible reduction in the price of such storage. There two general types of disk storage, hard and floppy, although cartridge disks are sometimes referred to as "a separate type of disk." All types of disks come in a variety of sizes, but the general principles for how the disks store information are the same regardless of type or size. A brief description of how disks store information will be given; this is followed by a description of available disk-drive systems, as well as what the future may hold in terms of disk storage.

Disk Media

Data are stored on disks in much the same manner as on tape, i.e., magnetically. However, there are several differences in the way the data are packaged on a disk, and with the advent of new recording techniques, there promises to be differences in the manner of storage as well. Data on a disk are stored as a string of bits, with each bit represented on the disk as the polarity of a magnetic field. The chapter on recorders discussed how information is stored on tape, and until recently similar techniques were used for disks. The strings of data on the disk are stored in concentric rings (Fig. 9.11).

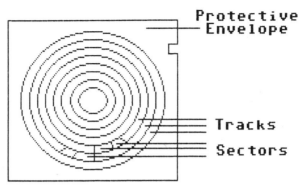

Figure 9.11.   Tracks and sectors on a floppy diskette.

Figure 9.11 shows that a disk is laid out in concentric rings called "tracks," with the tracks broken up into sectors. Different sizes and types of disks have different numbers of tracks. Each sector holds a given amount of data depending on the density of the disk, i.e., how tightly the data are packed into a sector. The combination of numbers of tracks and sectors and the density of the disk determines how much data can be stored on a given disk. These factors depend not only on media but on the hardware used to access the information on the disk. Regardless of what new technology is applied, the concept of using concentric rings to store data on disks seems likely to remain.

There are two basic types of media: rigid and soft (floppy). Rigid media are made of materials such as a specially treated ceramic that can store magnetic charges and is able to handle the stress involved with rotating at very high speeds. The hard disks are referred to as "platters." A *floppy disk* can be thought of as a "circular pancake" of magnetic tape. For the floppy disk to be used in a disk drive, the pancake is enclosed in a special envelope. Figure 9.12 illustrates how a floppy disk is constructed. Floppy disks are often referred to as *diskettes*.

Disk Drives

The information on disk media is accessed using disk drives. The types of disk drives take their names from the media that they use. For both hard and floppy-disk drives the principle is to read and write the data on the media as it is spun by the disk drive. In the case of the floppy-disk drive, the disk is spun at about 360 rpm, which means that a given section of the disk passes a fixed point in the drive about every 3 ms. In addition, an entire track passes by the same point every 3 ms. A hard disk, on the other hand, can spin at a rate of 3600 rpm, reducing the lag between arrivals times by a factor of 10 and increasing the rate at which the disk

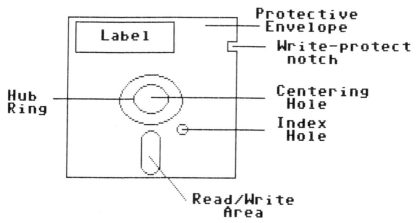

Figure 9.12.   External view of a floppy diskette.

passes by a given point by the same factor. As you may have guessed, these differences between floppy and hard disk drives have important implications with regard to their information-handling capabilities.

The disk read/write heads ride on a thin cushion of air just above the surface of the disk media. Unlike tape-drive heads, disk-drive heads are movable. Since the entire surface of the media is readily accessible to heads, unlike for a tape drive, it is relatively easy to randomly access the data on a disk. This accessability accounts for some of the popularity of disk drives over tape drives as permanent storage devices. However, the heads can only move perpendicular to the tracks on the disk. Since the disk is laid out as a flat surface with concentric rings of data, the data are accessed by moving the head to the track where the data are stored and then waiting until the desired sector passes underneath the head. At this time the magnetic information on the disk is either read or is altered by the head to reflect new data being stored on the disk. In order for this system to work, the disk head must be positioned properly and the data read at the appropriate time. This is done by having the tracks and sectors identified on the disk. The head reads the track and sector information in order to properly align itself. Since sectors come one right after the other on the disk, the disk is spinning, and the disk has to read information for positioning after it operates on each sector, which requires a slight pause as the drive decodes the positioning information. Disk sectors are not written (and hence read) consecutively, but rather are written in a leapfrog manner. The number of sectors between writes is referred to as the "interleaving factor," but is transparent to the user; the fact is included here only to aid in understanding the mechanics of how a disk drive works.

The implications of the aformentioned differences between hard and floppy drives now becomes apparent. Since the speed of accessing data depends on how fast data pass the head and how fast the head can get to the data, it is obvious that a hard disk has a clear advantage in both cases. The head in a hard disk will find the data faster and read/write the data faster. Of course, a hard-disk drive is also more expensive, so the need for rapidity of access and high data-transfer rates needs to be weighed against the differential in cost.

Another difference between floppy and hard disks relates to the accuracy with which the read/write heads can be positioned. For a hard disk, which is fixed in place, the accuracy is greater than for a floppy disk, which has to be mounted on a spindle every time it is used. (Since many computer media and devices are removable and in the past were generally mounted on spindles, "mounting" has become the jargon in computers meaning "to place media in or on a computer" or "to provide the computer access to a device.") In addition, hard media permit a greater density in terms of both tracks and sectors. These factors combine to permit much greater storage capacities for a single hard disk versus a single floppy disk. This is another factor that must be considered when weighing the cost/benefit ratio between the two types of storage devices.

Originally, floppy-disk drives had only one read/write head per disk. Recently it has become common for floppy disks to have heads on both sides of the disk. These drives are referred to as *double-sided disk drives.* Hard-disk drives can have many heads. This is possible because many hard-disk drives actually contain multiple platters, rather than the single disk per drive arrangement that is typical of floppy disks. An arrangement of eight heads and four platters in a single hard disk is not uncommon. The advantage of such an arrangement is greatly increased storage with no loss of speed of access.

Still another difference between floppy and hard disks is the portability of the media. Hard disks are usually fixed in place, whereas floppy disks can be transported from machine to machine. Cartridge disks are an exception to this. Cartridge disks are hard disks that are encased in a hard jacket in a manner similar to that for floppy disks. These were originally developed to handle the problems of capacity and portability. Having multiple disks effectively multiplies the capacity of the drive in the same manner as the multiple platters. The removability permits portability. A limitation of cartridge disks is that the maximum capacity is considerably less than that of fixed, hard disks.

There are also limits to the portability of floppy and cartridge disks. Recall that even if the disk fits into the disk drive, the data on the disk still have to be read by the disk drive. This leads to issues such as formatting, which will be covered in the next section.

Some of the preceding discussion probably sounds esoteric. So that the reader obtains a better understanding for how these issues impact on a computer user, how to use disk systems will be discussed before a brief discussion of expected developments in disk drives and media.

How to Use a Disk System

Disk systems are extremely easy to use as well as being a quick way to access and store data. With hard-disk systems there are no physical manipulations necessary to use the disk because all of that work is done internally. However, the original installation of the hard-disk system should be done by an expert. This is because both the hardware and the software have to be installed on the disk in the proper manner for the system to work, and this requires expert knowledge. As more stand-alone hard-disk systems are developed, this will be less necessary. To use the hard disk, one just turns it on. In some cases, as in UNIX systems, the use of the disk is unnoticeable ("transparent" in computer jargon) to the user. In other cases, the commands to use either a floppy- or hard-disk system are the same.

A floppy-disk system can usually be installed by the user if the floppy disk system is external to the computer. If the system is internal, then obviously a hardware expert is required to install the system. Using any kind of disk system requires software, i.e., the computer uses software to control the operation of the disk. This software is called, reasonably enough, the *disk operating system*, or DOS. Some computer systems have the necessary software internally, which is the trend in computer systems. For other systems, the DOS is on a disk and there is a short program in the computer that reads in the DOS. This small program is called a *bootstrap program* because it reads a program off the disk and starts that program, which in turns reads in the rest of the DOS. In effect, the computer is "lifting itself up by its software bootstraps" (a program reading in a program that reads in the DOS).

To use a floppy disk system, one must turn it on along with the computer and all other peripherals. If the computer contains the DOS internally, then the system is ready to go; if a particular program is desired then the disk with that program on it must be loaded into the disk drive and read. If the DOS is not located internally within the computer, then the disk containing the DOS must first be loaded into the disk system and read.

How to Load and Run Floppy Disks

A floppy disk drive has a top and bottom. Obvious, right? The bottom is the side of the disk toward which the disk drive door is closed. So what? Well, disk drives can operate on their side as well as flat, and knowing which side is the top is crucial to proper loading of a floppy disk.

These rules should be followed whenever loading and running a floppy-disk drive:

1. The label side of a floppy disk should always be facing toward the top of the disk drive when the disk is inserted into the disk drive.

2. The disk should never be inserted or removed when the drive is spinning and/or the head is active. This can damage the media and/or the drive. Some drives rotate as long as the disk is in the drive, but release this mechanism when the drive door is opened.

3. The disk should be inserted into the drive gently. It should be inserted until it can go no further. If a disk is inserted into a drive with excessive force, the disk can be crimped and damaged.

4. The disk-drive door should be closed gently but firmly, making sure that the door is completely closed and locked in place.

5. A disk drive should not be operated in a hot environment. The temperature inside of a disk drive is anywhere from 20 to 40 degrees warmer than the outside temperature. With a room temperature of above about 80°F, the chances of damaging the media or getting strange behavior from the disk drive increase dramatically. This is particularly true if the disk drive does not have a fan in the drive compartment.

6. If the DOS must be loaded from a disk, make sure that the DOS is on whatever disk is in the drive, or the system may "hang up," i.e., stop operating properly.

7. Keep dust and dirt out of the drive and off the disks. Dust covers for disk drives and containers for disks can save many headaches and lengthen the life of system and media. Although many disk drives now use both sides of the disk to store information, there are many drives that use single-sided disks. Keep in mind that the single-sided disk drive stores data on the side of the disk *opposite* the label, and thus this is the side of the disk that must be kept clean.

Some people recommend using a hole punch to make single-sided disks into double-sided disks. This can be done because all disks are originally manufactured to be double-sided. However, single-sided disks are the disks that failed to pass the certification tests on both sides. In addition, current disk jackets are designed to help keep the disk clean. Because the disk is designed on the assumption that it will always spin in the same direction, flipping the disk and using the other side reverses the direction and defeats the cleaning design by dumping all the collected dirt back into the open area in the jacket. My advice is not to use the hole-punch method to increase media storage capabilities. Buy double-sided disk drives if that kind of storage capacity is really necessary and your computer can use them.

8. While we are on the subject of disks, recall that formatting a disk

was mentioned earlier. Recall that data on floppy disk are organized in tracks and sectors. This organization is written on the disk. Unfortunately, as is common in the computer business, not all manufacturers use the same organization for their disk drives. Hence, it is necessary to format a disk (write on the disk the track and sector information) so that the disk drive can use it. A program that will do this for you is almost always provided as part of the DOS. A good practice is to format disks by the box, and when there are only two to three formatted disks left, format another box.

9. Make backup copies of every disk and every program. (Now where have you heard something like this before?) This rule cannot be overemphasized. Failure to heed this rule is the number 1 reason for "computer suicide."

10. Always have plenty of disks on hand. You will find that you never have enough. Remember that there will always be a ratio of almost two disks for every one work disk because of rule 9.

11. Like all other mechanical instruments, disk drives do wear out and break. Be sure to know where to take the drives before they break in order to reduce the lost time as much as possible. If it is critical that at least one drive be available at all times, then get a second drive. The second drive will also considerably reduce the time required to back up data and obviously expand the amount of storage immediately available, which can be very helpful when working with large data files.

12. Recall that disks are magnetic storage media just like tapes, and the same care has to be taken to keep them away from magnetic sources. Some magnetic sources are more apparent than others. For example, vacuum cleaners can do an excellent job of garbling or "cleaning" a disk or tape as well as the floor. A general rule is to store disks on a high place, preferably in a metal cabinet.

These rules will provide guidance when using floppy disk drives. It should be kept in mind that when all else fails, you can always read the manual. Unfortunately, in my experience floppy disk manuals are generally long on technical information and short on general user information. The intent of these rules is to help fill in the gaps and give some pointers with regard to everyday use that the manuals do not cover.

Processors and memory (core plus disk and/or tape) comprise the basic computer but are insufficient for people to use it. The "standard" computer includes two other peripherals in addition to what has been discussed here. These are terminals and printers. Terminals for many computers have the terminal in two pieces, a keyboard and a monitor. For this reason monitors will be discussed in the terminal section. There are many other peripherals, such as modems and A/D (analog-to-digital) converters, but these will be discussed when the applications using those peripherals are discussed.

Input Devices

There are a variety of devices that provide the computer with a way to receive input from the user. The most common form of input device is a *terminal.* Other input devices include *mice, joysticks, light pens, tracballs,* and special sensing peripherals such as *analog-to-digital converters.* This section will not discuss the special input devices, which have been discussed to some extent in other chapters, but will focus on those devices that the user directly manipulates to provide input to the computer.

Terminals

For the purposes of this discussion, "terminals" will be considered to be any combination of a typewriter-like keyboard and a monitor. There are many terminal configurations that fit this general definition. The keyboard and monitor portions of the terminal may be combined in one unit or they may be two completely separate components, such as is the case for many personal computers. Regardless of the configurations the basic components of keyboards and monitors remain the same, so each will be discussed separately.

Keyboards

Keyboards provide a means for entering alphanumeric data into the computer by pressing keys on the keyboard. A typical keyboard is laid out much like a typewriter keyboard, except that there are some special keys and some of the regular keys function slightly differently from the corresponding typewriter keys.

Each of the different types of keys are generally clustered in groups on the keyboard. The main clusters are the typewriter keys (letters and numbers laid out as for a typewriter), cursor keys, numeric keypad, and function keys. The characteristic pattern is for the typewriter keys to occupy the central portion of the keyboard, with the other key groups found to the side or above the typewriter keys.

When a key is pressed on a terminal keyboard, a character or string of characters is sent to the computer. Each key has some defined output. Most of the keys always have the same output, but some keys can be redefined. How many keys can be redefined depends on the design of the keyboard. We will expand upon this as we discuss each section of a "typical" keyboard.

The typewriter portion of the keyboard that contains the letters and numbers is usually laid out in the same manner as a typical typewriter. This layout is referred to as the "QWERTY layout," because of the letters in the upper left portion of the keyboard. There are alternative layouts available, although the only one that is at all common is the DVORAK keyboard, which is named after the inventor of the layout. The QWERTY layout is the traditional layout and was developed for mechanical typewriters, with the design criterion of keeping the impact hammers for most common keys as far apart as possible in order to prevent jamming. For computers, which do not have mechanical parts, this consideration does not apply; the DVORAK keyboard was developed to take advantage of this fact. The DVORAK keyboard was developed with the design criterion that the most common keys should be in the middle of the keyboard in order to increase the efficiency of use. The long history of the QWERTY keyboard has kept this keyboard as the most common, but the DVORAK keyboard is slowly gaining acceptance, especially with writers.

The key output for the typewriter portion of a keyboard is usually in the form of an ASCII character. ASCII (American Standard Code for Information Interchange) refers to a standard method of representing characters. Table 9.1 gives the ASCII definitions. There are "different" ASCIIs, which are dependent on the number of bits available to represent the character, but the most common for terminal communication is seven-bit ASCII. The seven-bit ASCII character code will be assumed in this discussion. The "CAPS" representation of characters in the typewriter portion of the keyboard would be the same regardless of the layout used on the keyboard. Note that there are definitions for the number keys as well as separate definitions for the capital and small letters, plus some "extra" definitions. Some of the extra characters are used to handle transmission of information such as signalling the beginning and end of transmission strings. Other extra characters permit special characters to be sent to the computer to signal special events. Also note that there are many more ASCII characters than there are letters and numbers. Although it is called "seven-bit ASCII", eight bits are transmitted to the computer; therefore there are potentially 255 characters available. Many of these extra characters provide limited graphics capability using only the available ASCII characters. This will be discussed in more detail later when monitors are discussed.

The cursor keys are usually arranged in a compasslike manner with the up-arrow key pointing toward the top of the keyboard, although occasionally the cursor keys are laid out in a row. The usual order for keys laid out in a row is to have the left and right keys on the left and the up and down keys on the right. The cursor keys are used to move the cursor in the direction indicated by the cursor key. The "cursor" is a pointer on the terminal monitor telling the operator where data will be input on the screen. On some keyboards, most notably the IBM-PC, there are some additional keys associated with the cursor keys, which are the HOME, END, PG UP, and PG DN keys. Many programs use these additional keys to make large cursor movements, with the regular cursor keys used to make small cursor movements.

The numeric keypad, which is a common feature on a computer key-

Table 9.1
ASCII Table

Character	Decimal	Character	Decimal	Character	Decimal
NUL	00	.	46	\	92
SOH	01	/	47	]	93
STX	02	0	48		94
ETX	03	1	49		95
EOT	04	2	50	ˉ	96
ENQ	05	3	51	a	97
ACK	06	4	52	b	98
BEL	07	5	53	c	99
BS	08	6	54	d	100
HT	09	7	55	e	101
NL	10	8	56	f	102
VT	11	9	57	g	103
FF	12	:	58	h	104
CR	13	;	59	i	105
SO	14	<	60	j	106
SI	15	=	61	k	107
DLE	16	>	62	l	108
DC1	17	?	63	m	109
DC2	18	@	64	n	110
DC3	19	A	65	o	111
DC4	20	B	66	p	112
NAK	21	C	67	q	113
SYN	22	D	68	r	114
ETB	23	E	69	s	115
CAN	24	F	70	t	116
EM	25	G	71	u	117
SUB	26	H	72	v	118
EXC	27	I	73	w	119
NP	28	J	74	x	120
GS	29	K	75	y	121
RS	30	L	76	z	122
US	31	M	77	{	123
[sp]	32	N	78	¦	124
!	33	O	79	}	125
"	34	P	80	~	126
#	35	Q	81	DEL	127
$	36	R	82		
%	37	S	83		
&	38	T	84		
'	39	U	85		
(	40	V	86		
)	41	W	87		
*	42	X	88		
+	43	Y	89		
,	44	Z	90		
-	45	[	91		

board, is arranged very similarly to that for a calculator except that the multiplication and division signs are generally not included. The purpose of the keypad is to permit rapid entry of numeric information and is laid out like a calculator for ease of use. On the IBM-PC, the cursor keys are in the numeric keypad and there is a key (NUM LOCK) that permits switching between the two functions for the keypad.

Another key group is the function keys, which are generally used to send a string of characters to the computer in order execute a function; hence the name "function keys." Most function keys are predefined, although there are programs that permit redefinition of the character string sent by the key. Most such programs create a separate memory area that is devoted to the function-key definitions. Some terminals have their own memory dedicated to function keys and hence can do the redefinition separate from the computer. These terminals are said to have programmable function keys.

Along with the above groups of keys, there are some special keys on a computer keyboard. The most common are the CONTROL, ESCAPE, ALT, and DEL keys. The CONTROL key, often shortened to CTRL or CTL or symbolized by ˆ, is generally used to send command sequences, sometimes referred to as "control sequences," to the computer and is used along with the other keys in the typewriter portion of the keyboard. The ALT key also is used in this manner. The CONTROL key modifies the output for an alphanumeric key by converting the ASCII output for the key into the lower 32 values. For example, ˆM is a carriage return, which is the same as ASCII 13, because M is the 13th character in the alphabet. The ALT key does the same but uses the upper part of the ASCII table. The ESCAPE (or ESC) key is usually used to exit from a mistake. The DELETE (or DEL) key is used to erase the character at the position of the cursor. This key is used with other keys to provide some simple editing functions in the keyboard although some terminals provide extensive editing capabilities in the terminal, independent of the computer.

Although a terminal keyboard seems to have many parts, such a device can be used by anybody who can hit a key and has the advantage that many people are trained to type. The computer keyboard has proved to be a very flexible input device for many different types of computers.

Monitors

The output of the terminal keyboard is typically displayed on a monitor as well as being sent to the computer. Monitors were discussed in chapter 6 in terms of some general rules for using monitors that are connected to video equipment other than computers. This section will expand upon that discussion and provide more technical information about monitors from the point of view of the user. The user may have to describe a project or problem involving the use of a terminal or video display to a programmer and should know enough about the technical aspects to define and discuss the problem.

Terminal monitors can be viewed in two basic ways: (1) as character-mapped displays suitable for text or (2) as bit-mapped displays suitable for graphics. Monitors can also be dichotomized as color versus monochrome. First, we will discuss the mapping issue and then discuss the issues of color and resolution.

Mapping can be illustrated by considering an alphanumeric character displayed on a monitor screen. The character can be considered either as a whole or in terms of each individual part that makes up the character. The wholistic view is the character-mapped view and deals with the display in terms of character-sized blocks. It is always the case, however, that the character is generated by a matrix of x bits by y bits. The bit-mapped approach would draw the character bit by bit. There are advantages and disadvantages to each way of displaying data, but the underlying reality is the same. Monitors display data as organized bit patterns.

The character-mapped display mode is often used to display text because it is faster to use predefined blocks of data for each character than to draw the character using rules. With the advent of faster and more powerful video processors, this speed advantage is decreasing to the point where it is not important for normal display purposes and so most terminals now use a bit-mapped display.

Why would a bit-mapped display be preferred? Mostly because of its flexibility. When the character is drawn, it can be drawn in any shape and so an infinity of shapes is available. With character-mapped mode, the character shapes are stored in ROM and each character set would require that the desired shape be preprogrammed into ROM. For other than very common character sets, this approach would eventually break down and become very expensive. Another advantage is the ability to easily combine graphics with text and display aspects of text such as underlining.

Bit-mapped displays raise the issues of resolution and color. Since bit-mapped displays are most useful for graphics, it might be thought that all monitors should be color monitors. In fact, color monitors currently suffer from a resolution problem and so are not best for some applications, most notably intensive text (including numeric entry) applications. For these applications a monochrome monitor is most appropriate. Monochrome monitors are inappropriately named for they are not single-color monitors. Monochrome refers to the fact that the text is in a single color. However, the background is in a different color, generally black, and there is control over the intensity of the display so shades of gray can be displayed using a monochrome monitor. The advantage of a monochrome monitor is resolution.

Monochrome monitors have a built-in advantage for resolution because of the manner in which color is displayed on a monitor. Color is displayed as the combination of the three colors red, green, and blue (RGB). This requires three outputs for every point on the display while the monochrome monitor needs only one (the background is simply the absence of any output). This permits a three-to-one advantage in display resolution for the monochrome system versus the color system for the same number of outputs to the screen.* Monochrome monitors are much simpler and cheaper because less electronic circuitry is required to decode the signal into its composite colors. Considerable improvements in color monitors are changing this situation, but monochrome monitors are going to be the resolution leaders for a while.

In view of the rapidly evolving nature of color displays, there will be a short discussion of different types of color displays in order to assist readers in determining which display might be best for their application. For computers, the use of color displays is closely tied to the resolution of the display in combination with the variety of color available to be displayed. This link is explained simply because the computer views color displays as bit-mapped information in memory. The color displays require a lot of information to be placed on the screen. Since such displays are bit-mapped displays, this information must be available for each bit on the display. If the display only requires one bit of memory (on vs. off) for each bit on the screen, the number of bytes of memory is the number of bits in the display divided by 8. For a high-resolution display of 750 horizontal bits × 350 vertical bits, this means over 32,000 bytes of memory. This would be the case for a high-resolution monochrome display. We will now do the same analysis for a color display.

For a monochrome display, each bit was simply "on" or "off." For a color display, each location represents a color. But each color is a choice among the colors available, and so the amount of information per location is determined by the number of choices. Recall that the computer does not see colors, it only sees codes. For example, if there are 16 colors, four bits will be required to unambiguously identify each color. The greater the number of colors, the more alternatives that have to be coded and so the more bits required for each location. Thus, the number of bytes required for a color display can be determined by calculating the number of bytes required for a monochrome display and multiplying that number by the number of bits needed to code the color options. For the color equivalent of the monochrome example given above, it would require 128,000 bytes

---

* There are two main types of color monitors: those that split the color signal into each of its three components (RGB monitors) and those that do not (composite monitors). RGB monitors will have better resolution than composite monitors because of the better control over how the color is mixed and presented on the monitor.

to provide a 16-color picture of equal resolution. For a really rich display with 4096 colors available, it would require about 400,000 bytes of memory. The complexities of display described earlier, combined with the larger memory and decoding requirements, account for the high cost of color displays.

Because of the computational and the display requirements associated with color displays, terminals that provide high-resolution color have been used most frequently as stand-alone terminals attached to mainframes or minicomputers. Interestingly, the development of personal computers with adequate color capabilities began with home computers such as the Commodore 64. It is only very recently that the more expensive computers are starting to provide better colors displays. The IBM-PC now has two color display standards in common use, the Color Graphics Adapter (CGA) and the Enhanced Graphics Adapter (EGA). The CGA standard has the same resolution as the Commodore 64, 320 horizontal bits × 200 vertical bits and looks very similar. With a 640 horizontal bit × 400 vertical bit mode, the EGA standard has four times the resolution. However, the best color is actually provided by two other machines, the Amiga by Commodore and the Atari ST series, with a slight edge held by the Amiga. If a powerful color computer at a reasonable price is the primary consideration, these two machines should definitely be considered. The Amiga also has an option for IBM compatability. If frequent IBM compatability is important, the EGA color system is a considerable improvement and should be considered; this is especially true if much text is going to be displayed, since high resolution makes a considerable difference in the quality of a text display.

Remote Terminals

Most of the preceding discussion has focused on issues that pertain to all terminals. For multiuser systems, the most common type of terminal is a remote terminal. As microcomputers become more powerful, multiuser systems will become more common; thus remote terminals merit a brief discussion.

Virtually all remote terminals consist of a separate keyboard attached to a monitor. Such terminals are generally classified as either *intelligent* or *dumb*. The term "intelligent" refers to the fact that the terminal is capable of executing commands independently of the computer to which it is attached (generally referred to as the "host computer"). Some terminals are specifically designed for graphics applications. Since there are over 50 terminal companies and literally hundreds of terminal models, it is usually possible to find the combination of price and performance that is appropriate for a particular application.

These are some aspects of remote terminals that are important for the user:

Size of Screen. In general, the larger the screen, the larger the character size and hence the greater the readability of the display for text. This interacts with the character display matrix size (see below).

Color of the Characters. Amber is generally regarded as causing the least eyestrain, but the terminal must have good contrast to take advantage of the better color.

Character Display Matrix Size. Character matrices are specified as the number of bits across by the number of bits down that are used to represent the character on the screen. In general, the more bits in the matrix, the clearer the character. The exception arises when the aspect ratio (the height/width) is not proper.

Screen Format. Most terminals display 80 characters across and 24–26 lines down. Some terminals can display up to 135 characters across with 24–40 lines down. The more dense character displays are useful for accounting and spreadsheet application and should be used only with terminals having a display screen of 14–19 inches.

Display Resolution. Applies to graphics terminals. Resolutions of up to 2048 × 2048 are available and are used mostly for engineering applications, such as circuit design. Again, the higher resolution should be used with the larger display screens.

Interface. Almost all terminals use a serial interface (i.e., information is sent bit by bit in a consecutive stream) and most use an x-on/x-off protocol (i.e., the manner in which communication between the host is controlled). Unfortunately, although these are standard interfaces and protocols, the standards permit considerable flexibility; therefore, the key here is to get the cable set up properly. Try to have the interconnection done by an expert.

Emulation. Recall from the discussion of ASCII that there are a number of control codes available to the terminal. How these codes are interpreted determines how the data end up on the screen. Some terminal definitions have become standard over the years, most notably Digital Equipment Corporation's VT terminal series, and many terminals made by other manufacturers will emulate that type of terminal to make the job of the person interfacing the terminal to the host computer easier. It is highly recommended that the terminal be able to emulate one of the later versions of the VT series or another common intelligent terminal.

Other. This depends on the application and includes such factors as keyboard layout, number of function keys, and compatability with particular graphics software.

Other Input Devices

In addition to keyboards, other input devices such as mice, joysticks, light pens, and tracballs also provide input to a computer. These belong to a class of input devices referred to as "pointing devices." They are especially useful with screen displays that have been programmed with these devices in mind. The first user interface that used pointing devices was designed over 10 years ago by Xerox Corporation. This interface is now used on several home/business computers, such as the Macintosh and the Amiga, but is just beginning to be used extensively. The primary reason for such slow application is that considerable programming is required to make such interfaces useful. The primary application for a pointing device is in graphics, such as for design and drafting tools. An example of the ease with which such interfaces can be used once the programming is done is to see a young child using a joystick or mouse to interface with "Turtle" graphics (a construct within the LOGO high-level programming language).

Pointing devices have also become very popular for applications involving handicapped users. A joystick has much less severe manipulation requirements compared with a keyboard, although text entry is generally slower. Another application area where such devices might be useful is in test situations where a joystick could be used to change the parameters of the test. This would be an expansion of the current use of a button for testing in audiology. Using a light pen to indicate choices on a menu for testing or analysis is another potential application.

The trend in the area of terminals is to have keyboards supplemented by pointing devices. Furthermore, some of the new high-resolution color systems may fulfill the needs currently met by monochrome systems. With resolution greater than that of a home TV and in combination with a CD-ROM and video digitization, high-resolution color systems serve as excellent rehabilitation tools. The most important stumbling block to the exciting applications and expanding capabilities of terminals is software development.

Hardcopy Output

Hardcopy output (output onto a sheet of paper) is a necessary part of any computer system. Hardcopy output is handled primarily by two types of devices: printers and plotters. Plotters have been discussed previously in connection with audiological, speech, and research instrumentation. The plotters for computers are the same, except that they are driven through characters sent to the plotter rather than through voltages sent to the axis drivers of the plotter. Since there is a trend for printers to take over the function of plotters, especially with the advent of the laser printer, and because the function and use of plotters has been discussed previously, only printers will be discussed in this chapter.

Printers

Printers come in many shapes, sizes, and capabilities; the range of capabilities has increased considerably recently. Originally terminals and printers were one unit; the teletype. The teletype, however, was soon split up into an input device, the terminal, and a separate hard-copy output device (the printer).

The first printers were only good for alphanumeric output and were slow. In addition, they frequently broke down because they were based on the typewriter mechanism and were not designed for the continuous printing that a computer can require. Soon printers capable of printing a whole line at a time were developed with speeds of 100 or more lines per minute. These printers were used in large computer centers and cost more than $10,000, which at that time was an even more impressive amount of money. While 100 lines/min sounds fast, it represents about 130 characters/s, which is the speed of an excellent typist. Of course, the printer does not get tired and can keep up this speed all day and night. There are printers currently available for less than $300 that provide speeds of 120 characters/s. While these printers cannot run day and night like the computer center printers, this comparison will give some idea of how printer prices and capabilities have followed the general trend in computer hardware for greater power at lower prices.

There are currently four major types of printer technology: impact, dot matrix, ink jet, and laser printers. Each of these types has advantages and disadvantages, and the weighting of these factors changes constantly. The intent here will be to review briefly each of the printing methods and to describe the most common applications for each type.

Impact Printers

Printers have been customarily described in terms of how the print head, the device that places the information on the paper, operates. Impact printers operate very similarly to typewriters. A hammer strikes a metal or plastic letter that impacts on an inked ribbon and transfers the letter to the paper. The letters are on little fingers arranged like the spokes on a wheel, and the mechanism in the printer rotates the wheel so that the hammer strikes the appropriate letter. Not surprisingly the wheels are called "print wheels."

High-quality impact printers yield a print quality identical to that of a typewriter. This feature has led to such printers being termed *letter-quality printers*. This term can lead to confusion. Not all impact printers can give high-quality print, i.e., print comparable to an office-quality typewriter. If this level of print quality is desired, be sure to see the printer in operation and get sample printouts for comparison purposes.

While impact printers offer high-quality print, they are slow. Speeds range from 10 to 60 characters/s. There is another aspect to speed, and this is related to how the location of the print head is determined. One method is to have the printer type from the beginning of the line to the end of the line regardless of the number of characters on the line. Another method, which is now the most common method, is called "logic seeking." This refers to the fact that the printer scans ahead of the character that it is currently printing, and if the next character is not on the same line, the print head is positioned to the optimal print location for the next line. Thus the print head travels to where there are characters to be printed rather than crossing empty space and wasting time. A printer without this feature is considerably slower than a printer with this feature.

Impact printers have another limitation. The characters available are restricted to those on the print wheel. If special characters are required, the print wheel must be exchanged for one that has the required characters, and it may be the case that no print wheel contains the desired character. This is not a severe restriction for general office correspondence, but may be a problem for special applications.

If the application requires letter-quality print, as for office correspondence, then this type of printer is probably the printer of choice. However, since most applications do not require such high quality print, dot matrix printers can be used.

Dot Matrix Printers

Dot matrix printers get their name from the fact that the print head is actually a matrix of wires (generally called "pins"). Groups of pins are selected from the matrix based on the required characters. This group of wires transfers the character to the paper in much the same manner as for an impact printer. Any group of pins may be selected and the resolution of the characters will depend on the number of wires in the matrix and the spacing between adjacent wires. The obvious benefit of a dot matrix printer is flexibility. That is, a character can be any combination of wires in the matrix. This allows not only the typical alphanumeric characters but special characters and graphics output. This flexibility is only limited by the number of wires in the matrix. The graphics output is available through a feature called *dot addressable graphics*, which refers to the ability to use any of the pins in the print head anywhere along the line being printed. Using this dot addressable feature, along with high-resolution print heads, can yield print quality that is very similar to that produced by impact printers.

Another feature of dot matrix printers, which may not be so obvious, is their speed. Commonly available dot matrix printers, in the same price range as the impact printers, have speeds from 80–350 characters/s. To put this in perspective, this speed difference can mean the difference between a document being printed out in 1 hour with an impact printer or in 8 minutes with a dot-matrix printer.

Dot matrix printers are the most common type of printer because of their flexibility, speed, and price. However, they share a common drawback with impact printers, and that is noise. Having a printer next to you is convenient but noisy. Two newer technologies are being developed to provide even more flexibility and speed than dot matrix printers and to try to solve the noise problem. These are the *ink jet* and *laser printers* discussed next.

Ink Jet Printers

Ink jet printers are very similar to dot matrix printers except that they spray a jet of ink from the pins to transfer a character to the paper rather than having the pins impact on a ribbon. In all other respects except one, they operate on the same principles and have the same advantages as dot matrix printers. The exception is noise. Ink-jet printers are very quiet. When they operate, the only sound is the swish of the print head.

It should be noted that ink jet technology is still improving and the quality of the print and the mechanics of delivering ink from the reservoir to the paper is still being worked out. Ink-jet printers could have the capability of delivering close to impact-quality print, but remember that the ink-jet print head has the same characteristics as a dot matrix print head; therefore, the same limitations with regard to resolution apply.

A new type of printer has been developed recently that has the potential for replacing all of the above printers. This printer represents the application of laser technology to printing.

Laser Printers

The term *laser printer* sounds like space technology, but the basic principle is actually quite simple. A laser is just a focused, thin pencil of light. By changing the location that the pencil is focused, the laser "writes" on the paper. It is quiet because there is no impact. In addition, there is no possibility of an ink spill. Perhaps the most exciting fact of all is that because the laser is just like a pencil (or a paint brush), it is theoretically possible to produce graphics of the same quality as hand-drawn art. For the same reason, i.e., the laser can "write" continuously, it should be possible to produce print comparable with that of a typewriter. Interestingly, the print speed of such a printer is incredible; its speed is in the thousands of characters per second. In effect, laser printers offer the best of both worlds.

All of the aforementioned features are available today, but are extremely expensive. Although laser printers can cost below $4000, the features listed here cost above $12,000. This price has restricted such powerful printers to large companies and small businesses that can justify such cost. When the price drops below $3000, all but home users will be able to employ such printers; if the price drops below $500, the expectation is that almost every printer will be a laser printer.

Now that all of the hardware necessary for a computer system has been described, it all needs to be put together. In general this is straightforward, but there are aspects that can be difficult. Before discussing actually putting together a system, there is another area which must be discussed, namely, *software*, which is what makes the hardware work.

Software

Software is the "fuel" that makes computers run. A computer without software is like a car without gas. Just like different kinds of cars with different kinds and levels of power need different kinds of gas, different kinds and levels of computers need different kinds and levels of software. The intent of this section of the chapter is to introduce and briefly describe various types of software. The next section will then apply what we have learned about hardware and software by showing in a limited way how to build computer systems for applications. The emphasis will be on how to use hardware and software, rather than a recommendation for specific hardware and software packages.

Software can be categorized in several ways; there is no claim that the categorization employed here is the only way to do it. However, the categories have been commonly used by others, and hence should be understood before trying to communicate software needs. The categories of software that will be discussed here are operating systems, utilities, languages, and applications software. Applications software will be further subdivided into word processing, spreadsheets, database management, graphics, and video games.

Operating Systems

The hardware portion of this chapter pointed out that there are many parts to the computer besides the processor itself, which is just the "brains" of the operation. The processor has to have some means of telling the rest of the system what to do. The *operating system* software is how the processor controls the system. It links the processor to the various parts of the computer system and controls the operation of those parts in a coordinated manner. The operating system software underlies all other software in the system; without some type of operating system software, a computer system is nonfunctional.

There are many different operating systems. Some of these are nearly invisible to the user because they are not labeled as such. For example, in some home computers the operating system is incorporated into the system itself rather than existing as a separate piece of software apart from the machine. That is, the software is in a ROM, which is activated when the machine is turned on. In fact the trend is to include even very sophisticated operating systems in ROM in the machine because of the ease of use and the decreasing cost of ROM chips.

Most sophisticated operating systems currently exist apart from the machine, and even for ROM-based operating system machines it is possible to load alternative operating systems into the machine. This requires that there be some means for getting the operating system software into the machine. Recall that the operating system is the control software for the system and without it, there is no control. So how does the operating system get into the machine if it isn't already there in ROM? The answer is that there is a very short piece of software in ROM, which is activated when the machine is turned on and which loads part of the operating system into memory and turns control over to this software, which in turn loads the rest of the operating system into memory and activates the operating system. As mentioned previously, due to the nature of this operation, which is akin to lifting yourself by your own bootstraps (a piece of software loads in a piece of software, which loads in another piece of software, etc.) the software in ROM is called the *bootstrap program*. This operation occurs regardless of the origin of the operating system software.

There are several major operating systems in the field, but since the primary focus of this chapter is towards the smaller user, the mainframe operating systems will be ignored. However, be aware that many of the principles discussed here, and at least one of the operating systems (UNIX), can be applied to the mainframe systems. The three operating systems that will be used for examples in this chapter are CP/M, MS-DOS (PC-DOS), and UNIX.

Each of these operating systems will be briefly described. Then how to use an operating system, with examples from each system, will be covered. This will be followed by the discussion of applications.

CP/M

Control Program/Microprocessors (CP/M) was the first operating system for microcomputers that gained widespread acceptance. The reasons were that it operated on a variety of manufacturers' machines, it was relatively powerful, it did not consume a lot of memory, and modifying the operating system for the computer system configuration was far easier than in the past. The major disadvantage is that the CP/M operating system was designed for 8-bit systems and has not been suitably modified for the more powerful current processors. However, keep in mind that if the computer does the job desired, the number of bits in the processor is irrelevant. This issue will be discussed throughout this section.

There are three parts to CP/M: CCP, BIOS, and BDOS. The command control processor (CCP) is the part of CP/M that interacts with the user.

The basic input/output system (BIOS) is the part of CP/M that sets up the relations between the hardware components of the computer system and operating system. The basic disk operating system (BDOS) is the part of the system that controls the flow of information to and from the disk system. Figure 9.13 illustrates the functions of the various parts. The CCP and the BIOS are modifiable by the user as long as certain conventions are followed. In fact, it is necessary to set up the BIOS specifically for a particular system. The memory not allocated to these three sections is available for programs and is referred to as the *transient program area*, or TPA. Figure 9.14 shows a memory map for CP/M in a 64K computer.

The CP/M system operates by having some basic disk operating system functions available at all times and having other functions available as separate programs. The other programs necessary to make up a complete operating system are included as part of the package. That is, CP/M is not a single program, but actually is a collection of programs that provide a complete programming environment. The intent of the developers of CP/M was to produce a powerful enough operating system to develop software, while still keeping it small enough for the 8-bit systems of the time (1970s). This meant the system software had to fit into a 64K machine (a 24K machine was the minimum configuration) while still leaving enough room for other software. It was also the case that, as the operating system capabilities were expanded in succeeding versions, compatibility with previous versions was maintained to a great degree. This meant that

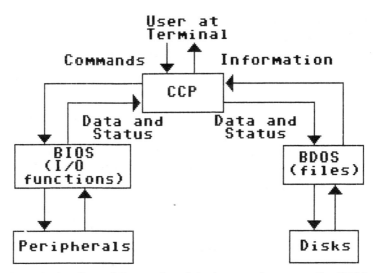

Figure 9.13.   Control flow and modules in operating system for CP/M.

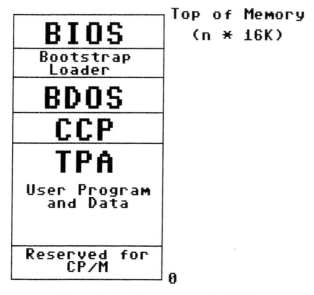

Figure 9.14. Memory map for CP/M.

software developed under an early version of the operating system would run on a later version. Given these goals, CP/M has to be considered an outstanding achievement.

The CP/M system is not a perfect operating system. Primary shortcomings in CP/M include a poor program editor, ambiguous error messages, poor error handling, and poor documentation. Most of these deficiencies have been addressed by others with programs such as powerful program editors, new CCPs that give better error messages, and a plethora of books that explain CP/M and how to use it.

MS-DOS (PC-DOS)

The Microsoft disk operating system (MS-DOS) became popular with the popularity of the IBM personal computer, which used the operating system under the name PC-DOS. MS-DOS has many similarities to CP/M 3.0 (the newest version of CP/M), but has some added features. The basic concepts underlying the operating system have remained, but the system assumes a much larger memory space and has taken advantage of this space. In addition, some UNIX features, most notably a treelike subdirectory structure, have been incorporated into the system. MS-DOS has a BDOS and a BIOS, just like CP/M; MS-DOS also autoboots a program called *Autoexec. Bat* when it is booted off the disk, just as CP/M will if configured to do so. MS-DOS also uses a command line interface to the user, and hence the transition from CP/M to MS-DOS is relatively easy.

Given the considerable similarity between MS-DOS and CP/M, there is not much need to expand upon the description of the system, except for the directory structure, which is quite different from CP/M and very similar to UNIX. When information is stored on a mass storage device, there has to be a way for the operating system to find the information when it is requested by the user. Information is stored in files, which are simply groupings of information under a single label (file name). Operating systems access information on the mass storage device via the file name. In order to use the file name to bring up a file, the system stores the location of the data long with the file name in an area on the mass storage device called a *directory*. The directory is much like a building directory that lists, next to the name, the location where that person or company might be found. Since disks are the most common mass storage device, the rest of this description of directories will be restricted to disk directories.

There are two common ways of handling directories. The first is to store the physical location of the file on the disk with the file name. The size of the file will also be indicated. There is a limit on how big a file may be accessed in this manner because the allocation of space to store file size in such a directory will be limited to conserve space. This makes sense on a small disk because there isn't much room on the disk anyway. This is the type of directory used by CP/M. Recall that CP/M was developed on machines with limited memory. It was also the case that the original disk drives had small capacities as well (on the order of 90 kilobytes). With the advent of larger disks (up to several megabytes), it was necessary to modify the directory system to accommodate the large files that were possible. The strategy was developed to add an indicator of where the next section of the file was located if the file was too large for a single directory entry. Thus a single file name that referred to a very large file could have multiple entries associated with it. While this file directory system works, it has some deficiencies; the most obvious of these is that if you have a large number of files on the same disk there is no easy way to organize them. The UNIX operating system, described in the next section, utilizes a directory structure that permits this organization and still permits efficient location of a file.

The directory structure made popular by UNIX and adopted by MS-DOS is a treelike directory structure. In this directory system there is not only a main directory but it is possible to set up subdirectories as well. Directories are treated by the system as file names, but rather than pointing to the location of a file on the disk, the directories point to the location where the file names are stored. The file name entries are then like the CP/M structure described previously.

It is easy to see how this type of directory structure can help organize a system. An analogy might be putting companies with similar activities on the same floor of a multistory building, with companies having different activities on different floors. The floor could be labeled with the activity predominant on that floor. This would obviously speed up the task of finding a company that engaged in "activity x" because it would not be necessary to go through every name in the building directory to find the "activity x" companies. The same thing would apply to the computer directory. All files having to do with a particular client could go into a single subdirectory, and particular sets of clients could be grouped in a subdirectory, and so on.

The main advantages of the MS-DOS operating system are that it is used on a very popular computer, the IBM PC, so there is a great deal of software available for the operating system; it is familiar to CP/M users, and so the transition is relatively easy; and it takes advantage of a larger memory space than CP/M. It suffers from some of the same problems as CP/M relative to ease of use and is a single-user system. A system that addresses the single-user issue and is more powerful than MS-DOS is the UNIX system, which is described next.

UNIX

Bell Laboratories originally developed the UNIX operating system for their scientific environment. The nature of the operating system reflects this environment. It is very sophisticated and is comprised of a very large number of programs that can be linked together. The facility for linking these programs together and, in effect, programming the operating system is an integral part of UNIX. This capability of any person creating their own private environment that is most comfortable for their own use is unique among major operating systems. Virtually anything in UNIX can be changed. In addition, because of the assumption that technical users would be using the system, there are very few restrictions on what an individual user may do. These are all very great advantages in a scientific and technical environment. They also provide tremendous opportunities for customizing the operating system for particular environments.

The major drawback is that UNIX in its raw form appears somewhat intimidating. This is a misconception based on the fact that UNIX has an extremely large number of commands. Rather than emphasizing the flexibility provided by this rich command structure, the complexity has been emphasized. In actuality, UNIX is at least as user-friendly as CP/M or MS-DOS in its raw form, and is far more easily customized for the individual user. In fact, a learn mode is built into UNIX, which is not provided by other operating systems.

UNIX was originally developed on mainframe and minicomputers. It has only recently become available on microcomputers. However, if imitation is the sincerest form of flattery, then it should be recognized that the MS/PC-DOS operating system borrowed from UNIX when it was developed, and that each successive version of PC-DOS becomes more like UNIX. It appears that UNIX will become the de facto standard for operating systems in the future, although it may have many names. There are several reasons for this, some of which have already been described.

UNIX is a multitasking operating system. This means that UNIX was created with the idea that several programs would be operating simultaneously. This has the advantage of supporting multiuser capability, i.e., more than one user operating the computer simultaneously. Both MS/PC-DOS and CP/M were created as single-user operating systems although multiuser versions exist or are being developed. Other reasons for UNIX popularity: portability (the capability to write programs on one computer and use them, essentially unchanged, or another computer); malleability (UNIX is easily modifiable for environments or users); major vendor support (AT&T was the original developer of UNIX and continues to provide support. IBM is also supporting UNIX.); the increasing power of microcomputers is making it possible to support such a system on a desktop computer; and finally, maturity; i.e., the UNIX operating system has been extensively developed and has been around long enough for there to be experts in its use and for many of the "bugs" in the operating system to be eliminated.

UNIX actually consists of several layers. The general structure is illustrated in Figure 9.15. The *kernel* is the only portion of the operating system that is critically dependent on the hardware. All the other layers (*system calls, shell, utilities*) are written in such a way that they do not differ. The user interacts with the computer at the shell or utility program level. If the user-written utilities and application programs are written properly, they will also not change from machine to machine. This has the obvious advantage of a uniform user interface for any machine using UNIX, at least when one of the original UNIX shells is used.

The structure of UNIX means that software is written at different levels and that the different levels interact (Fig. 9.16). The user will not be writing software at all these levels. However, UNIX is set up in such a way that it is easy for the user to operate at the application or user-written utility level because all parts of UNIX are programmable. You can even combine commands into a simple program, and as long as you remain "logged on," you can recall these *command strings* at will. Even better, command strings can be easily placed in a file, can be given a name, and made interactive so that, in effect, new "commands" are created. These new commands are referred to as *shell scripts*. While they are similar in concept to "batch" or "submit file" in MS/PC-DOS or CP/M, respectively, they are far more powerful. This improved capability results partly because there are many

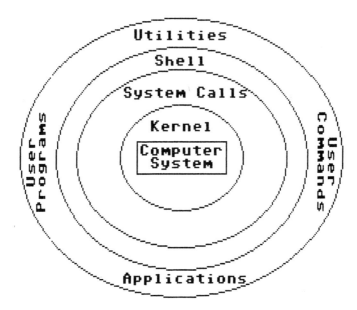

Figure 9.15.   Organizational structure of UNIX operating system.

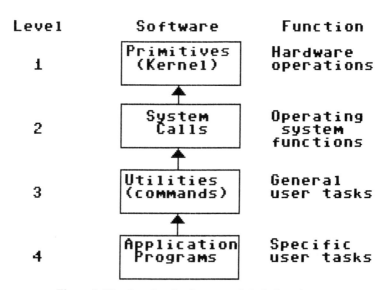

Figure 9.16.   Levels of software and their functions.

more functions provided for use in the shell scripts (virtually anything in Unix can be used) and partly because of the larger number of building blocks in Unix.

Unix also introduces another aspect of operating systems that is not present in MS/PC-DOS or CP/M, and that is "logging on." Unix is a multiuser operating system, and in order for the operating system to handle everybody's programs properly, it must be able to identify each user. It must know this in order to schedule everybody and prevent conflicting use of individual programs or computer resources. The system also has to have at least a minimal level of security so that users operate with their own programs and not those of another user, at least not without their permission. Unix does both of these tasks, identification of user and the first level of security, through the log in process.

The log in process is a legacy from mainframe computer operating systems. The user sits at a terminal and enters a word, usually some form of his or her name. The computer responds with a request for the "password." The password is supposed to be known only to the user. For each user there is a unique user name-password combination. It is recommended that the password not be a common word and that it be split into two parts, with the two parts separated by a nonalphabetic character such as a slash or dash. If the password and user name are correct, the computer gives the user access to the machine, otherwise the user is not permitted to use the computer. At this point the user is "logged in."

Once the user is operating the computer, regardless of the operating system, there are several ways to proceed. In general, the user will either be giving commands to perform specific tasks or will be employing applications software. If the user is a programmer, then any of several programming languages may be employed. Here again, the hierarchy of use is encountered. In this case, programming languages represent the kernel and system call levels, as well as providing the means for generating the applications programs. Unix extensively use shell scripts for many applications, whereas the other operating systems will use programming languages. There are many applications areas for computers. These include word processing, database management, data analysis, project planning, games, and programming. These application areas will be discussed briefly, starting with programming because that is the basis for all the other areas. In addition, some introduction to programming principles will aid in using programs in other application areas.

Programming

Programming involves writing software to solve a particular problem. As will be seen from discussions on various application programs, the concept of programming extends beyond the use of programming "languages" such as BASIC or C. Programming occurs at each of the software levels described earlier. This view of programming means that every user is a programmer. It is important to approach computer use this way because it will maximize the utility of the computer. While there are some areas where only a programmer will operate, users should realize that it is not necessary to have the title of "programmer" in order to effectively use a computer.

The programmer usually uses one of several programming languages to program the computer to perform the required tasks. There are two important considerations for the programmer before actually writing the software. These are the definition of the problem and the selection of the programming language. Failures in these areas will lead to increased cost and time and, occasionally, complete failure.

Defining the Problem

Whenever a computer is to be used to solve a problem there are some simple questions that need to be answered prior to programming the application. The first question is whether a computer should be used at all. This may seem like a trivial question, but many times tasks are computerized that could have been done as well or better manually. For example, computers are frequently touted for maintaining calendars. For a programmer or user who is frequently at the computer anyway this may be reasonable, but for most people the need to turn on a computer in order to use a calendar is a waste of time. It is also not very easy to carry around a computer in order to check your schedule.

This example also illustrates the interaction between the definition of the application and available hardware. The appropriateness of doing an application frequently depends on what hardware is available. When computers are small enough to fit in a pocket, powerful enough to maintain multiyear calendars, and become extremely cheap, then it will make sense to use a computer for personal scheduling. Hardware requirements for other applications must always be considered in the environment where the task is to be performed. The environment includes not only physical space requirements, but also characteristics of the personnel. Some applications can be done only if there are a lot of personnel with extensive computer experience, whereas other applications require personnel with almost no experience. These physical and personnel requirements must be considered as part of the definition of the problem.

Another aspect of problem solving with computers is the determination of the key components of the problem. This involves getting the perspective of all users and a description of the task to be performed. The expected outcome of all this work is a written software specification if the work involves only software, or a system specification if both hardware and software are required. Such a specification describes the software/hardware to be used for each task and a rationale for each choice. The specification should be shared with users as it is being developed. There is a twofold advantage for doing this. First, the specification provides a blueprint. Second, and most important, it ensures that the problem has been well thought out.

Part of the specification will undoubtedly be the selection of the computer language(s) or application software for the task. This is an important choice because computer languages and applications software, like hardware, have strengths and weaknesses. Some computer languages and applications software packages will now be described briefly to give some idea of what is available and how it may be applied. The packages will be described in general ways in terms of certain applications areas. There will be no attempt to be complete as there are literally thousands of software packages available for either CP/M, MS/PC-DOS, or Unix.

Programming Languages

There are many programming languages available for all levels of computers. Programming languages are used to program applications software. In general, languages are split into two levels: machine level and higher level. The machine level languages are usually faster and are closer to the type of information that the computer uses, whereas high level languages use a more language-like syntax that will implement many machine language instructions with a single command.

Machine Level Languages

Although programming originally started by actually inputting the ones and zeros of the binary system, which is the computer's language, this is not done anymore. Machine level languages are now more properly referred to as *assembly languages*. Assembly language is a programming language that substitutes a *mnemonic* for a particular instruction to be executed by the computer. It should not be assumed that all assembly languages are alike, although there are many similarities.

The various assembly languages are machine specific. That is, each assembly language is designed to implement only the instructions for a particular central processing unit (CPU). Thus assembly language for a Z80 CPU (used for CP/M) will be different than that for an 8088 CPU (used for MS/PC-DOS) or a 68,000 family CPU (frequently used for microcomputer implementations of Unix). There may even be differences between assembly languages for the same CPU. For example, assembly languages for the Z80 CPU can use either Intel or Zilog mnemonics. The same is true for all levels of computers.

There are two steps required for using assembly language. First, the assembly languages instructions have to be written into a program. This step is referred to as *coding*. The second step is to convert the assembly language mnemonics into the binary language of the computer. This step is referred to as *compiling*, although this is frequently broken into the three steps of compiling, linking, and loading. The compilation in this case converts the code into an intermediate form of binary coding, which is hex coding. At this point the program is referred to as an *object module*. Linking combines many object modules into a single module, which is used by the loader. The loader takes the linked object module and converts it into the binary language of the computer and in a form that the operating system can load the program and run it, hence the name. Different assembly languages may handle these steps in different ways, combining or separating them. But all of these steps must be done to get to the final product, which is an application program that the user loads and runs.

Assembly language is used to obtain the maximum speed from the computer. The main disadvantage of assembly language programming is the time and cost of implementing an application that uses this level of language because each machine instruction has to be specified separately. Most applications require thousands of such instructions and thus take a long time to generate the programs. For some applications there is no other choice. Such applications are those that require very high speed, such as generating acoustic signals by computer or capturing acoustic signals by computer.

High-Level Languages

High-level languages are languages that comprise instructions that are in effect small machine-language programs. The mnemonics employed in high-level languages are more like natural language and describe broader actions than for assembly language. For example, to print a character on the screen in assembly language would require several lines of code that would consist of instructions such as LDA, STA, and OUT; whereas in a high-level language a single line using an instruction such as PRINT would be sufficient. The primary advantage of high-level languages is that they can be coded more quickly and are easier to debug. The disadvantage is that they are generally much slower than assembly language.

There are two major types of high-level languages: interpreted languages and compiled languages. The labels refer to the manner in which the language is converted to a usable program. That is, a particular language is not always an interpreted or a compiled language, but some languages are more commonly one or the other. An example of a language that is usually interpreted is Beginner's All-Purpose Symbolic Instruction Code (BASIC). An example of a language that is usually compiled is *C*.

An interpreted language is a language in which the commands are examined by the computer and converted to machine language as the computer encounters the instruction. This means that the computer scans the program from the beginning to the end and examines each instruction in turn for possible execution even if the program says to go to a specific part of the program. Many microcomputers now have BASIC interpreters in ROM so that the user has a computer language available when the computer is turned on. The two advantages of an interpreter are ease of use because programs can be executed immediately and the speed with which simple applications can be programmed. The two disadvantages are inferior execution speed (recall that the program must scan in a serial manner each time it needs to hunt for a program line) and the difficulty of debugging the code because most BASIC interpreter use line numbers to refer to parts of the program that perform a certain function rather than using a meaningful name to designate the function.

Compiled languages are languages that are developed in a manner similar to that described for assembly language, but the syntax of the language is high level. An example of a compiled language is C, which is the language used to write the Unix operating system. When using a compiled language, the programmer writes the program using a program called an "editor." The editor program is an application program designed for the entry of text, usually programs. The text form of program then follows the compilation steps of compiling, linking, and loading described previously for assembly language. The advantage of a compiled language is speed (because the program that is loaded is actually a machine language program that does not have to serially scan program lines) and ease of debugging. The use of proper programming technique (i.e., coding and testing one module at a time) combined with the fact that programs and subprograms can have meaningful names rather than line numbers, makes debugging much easier. The disadvantages of compiled languages compared with interpreted languages are that the programs are more difficult to code and simple programs take longer to code. As the programs get longer and more complex, these disadvantages become less important than the advantages; most long and complex programs are written with a compiled language.

The differences between interpreted and compiled languages are starting to get blurred because of the increasing speed and power of microcomputers, which improves the speed of interpreted languages and the restructuring of interpreted languages to include meaningful subprogram names and other features that were formerly found mainly in compiled languages. An example of this philosophy is the BASIC interpreter on the AMIGA microcomputer and the C interpreters that are now available.

An advantage of high-level languages in general is their portability. This is true for both interpreted and compiled languages. That is, the text form of the program can be transferred from CPU to CPU and be used essentially unchanged. The emphasis here is on CPU because different brands of computers may have the same CPU, and it is the CPU that is important to programmers because it determines what instructions can be executed by the computer. This is in contrast to assembly language, which is specific to a particular CPU. This portability is not perfect, and there are frequently small changes that must be made. In addition, some languages are more easily transportable than others. For example, *C* is generally more transportable than BASIC because there are so many more forms of BASIC than of C.

There are also languages that are referred to as *fourth-generation languages* (4GL), but these are more closely related to applications software than what is traditionally thought of as programming languages. The ideal is to reach fifth-generation languages, which will permit the user to use normal conversational language and enable the computer to generate the necessary applications software from the user's commands. Although there is a lot of effort currently being expended to create such languages, it may be 5 to 10 years before the first fruits of such labors will be available at all. Even 4GL is still in the early stages of implementation, and then only in mainframe environments.

Applications Software

Applications software is not a single type of software, but is generally classified in terms of area of application. The application areas considered here are word processing; spreadsheets; database management; graphics; clinical office management, which includes some of the above areas; and laboratory research. In addition, there are different levels of applications software. The packages residing on mainframe computers generally have more features than those on smaller computers and are also capable of handling larger tasks.

Two general comments with regard to application programs: One, there is no single application program in any application area that can cover everybody's needs. Two, a good idea for saving on costs is to carefully define your needs and to read several reviews in reputable magazines before purchasing any software.

Word Processing

Word processing programs deal with text manipulation, which includes both the entry and output of text. Different programs have different strengths in each of these areas. In addition, some programs have extra features that may be useful for particular users. Their ability to replace typewriters for many applications has made word processing programs the major reason for the increasing use of microcomputers in business.

There are still some applications for which typewriters remain useful, such as filling out single forms or typing addresses for a single envelope. These tasks could be done with a microcomputer, but they would be extremely tedious and take much longer than necessary. There are good examples of the fact that computers should be used appropriately and that just because something *could* be done by computer doesn't mean that it *should* be done by computer.

Some of the features of word processing programs are the ability to change text easily, to check spelling, to prepare tables of contents, to format documents, and to index. Not all programs can do all of these tasks, and word processors should not be selected for the number of their features, but for their appropriateness to the application. For example, if the main requirement is text entry, then the word processor should be easy to use and fast. If the application is a text book, then a broader range of features is required such as tables of contents and indexing. As for all software, try it before buying it.

There are some terms associated with word processing that should be known. The first is *WYSIWYG* (what you see is what you get). The term refers to word processors that show on the screen the text formatted in the same form as it will be on the paper when it is printed. This term was made popular by a word processing program called Wordstar, which is probably the most famous and well-known word processing program and was the first program to use this approach. Most current word processing programs use this approach in one form or another. Unfortunately, not all word processing programs that advertise themselves this way are exact in the relation between screen and paper; therefore this feature should be checked if it is important.

A second term is *word wrap*. This refers to an operation during the text-entry process. As words are entered on the screen, the computer program checks to see if the word extends beyond the right margin. If it does, the location of the word is adjusted to begin on the next line. This feature is very important for text entry as it makes the text readable. Almost all word processors have this feature. For computer program entry, however, this feature should be disabled because it may cause errors in the program with inappropriate breaks in the line.

Most of the previous discussion has focused on word processors for entering documents such as manuscripts and letters. There are also word processors that are designed for entry of computer programs. These word processors are called *text editors* because the focus of these word processors is not for formatting paper printout. Such text entry programs were traditionally referred to as "editors," and that is the source of the present name of text editors. Some of these programs are optimized for the entry of a particular programming language and are occasionally included as part of a programming package. These packages have such features as checking the syntax of the code as it is being entered, interacting with compiler to point to errors, and formatting the text on the screen as it is entered so that proper indentation or other aspects of form are employed. Many computer users have both word processors and text editors available. Some word processors, such as Wordstar, have specific modes for each application.

Spreadsheets

Spreadsheets are probably the major application program that made microcomputers so popular with business, as they are especially suitable for financial analysis and yet are relatively easy to use. While financial analysis programs existed on large mainframes, these programs were difficult to learn and use. When spreadsheet programs were developed for microcomputers, the programs were purposely made much easier to use because the user was assumed to be much less sophisticated than the user of mainframe packages. The best known and most popular program in this area is Lotus 1-2-3, which is primarily a spreadsheet although it also has some database and graphics capabilities.

A spreadsheet can be viewed as a matrix of cells. Each cell contains either text, numeric data, or a formula. The contents are labeled by the cell name, which is either row-column format (r1c1 would be row 1, column 1) or Visicalc format (rows are numbers and columns are letters: A1 is column 1, row 1). Visicalc was the first popular spreadsheet program.

Spreadsheet programs permit calculations to be made and displayed easily. For example, a cell can contain a formula that says take the content of cell r3c4 and multiply it by the content of cell r5c6. The result will appear in the cell with the formula. Whenever the content of either of the referenced cells is changed the result is immediately changed. This permits easy manipulation of numbers and the investigation of "what if?" scenarios. Thus, spreadsheets are especially useful for models. One caveat to this is that the spreadsheets, while reasonably fast calculators, are doing a lot of work in addition to calculating, and if the calculations are going to be very complex, it may be better to use a dedicated program rather than a spreadsheet.

Spreadsheets are excellent for many applications, ranging from statistics to managing the financial affairs of an office. In fact, because spreadsheets have been used by businesses longer than by clinicians, there are many excellent packages that tie into spreadsheets for managing the financial aspects of a business. Thus, this type of package may be very useful to a consultant or to a small clinical office.

Spreadsheets are also excellent for data summary and analysis in a research environment. The layout of data in matrix form according to test conditions is a natural for spreadsheets. The ability to be able to enter data and watch the summary statistics, such as mean and standard deviation (which are built in functions in almost all spreadsheets), change as the data are entered is great for analysis. The spreadsheet also permits what-if analyses, such as regrouping subjects, and allows easy sorting of data according to performance. It is recommended that a spreadsheet package with graphics be used because the ability to display various data and scenarios is very helpful for online data analysis.

Database Management Systems

Spreadsheets are very useful for numeric data, but they do not handle textual data or the relations among textual data very well. Database management systems (DBMS) have been developed to fulfill the need to handle this type of data. Database managers fall into two general classes: file managers and relational databases.

File managers and relational databases differ mainly in the way they handle data files. File managers can only deal with one file at a time, whereas relational databases can access and use information from more than one file concurrently. File managers are extremely useful for pulling information from single-file databases, such as mailing lists and bibliographic files. However, they are not as good in applications such as relating similar information that may be stored in several files, e.g. when the same patient's name is found in various files pertaining to his her medical record, financial information, or participation in a research study or a donor program. For this latter case, select a relational database that can automatically add information to a report from all files simultaneously by setting up a "relationship" among the files. The files must have something in common, such as an identification number, in order to do this.

These are some questions that should be asked when deciding if a database is necessary or what type of database features to purchase.

1. Is a file manager sufficient for the application, or is a relational DBMS required?

2. What is the maximum number of fields per record in the database package? This is not a critical matter as long as it meets some minimum criteria such as 255. (The reason is that if the number of fields exceeds this criterion, there are too many fields in the record and the fields should be broken up into separate records.)

3. What is the maximum length of a field? This should only be considered if lengthy textual information will be contained in the database.

4. What is the maximum storage capacity of the database? This has to be considered in the context of the storage capacity of the system being

used to contain the database. For example, a 2-billion record capacity for the database program is meaningless on a 680,000 byte floppy disk system.

5. How many files can the DBMS access concurrently? This is an important question because it impacts both speed and flexibility of operation of the DBMS.

6. Is the program copy protected? This is important because you should be able to easily make a working copy of the program disk. The original should be kept in a safe place. Keep in mind that copying the software on any machine other than your own is illegal.

7. Is data field masking a desirable feature? Its flexibility allows easy-to-use input formats for input screens to be created.

8. Is indexing an important feature? The assignment of key words is important for large DBMS applications because it impacts the speed of searching through database. In order for indexing capability to be useful, it should be possible to key within records as much as desired.

9. Is sorting capability important? This is done so often that it should be done well.

10. Can the data within the database be converted to other formats? It should be possible to put data in a form readable, and hence usable, by other programs such as word processors or spreadsheets.

11. What is the menu capability? This capability can be overrated. However, the database package should be flexible, that is, the DBMS should be able to create custom menus that permit short cuts by sophisticated users of the system.

12. Is it possible to access data in an informal way? This capability is referred to as a *query language* and should be as English-like as possible. In addition there should be good flexibility in the language, that is, only being able to search for records rather than fields within the data base is not desirable. This will probably relate to question 7 because it may be impossible in some packages to actually write a query program using the language of the DBMS. However, it is far more desirable for this capability to be present in the system.

13. Is the DBMS able to generate good input screens? Here the power of the screen generator and the flexibility of the DBMS language, if the system has one, must be traded off. The trade-off arises because it may be possible to write great screen management programs with the database language, but the amount of time it takes to write the programs must be related to the amount of time saved by the screens.

14. What are the workspace requirements? DBMS systems take up a lot of room and the hardware must support it. This requires knowledge of whether the DBMS uses fixed or variable length files. Variable length DBMSs will typically use less space. This should not be a major consider-

ation in picking a database unless the available storage is a real problem. It is usually better in the long run to buy more storage for the DBMS of your choice than to buy a lesser package and "shorehorn" it into available space.

15. Does the DBMS generate good reports? Report generators have to be considered in the same manner as screen generators in item 13. That is, there will be the same trade-off between power and flexibility relative to time savings.

16. Do you have a library of preset input and output screens or reports? These are very useful for both programming and application purposes.

17. Can batch processing be used? Batch processing, which is the ability to process routine tasks without the user being present, is required. The reason is the amount of time (usually several minutes and occasionally hours) that database analyses can take. This capability can apply to subsets of analysis. For example, you enter three items, give one command, and away it goes.

18. Is it programmable? A programming language is a highly desirable feature if versatility is required; otherwise, it is not as important. Unfortunately, Murphy's law requires that versatility will always be necessary.

19. How good is the documentation? The program documentation must be clear, at least to a programmer. Users seldom, if ever, use the original database documentation. However, application documentation prepared by the people in charge of training users on the DBMS must be readable by anyone.

20. What are the security procedures? Security procedures with multiple levels are an absolute requirement. This does not mean 300 levels of password protection are required. Three would probably be sufficient, with one of these being at the system manager level.

Graphics

Graphics is an application area that has recently grown significantly and promises to advance much further. The impetus comes from the fact that graphics are great for communication. Graphics packages on computers have the same potential for replacing much redrafting that word processors have already demonstrated in replacing retyping. In addition, the newer software has considerable flexibility and can even work in color. It must be cautioned that graphics are one of the most expensive applications of computers because considerable processing power and sophisticated programming is required. Some newer computers such as the Apple Macintosh or Atari ST, and especially the Commodore Amiga were designed with graphics in mind and are fairly inexpensive.

Integrated Software Packages

Integrated software packages, which combine modules that do each of the tasks described above, provide the potential for doing all of these tasks from a single program. It has been discovered that the integrated programs do not do as well at the individual aspects of spreadsheets, DBMS, etc., as dedicated packages, and so interest in this software has waned. However, limited integration, that is, packages that focus on a particular type of task such as spreadsheets and provide other somewhat limited capabilities, have remained popular. The best example is Lotus 1-2-3, which has often been called the first integrated package although it is really a spreadsheet with limited integrated capabilities.

Although the trend has moved away from integrated software packages, it has not rejected integrated environments. These newer environments, which try to mimic a desktop and use icons to indicate tasks, have slowly begun to be popular. Discussion of these environments could belong with the section on operating systems, but these environments are really application programs that run automatically and serve as an interface to the operating system for the user. This distinction is not always apparent, but in a well-designed system the user can operate at either the operating system level or the integrated environment level. For such an environment to succeed takes a lot of processing power and sophisticated programming, and it is only recently that such power has come to microcomputers. Xerox is frequently credited with creating the first such environment, but other companies have ended up popularizing it.

How to Apply a Computer to Your Life

The software packages described here provide tools for many applications. In addition, custom software can provide tools for applications that do not have such widespread use, and much laboratory software falls into this category. Some of the application areas where computers can make a considerable impact are summarized here:

1. Clinic:
   Recordkeeping;
   Observational research;
   Report preparation.
2. Laboratory:
   Control of experiments;
   Generation of stimuli;
   Analysis of stimuli;
   Data analysis;
   Article preparation.
3. Classroom:
   Computer-assisted instruction (CAI);

Recordkeeping;
Preparation of class materials.
4. Business:
Recordkeeping;
Financial Analysis,
Presentation materials;
Report preparation.
5. Mathematical:
Statistics;
Modeling;
Simulation.
6. Home:
Recordkeeping;
"Remote" control of appliances;
Entertainment;
Education.
7. Games:
Educational;
Arcade,
Adventure.

It can be seen that there are many applications for computers, but the areas of most interest here are the clinical and research applications. Two systems will now be described that might be appropriate for each of these applications areas. The first will be a clinical system in a clinical practice situation outside of a university. The second will be a laboratory system.

Clinical Computer System

A clinical computer system needs to be able to do the several tasks that are performed in every clinic: scheduling patients, test administration, diagnostics, rehabilitation, data management, inventory control, financial management, and word processing. All of these tasks could be handled with a single system or several systems. Each task and its requirements will be discussed in turn, and the resulting system will then be described.

Many new audiometers have computer interfaces. The interface could actually control the audiometer, but at this time it is more likely that it provides access to the settings of the audiometer. This permits the direct collection of audiometric data from the test session. This information could either be output in a report and/or be placed in a database. In either case the data must be brought into the computer and then placed in data files in a format that is accessible to the word processing and DBMS programs. This also impacts the choice of word processing and DBMS software.

Based on the audiometric data, a complete report including history information gathered during the patient's first clinical visit could be printed out for the use of the clinician to aid in diagnosis and to provide a report for the patient's file. This means that the hardware should include a letter-quality printer and word processing software with merge capabilities or a DBMS with good report-generating facilities.

This kind of choice between using a word processor or a DBMS or even a specially written program is typical of application software decisions. It is frequently the case that there are several ways to solve the problem, including not using the computer at all. In general, such decisions are made based on cost, but both long-term as well as short-term costs need to be considered. For example, the office may already have a word processor that it would like to use for generating the reports. However, as a practice grows the need for a DBMS will become greater. Therefore, it may be wise to get the DBMS now and start inputting data and generating reports although the real payoff may be 2 to 3 years away. An additional consideration is the eventual conversion cost if a DBMS is installed after using a word processor system combined with a manual data management system. The trick here is to project what your needs will be 3 to 5 years "down the road." The 3 to 5 year timeframe is based on the typical life cycle of computer hardware and software.

The clinical computer system would also be used for financial management. There is clinical practice software available for several different computers. It is always wise to check out this software before deciding that the situation is unique and requires a specially written software package. Such packages are almost always more expensive than they seem and it is better to enhance an existing package than to write a new one from scratch. This does not mean that it is never necessary to have software written; it is frequently necessary. The point is that building from the ground up is almost always unnecessary and is always very expensive.

Word processing has already been mentioned, but this is one piece of software that should always be purchased for a clinical system because it will be the most used piece of software. A piece of software that may not be used as much is the spreadsheet. While these are great tools for budgets, the clinical package may already contain these capabilities, and so a spreadsheet may be unnecessary.

Note that the previous discussion has focused on software. The software necessary to do the job must always be considered first. In fact, the first step to designing this clinical system was to describe the tasks that had to be performed without regard to how they might be done. For each of the tasks described here, one solution is to use a manual system. For example, if a very efficient manual system already exists for appointment scheduling and is easy to train as well as use, then there may be no need to computerize the appointments.

The first two steps involved in designing a computer system for the clinic, namely, describing the tasks to be done and the software available to do it, have not been done. It is time to describe the hardware. First, there is the basic computer. This could be almost any computer; the power of the computer depends on the size of the practice as seen 3 to 5 years in the future. For many practices, there will only be a need for one computer, which would be used by the receptionist/typist/records person. A simple personal computer with a good quality monitor could be used, as long as there was not a lot of input from multiple devices such as audiometers and other test equipment. If that is the case, then the computer either needs to be "multitasking" (capable of doing more than one thing at a time without getting confused) or "multiuser" (simultaneous use by more than one user). The difficulty here is that no software currently exists to take advantage of the fact that a multitasking computer costing less than $2000 is available. It should be noted that if a multitasking or multiuser system were to be employed, a hard disk would be required. Even for the case where an individual personal computer is being used, hard disks have become cheap enough that justifying their cost is easy.

Thus a minimum system would consist of a single personal computer with a hard disk. The need for a good-quality monitor cannot be overemphasized. The computer may be used as much as 4–8 h/day and a poor monitor will cause eyestrain and a host of other ills. Good monitors are cheap and a good buy. The minimum software would be a word processor with a mail-merge capability to handle mailing lists and billing if all other tasks such as billing and recordkeeping are done manually. A clinical software package should be considered strongly, but if the decision is made to create some software, it should be done on top of DBMS and spreadsheet packages that can *easily* share data with each other and the word processor. This does not mean you must get an integrated software package. Separate spreadsheets (with graphics), DBMSs and word processors can be used with one another although they are not an integrated package. The advantage of using the most popular packages is that they do have a lot of application overlays available. In fact, there is software that can help integrate different packages, even from different vendors. The key decision that needs to be made first is what to automate; then you can pick the software to do it. After that choose the hardware.

Research Computer System

A research computer system can only be designed based on the type of research being done. While there are some generic tasks that are performed in clinics and in research laboratories, the degree of overlap is greater between clinics than it is between laboratories. The focus here will be on the more generic parts of a research laboratory for human research into speech and hearing.

Some of the tasks done in a speech and hearing laboratory are word processing; data management; generation and acquisition of acoustic signals; signal analysis and manipulation; control of external devices; project planning; and data analysis, which might include graphics. The word processing tasks include article preparation, proposal writing, and communication with subjects. One of the primary purposes of a laboratory is to generate data, which requires a good data management system. This can be accomplished either with DBMS or spreadsheet software, or some combination of the two. The generation and acquisition of acoustic signals, from simple sounds to speech, is generally handled by user-written software. However, this software must be compatible with the data management package(s). It must also be compatible with the software used to analyze and manipulate acoustic signals. There is software available to do this, but they run on supermicrocomputers and minicomputers because of the power required.

Control of external devices will usually be done with a combination of user-written software and software supplied by the manufacturer of the device. The need to write special software because of special needs means that the laboratory system will require good software-development capability. This means both good editors and compilers and the hardware to do the process efficiently. Software development is one of the strengths of the UNIX operating system and may be one reason why it is so popular in a laboratory environment. Project planning software is readily available and can be done either with spreadsheets and/or with project management and planning software packages. Data analysis is another major laboratory activity; this would be done with the packages mentioned for data management and with a good statistical package. Whatever software is employed, some reasonable graphics capability must be included because so much data analysis is graphical, especially in the early stages or in studies with few subjects. Spreadsheets with graphics capability are good for this application.

Recall that many, if not all, of these tasks can be done manually as well. It should be noted, however, that almost nobody does either experimental control of signal generation and acquisition manually. It is simply too cumbersome, inefficient, and inflexible. Statistics are another area in which computers have proved to be useful because of the sheer mass of calculations that need to be performed.

The hardware portion of the system is dependent on how many of the aforementioned tasks are going to be performed on the computer. One possible configuration is to have a supermicrocomputer available to do signal acquisition and analysis as well as handle some of the data management. Another computer, a personal computer linked to the supermicrocomputer, could serve as a test station and do the actual test, with the data going to the main computer. This way, additional test stations could be implemented easily and the power necessary to do signal analysis, data analysis, and signal manipulation would not have to be duplicated and would be available to all systems. The software development would mostly be done on the main system because the tools for software development are generally more advanced on such systems.

The preceding description of a main supermicrocomputer surrounded by test station "micros" would suggest that the main system be a multiuser system. Another possibility is to use a network. The reason for the emphasis on interconnection is to assure communication and easy data transfer capabilities for all machines. The network alternative should only be approached by those with considerable technical resources and a lot of patience because networks are still a fledgling art. Multiuser systems, on the other hand, have been around for a while and are implemented much more easily. A third possibility is to use isolated microcomputer test stations. If there is only one test station, this might be very appropriate. However, some of the functions, such as sophisticated signal analysis and manipulation will have to be done elsewhere because the software is not readily available for microcomputer. If these functions are not required, then a single-user microcomputer test station would be very appropriate.

Management, Maintenance, with Training

The focus up to this point has been on describing the computer tools, both hardware and software, necessary to get the job done. However, no description of computers would be complete without a discussion of maintenance. Before a computer system is purchased, costs for "the care and feeding" of the machine and plans for maintenance of the data should be considered. Some pointers will be presented next concerning maintenance, management, and training practices.

There are several kinds of costs associated with a computer other than the obvious costs of hardware and software. First, there is the maintenance cost, which applies to both the hardware and the software. The hardware is just like any other machine; it breaks down regularly. Software has bugs that have to be either fixed or updated. Therefore, a fund should be budgeted just for maintenance of hardware and software prior to purchasing any computer system.

Second, there is a hidden cost associated with acquiring the computer, especially if it is the first computer. This is the indirect cost in time required to install the machine and learn how to use it. Time is literally money, and the time necessary for installation and learning the system must be planned. In some cases, training may be necessary, and the cost of the trainer must be borne, even if it is somebody already on the staff.

Third, there is the potential cost of a computer programmer, which is a necessity in a research environment, but could also be required in a large department. The programmer would be responsible not only for program development but also maintenance of the machine.

Fourth, the need to maintain the data must be considered. *All data should be backed up regularly.* It takes time and people to do this, but the alternative cost is the loss of all the data. If the amount of data to backed up is large, a tape drive may be appropriate. Using floppy disks to back up files on a hard disk is fine if the backup is done every day on files that have been added and if appropriate records are kept of the directories on the floppies, but such a system can become unmanageable. It is helpful to print out a directory for the backup diskette whenever it is changed and put the directory printout in the diskette envelope.

Data maintenance also includes cleaning up the system from time to time. This is especially important for hard-disk systems. Data on a hard disk will grow without bound if not managed carefully. Files that are very old and not used must be removed from the system. Occasionally large data sets will have to be swapped on and off the disk. The directories of what is on the disk must be maintained. This takes time, often a lot more than is expected. However, it must be done, or someday there won't be room for that critical file that must be saved and the system will hang and the file will go bye-bye.

Finally, consider the management cost of a computer. Somebody will have to be responsible for the machine(s). Since it is likely that the machine(s) will become important to the users as more and more data are stored on the machine, somebody has to make sure that all the tasks described here are performed and that the system remains in good working order. In a very large organization, there will be a data processing department to take care of this, but in most cases in the speech and hearing field such departments are not available or do not take responsibility for individual computer systems. The person who will be in charge should be known *before* the system is acquired, not appointed as an afterthought.

Chapter Summary

This chapter has covered a considerable amount of subject matter. The chapter began by discussing logic and how this was applied to modular programming equipment. Both logic and analog modules were discussed, and how to program them was shown along with some examples. The chapter then covered the building blocks of computers such as architecture, memory, and peripherals. Each section discussed some of the theory of operation and also how they were put together to form a computer. Next, software was discussed both in general terms, such as operating systems and computer languages, and in specific terms, such as application software packages. In addition, a clinical system and a research system were discussed in terms of describing how to design a computer system for these particular situations. Finally, the chapter presented a cautionary note emphasizing the need for budgeting time and money for management, maintenance and training before a computer system is purchased.

Modular Programming Equipment

Introduction

*T*his lab is based on the program described in chapter 9. Either of two modular programming systems, the Grason-Stadler system (which is no longer made) or the Coulbourn system, may be used. This lab will take some time, so be patient and check the logic carefully if something fails.

Method

Using the logic diagram shown in Figure 9.7 and the analog diagram shown in Figure 9.8, program the modular logic. Attach a signal generator to the input of the analog electronic switch and an oscilloscope to the output of the amplifier. Set the signal generator to output a 1 volt sinewave at 1,000 Hz. Set all timers to 1 s. Start the programmed sequence by touching the input of the timer to ground. An alternative method is setting up a logic switch to turn the program on or off and to use that to start the program running.

Results

Prepare a block diagram of the program for both analog and logic modules. Record the time course of the sinewave output as shown on the oscilloscope. Record the duration of signal on and of signal off. Do this for at least three sets of timer settings. Do the same for the logic signals. These recording should be done at the time outputs. Recall that the logic waveforms are 12 volts. Verify that the oscilloscope tracings match the expected time course based on the program.

Discussion

Discuss the programming in terms of ease of setup and debugging. What was the effect of modifying the timers on the integrity of the program? How hard would it be to switch between more than one program at a time? Were there any special problems in doing the programming?

14

Microcomputer Laboratory

Introduction

*T*his laboratory exercise depends upon the availability of equipment. There are several alternatives for the lab. The first is to write a simple BASIC program. The program should have some calculations and at least one branch. It would be best to assign a task for the computer to do. A suggestion is to ask the computer to give a particular answer to a user depending upon the letter in the first name of the user. The ASCII value of this letter is then reported back to the user, and the result of this value multiplied by a random number is also reported back. This will give a feel for how fast a computer can do a complex calculation as well as how it can make a decision based on input from a user. Such a program is shown in Appendix C, but it should be saved as an answer sheet because the program has already been debugged.

The second possibility is to do a microcomputer demonstration. This can range from doing an audiometer simulation to doing speech recognition and production. The demonstration will be determined by the availability of equipment and ideally would be done on two different levels of computer to give some idea of what is meant by computer "power." The program mentioned above could also be used for demonstration purposes, but would have to be modified to demonstrate differences in computer speed.

A third possibility is to provide a simple application using an application package, such as a spreadsheet, and to allow people to use it. The only limit on what can be done in this lab is time and availability of appropriate hardware and software. If a software or application lab is employed, be sure to allow plenty of time for the minimum necessary learning required to do the program or to use the application package. A most important requirement is that this lab be heavily supervised. Take advantage of the instructor, but don't be afraid to try things first. Remember that a computer is logical but not intelligent, at least in the classical sense. (Perhaps the instructor or mainframe will have ELIZA around. ELIZA is a simple demonstration of artificial intelligence and is fun as well.) It is very difficult to break a computer from the keyboard if appropriate safeguards have been taken with regard to user access to certain commands. ENJOY!!!

SECTION III

A

How to Write a Lab Report

The first rule on a laboratory report is to be clear and concise. Verbiage is not only unnecessary, it is unwanted. The proper form is essential in the lab report because it both organizes the writer and makes it easier for the reader to understand what was done and what it means. The purpose of a lab report is to communicate.

When you have completed an experiment, you will have to communicate the results to others. In order to do this you will have to be well-organized. You can assume that the reader will have the same level of technical competence as yourself. You can also assume that the reader will be busy. While fanciful literature is not required, good grammar will make the reading considerably easier and will be appreciated by the reader.

The reader's burden can be lightened considerably if reports are put into standard form and style. Such forms have evolved in the professional journals of all scientific disciplines, and authors and readers have learned to make use of them. You will be required to use some of the format dictated by the American Psychological Association that is used with minor modifications by many journals in the field of speech and hearing. Most important is the content and clarity of your reports, but this is affected by how well you observe the fundamentals of proper form.

Journal articles typically employ the past tense and the third person; for example, "The experimenter started the clock 20 seconds after the subject pressed the button" is correct form, whereas, "I started the clock 20 seconds after the subject pressed the button" is incorrect. Your writing should not be elaborate and flowery: simple declarative sentences are best. All reports should be entered neatly in ink in a lab book.

A report usually contains the following major sections: abstract, introduction, method, results, discussion, references, and appendix. The content of these major sections is outlined next.

Abstract. The abstract is essentially a summary of the report. It should contain a brief description of the problem area, the method, the results, and the conclusion. When writing the abstract, remember that many people read this section to find out if the experiment is within their own area of interest and to determine whether they should invest their time in reading the whole report. Many fine reports have gone unread because authors have provided a careless abstract of their work. The length of the abstract should be limited to 200 words. As a guide, you might attempt to construct the abstract by reducing each section of the report to one or two sentences.

Introduction. The introduction describes the purpose of the experiment and why you did it the way you did. It does not need to be lengthy, but the rationale for your experiment should be clear. The introduction should contain the reasons for conducting the study and a statement of the specific hypotheses to be tested, if any. In journal articles, references to previous work would also be in this section.

Method. The method section is frequently subdivided on the basis of the subjects (if any), the apparatus, and the procedure.

The subject section describes the characteristics of the subjects who participated in the study. All *pertinent* characteristics should be described. For example, an extensive description of learning capabilities would not be appropriate for most speech production studies.

The apparatus section should include a description of the functional aspects and relevant dimensional data concerning the apparatus. That is, you should describe the apparatus in terms that are easily recognizable to others. Frequently, model numbers are used to describe individual pieces of equipment and block diagrams are used to help describe the experimental setup.

The procedure section describes how the experimenter did the experiment. The experimental design and all other techniques and operations performed by the experimenter should be described. Describe what you actually did, especially if it deviated from some protocol. This information will be helpful to the reader and may explain unusual data or data that turned out differently from those of others.

Results. The results section should contain enough data to justify the conclusions. The findings will be presented in the form of tables, figures, and words. In general, this section should include only the major trends shown by summarized or derived data as described by measures of central tendency, dispersion, and statistical tests. Raw data are usually placed in an appendix. However, if the data are not such that derivations are possible or desirable, then raw data are presented in this section. In addition to the figures and tables, a results section *always* contains a written description, not an explanation, of what an intelligent reader might see in the data. The results of any statistical tests of significance are reported in order to lend support to the reliability of the description.

All tables and figures *must* be clearly labeled and *must* be given a title and a legend.

Discussion. Explain what the results mean, for example, what hypotheses they confirmed. Be careful not to overextend your results and claim or try to explain too much with them. Do not get philosophical.

The discussion section should also consider how a better experiment might be conducted; discrepancies, inconsistencies, and sources of error should be considered. Finally, this section may contain a discussion of new issues raised by the data of the experiment.

References. If you have references cited in the report, these go at the end in a separate section titled "references." These are typically cast in a standard format recommended by the American Psychological Association.

Appendix. As mentioned, this section contains the raw data, if they were not reported in the "results" section.

B

Insertion Gain Instrumentation

A longstanding problem in audiology has been the difficulty of determining the gain that a hearing aid actually provides to the patient. The use of a calibrated cavity to measure the output of an audiometer was discussed in the chapter on audiological instrumentation. A similar method has generally been used to measure hearing aid performance. The only difference was that the cavity was smaller to account for the smaller airspace between the end of the earmold and the tympanic membrane as opposed to the case of an open ear. The Knowles Electronic Manikin for Auditory Research (KEMAR) was also developed to try to help with this problem of estimating "true" hearing aid gain and response. The variability in earmolds combined with the variability in ear canal geometries made the above methods somewhat unreliable in estimating the gain response a particular individual received from a particular hearing aid.

It has long been known that the best way to measure the response of a hearing aid is to measure it in the ear of the person with the hearing aid in place. Such a measurement is referred to as an "in situ measurement." A very recent development in instrumentation now permits exactly that measurement. These instruments are referred to as *insertion gain instruments*. While not perfect, such instruments promise to make the task of fitting a hearing aid much more accurate, reliable, and more beneficial for the patient or client.

Theory of Operation

The insertion gain instrument measures the sound pressure level in the ear canal using a probe microphone. By comparing the response to a known signal before and after a hearing aid is inserted into the ear, the instrument can calculate how much gain the hearing aid is providing at each frequency. This enables the clinician to determine if the actual gain function matches the desired gain function.

These instruments are similar in many ways to spectrum analyzers, with the measurement target being the sound in the ear canal. Just as for a spectrum analyzer, there are two major approaches to determining the spectrum of the sound in the ear canal. The first is the frequency scanning method, and the second is the FFT method. Both were described in chapter 8, and that section should be reviewed for descriptions of the two techniques. An aspect of the measurement that pertains to this particular measurement was not discussed at that time. It is the need to deal with sound reflection.

When measuring with either analysis method, you must present a signal to the ear. The signal is presented from a loudspeaker and goes not only to the ear but also towards any other surface in the room. These sounds can be reflected toward the ear with a delay proportional to their distance from the ear and the speaker. For example, if there is a surface 3 feet away from the ear and the speaker, the sound has to travel about 6 ft and at approximately 1 ms/ft will arrive at the ear 6 ms after it left the speaker. If the target ear is 3 ft from the speaker then the reflected sound will arrive 3 ms after the original sound (6 for the reflected, −3 for the original). If a scanning algorithm is employed, the scanning filter must have moved sufficiently in frequency in those 3 ms for the reflected signal to be out of the passband of the analysis filter. For the FFT, the time window for analysis must be such that it does not include the reflected sound. This must be kept in mind when doing analysis with these instruments.

Use of Insertion Gain Instrumentation

The use of an insertion gain instrument is very simple. There are three major steps required to make the measurements. The first is equalization, the second is obtaining the open ear canal response, and the third is obtaining the aided response. For all measurements there should be no surface closer than 1 meter from the patient.

The equalization curve is intended to measure the system response in the region of the patient without the ear canal effects. To make the measurement, place the probe microphone on the cheek of the patient and secure it with tape. If it is possible, use nonallergenic tape. Record the response and then select the equalization function. The equalization will then be done.

The second step of obtaining the open ear canal response is done next. The probe tube of the microphone is inserted into the ear canal. It should be inserted to a depth sufficient that it will extend beyond the tip of the earmold for a hearing aid. Use the probe tube ring to mark the point along the probe tube at the edge of the entrance to the ear canal. Be sure to do this in a well-lighted situation in order to verify that the tip of the probe tube is not flat against the side of the canal or against the tympanic membrane. Record the response and store it.

The third and final step for determining insertion gain is to now place the hearing aid (or earmold if it is a behind-the-ear aid) into the ear canal, keeping the probe tube in place. This can be checked by checking the location of the probe tube marker ring. Record the response and store it. The insertion gain calculation can now be made by the instrument subtracting the open ear response from the response with the hearing aid. This calculation should now be selected, and the resulting insertion gain curve should be stored.

It should be possible to display any (or all) of three functions: the open ear response, which is sometimes called the ear resonance curve; the response with the hearing aid; and the insertion gain function. The first two curves will be in decibels sound pressure level. The last curve is a relative curve and will be in decibels. A negative value on the insertion gain curve means the hearing aid actually attenuated the signal for that frequency.

Cautionary Notes

The insertion gain instrument promises to be a powerful tool for clinicians and researchers. There will be a number of such devices available. Before selecting a device, it is best to verify that it will yield accurate information and that it is appropriate for its application. There are also some cautions that must be observed in its use.

The main criteria for selecting an insertion gain instrument are accuracy, reliability, and appropriateness. If these criteria are met, then price can become a factor. The validity of the results from an insertion gain instrument can be checked by comparing the instrument results in KEMAR with the known results for KEMAR. The reliability can be checked by making multiple measurements. This should include removal and reinsertion of the probe tube microphone. The instrument should make it easy to do reliable measurements. The appropriateness of a particular model to the application is mainly a matter of ease of use and training, as well as the sophistication required. In a clinical situation the instrument must be very easy to use, not easily breakable, and should make the basic measurements of unaided, aided, and insertion gain functions. For a research situation, greater sophistication or the ability to easily add functions not originally anticipated may be important.

There are some other cautions:

1. If there are two instruments made by the same company, they should give the same results for the same measurement. This should also be true across models.

2. Be aware that the tube for the probe microphone may be crimped when the hearing aid is placed in the canal. If strange results are observed, it may be necessary to repeat the series to ensure the results are correct.

3. Do not hesitate to repeat measurements. This is a new type of instrument and there is a lack of clear data on some important issues such as sound leakage into the tube from other sources and the influence of bends and crimps in tubing.

4. There may be some problems with scanning filter speed in some instruments. That is, the scanning rate may be such that reflections are being analyzed or that the filter and signal are not in synchrony.

5. Be aware of the limitations in resolution for FFT instruments. If the FFT is done every 100 Hz, then energy at any intermediate frequency may be ignored. The key to remember is that the FFT is not generating a continuous analysis function across frequency, but rather a discrete analysis function at selected points across frequency.

Finally, check the literature regularly. This is a good example of when following the research literature can yield clinical rewards. It is a good general rule to do this for all instrumentation, as there are new findings about what instruments do and how to use existing instruments on a regular basis.

C

Basic Program for Quiklab 14

```
100 REM PROGRAM FOR QUIKLAB 14
150 REM This program is designed to ask for the first name, take the
200 REM ASCII value of the first letter of the first name, then
250 REM ask a question based on that value and then
300 REM print out that value and that value multiplied by a
400 REM random number.
500 REM This is written in a "generic" BASIC, which should
600 REM work on most machines.
1000 DIM A$(30): REM permits a 30-character first name.
1010 PRINT "ENTER YOUR FIRST NAME";
1020 INPUT A$
1030 IF LEFT$(A$,1) > "L" AND LEFT$(A$,1) < = "a" THEN 1050
1032 IF LEFT$(A$,1) > "1" THEN 1050
1035 PRINT "THE FIRST LETTER OF YOUR NAME IS";LEFT$(A$,1)
1040 PRINT "THE FIRST LETTER OF YOUR FIRST NAME IS LESS
       THAN L"
1045 PRINT "THE ASCII VALUE OF THE FIRST LETTER IS";
       ASC(LEFT$(A$,1))
1047 PRINT "THE RANDOM VALUE IS";ASC(LEFT$(A$,1))*RAN(0)
1049 GOTO 1200
1050 PRINT "THE FIRST LETTER OF YOUR NAME IS";LEFT$(A$,1)
1052 PRINT "THE FIRST LETTER OF YOUR FIRST NAME IS
       GREATER THAN L"
1055 PRINT "THE ASCII VALUE OF THE FIRST LETTER
       IS";ASC(LEFT$(A$,1))
1057 PRINT "THE RANDOM VALUE IS";ASC(LEFT$(A$,1))*RAN(0)
1200 PRINT "DO YOU WANT TO DO IT AGAIN? (Y OR N)";
1210 INPUT B$
1220 IF B$ = "Y" OR B$ = "y" THEN 1010
1230 IF B$ = "N" OR B$ = "n" THEN 1240
1235 GOTO 1200
1240 END
```

Index

Page numbers in *italics* denote figures; those followed by "t" denote tables.